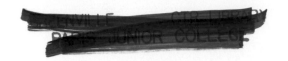

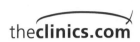

theclinics.com

NURSING CLINICS OF NORTH AMERICA

Diabetes

GUEST EDITOR
Gail D'Eramo Melkus, EdD, C-NP, CDE, FAAN

December 2006 • Volume 41 • Number 4

SAUNDERS

An Imprint of Elsevier, Inc.
PHILADELPHIA   LONDON   TORONTO   MONTREAL   SYDNEY   TOKYO

W.B. SAUNDERS COMPANY
A Division of Elsevier Inc.

1600 John F. Kennedy Blvd., Suite 1800, Philadelphia, PA 19103-2899

http://www.theclinics.com

NURSING CLINICS OF NORTH AMERICA Volume 41, Numbe
December 2006 ISSN 0029-6⸴
Editor: Ali Gavenda ISBN 1-4160-381

The ideas and opinions expressed in *Nursing Clinics of North America* do not necessarily reflect those of
Publisher. The Publisher does not assume any responsibility for any injury and/or damage to persons
property arising out of or related to any use of the material contained in this periodical. The reader is
vised to check the appropriate medical literature and the product information currently provided by
manufacturer of each drug to be administered to verify the dosage, the method and duration of admi
tration, or contraindications. It is the responsibility of the treating physician or other health care pro
sional, relying on independent experience and knowledge of the patient, to determine drug dosages a
the best treatment for the patient. Mention of any product in this issue should not be construed as endo
ment by the contributors, editors, or the Publisher of the product or manufacturers' claims.

Nursing Clinics of North America (ISSN 0029-6465) is published quarterly by Elsevier Inc., 360 Park Ave
South, New York, NY 10010-1710. Months of issue are March, June, September, and December. Busin
and Editorial Offices: 1600 John F. Kennedy Blvd., Suite 1800, Philadelphia, PA 19103-2899. Customer S
vice Office: 6277 Sea Harbor Drive, Orlando, FL 32887-4800. Periodicals postage paid at New York,
and additional mailing offices. Subscription price per year is, $116.00 (US individuals), $216.00 (US in
tutions), $187.00 (international individuals), $259.00 (international institutions), $160.00 (Canadian ind
duals), $259.00 (Canadian institutions), $61.00 (US students), and $94.00 (international students). To rece
student/resident rate, orders must be accompanied by name of affiliated institution, date of term, and
signature of program/residency coordinator on institution letterhead. Orders will be billed at individ
rate until proof of status is received. Foreign air speed delivery is included in all *Clinics* subscription pri
All prices are subject to change without notice. **POSTMASTER:** Send address changes to *Nursing Clin
Elsevier Periodicals Customer Service, 6277 Sea Harbor Drive, Orlando, FL 32887-4800. **Customer Serv
1-800-654-2452 (US). From outside of the US, call 1-407-345-4000.**

Nursing Clinics of North America is covered in *EMBASE/Excerpta Medica, Index Medicus, Social Sciences C
tion Index, Current Contents, ASCA, Cumulative Index to Nursing, RNdex Top 100,* and *Allied Health Literat
and International Nursing Index (INI).*

Printed in the United States of America.

GUEST EDITOR

GAIL D'ERAMO MELKUS, EdD, C-NP, CDE, FAAN, Professor and Independence
Foundation Professor of Nursing, Yale University School of Nursing, New Haven,
Connecticut

CONTRIBUTORS

SANDRA BENAVIDES-VAELLO, RN, MPAff, Doctoral Candidate, School of Nursing,
The University of Texas at Austin, Austin, Texas

DIANE BERRY, PhD, CANP, Assistant Professor, School of Nursing, University of North
Carolina at Chapel Hill, Chapel Hill, North Carolina

CATHERINE A. CHESLA, RN, DNSc, FAAN, Professor, Department of Family Health
Care Nursing, University of California San Francisco, San Francisco, California

DEBORAH A. CHYUN, PhD, RN, FAHA, Associate Professor of Nursing, Yale University
School of Nursing, New Haven, Connecticut

IRENE COLE, RN, MS, CDE, Doctoral Student, Department of Family Health Care
Nursing, University of California San Francisco, San Francisco, California

MARJORIE CYPRESS, MSN, C-ANP, CDE, Doctoral Candidate, University of New
Mexico College of Nursing, Albuquerque, New Mexico

JAMES A. FAIN, PhD, RN, BC-ADM, FAAN, Dean and Professor, College of Nursing,
University of Massachusetts Dartmouth, North Dartmouth, Massachusetts

MARTHA M. FUNNELL, MS, RN, CDE, Michigan Diabetes Research and Training
Center, University of Michigan, Ann Arbor, Michigan

ALEXANDRA A. GARCÍA, PhD, RN, Assistant Professor, School of Nursing,
The University of Texas at Austin, Austin, Texas

TIFFANY L. GARY, PhD, Assistant Professor, Department of Epidemiology, Bloomberg
School of Public Health, Johns Hopkins University, Baltimore, Maryland

MARGARET GREY, DrPH, FAAN, CPNP, Diabetes Trial Coordinator and Dean
and Annie Goodrich Professor, Yale University School of Nursing, New Haven,
Connecticut

FELICIA HILL-BRIGGS, PhD, ABPP, Assistant Professor, Department of Medicine,
Johns Hopkins University School of Medicine, Baltimore, Maryland

CAROL J. HOMKO, RN, PhD, CDE, Assistant Research Professor, Departments of Obstetrics and Gynecology and Medicine; and Nurse Manger, General Clinical Research Center, Temple University School of Medicine, Philadelphia, Pennsylvania

SARAH L. KREIN, PhD, RN, Research Investigator, VA Ann Arbor Healthcare System, Center for Practice Management and Outcomes Research; Department of Internal Medicine, University of Michigan Medical School; and Michigan Diabetes Research and Training Center, University of Michigan, Ann Arbor, Michigan

JARIM LEE, BA, Research Coordinator, Section on Behavioral and Mental Health Research, Joslin Diabetes Center, Boston, Massachusetts

GAIL D'ERAMO MELKUS, EdD, C-NP, CDE, FAAN, Professor and Independence Foundation Professor of Nursing, Yale University School of Nursing, New Haven, Connecticut

DAVID K. MILLER, RN, MSEd, BSN, BC, CDE, President, Health Education and Life Promotion, Hope, Indiana

JOHN D. PIETTE, PhD, Career Scientist and Associate Professor of Internal Medicine, VA Ann Arbor Healthcare System, Center for Practice Management and Outcomes Research; Department of Internal Medicine, University of Michigan Medical School; and Michigan Diabetes Research and Training Center, University of Michigan, Ann Arbor, Michigan

CARMEN D. SAMUEL-HODGE, PhD, MS, RD, Research Assistant Professor, Department of Nutrition, Schools of Medicine and Public Health, University of North Carolina at Chapel Hill, Chapel Hill, North Carolina

ANNE H. SKELLY, PhD, RN, CS, FAANP, Associate Professor of Nursing, School of Nursing, The University of North Carolina at Chapel Hill, Chapel Hill, North Carolina

GERALYN R. SPOLLETT, MSN, ANP, CDE, Nurse Practitioner and Associate Director, Yale Diabetes Center, Yale University School of Medicine, New Haven, Connecticut

DONNA TOMKY, MSN, C-ANP, CDE, Nurse Practitioner, Division of Endocrinology and Metabolism, Lovelace Sandia Health Systems, Albuquerque, New Mexico

KIMBERLY TROUT, PhD, RN, Assistant Professor, College of Nursing, Villanova University, Villanova, Pennsylvania

ANDREA DANN URBAN, MSN, APRN, CDE, Diabetes Trial Coordinator, Yale University School of Nursing; and Nurse Practitioner, Yale Pediatric Diabetes Clinic, New Haven, Connecticut

KATIE WEINGER, EdD, RN, Investigator, Section on Behavioral and Mental Health Research, Joslin Diabetes Center; and Assistant Professor of Psychiatry, Harvard Medical School, Boston, Massachusetts

ROBIN WHITTEMORE, PhD, APRN, Associate Professor, Yale University School of Nursing, New Haven, Connecticut

LAWRENCE H. YOUNG, MD, FACC, FAHA, Professor of Medicine, Section of Cardiovascular Disease, Department of Internal Medicine, Yale University School of Medicine, New Haven, Connecticut

CONTENTS

The incidence and prevalence of diabetes is increasing worldwide. National recommendations for screening and diagnosis of diabetes, hypertension, and dyslipidemia provide a basis for early detection, treatment, and intervention that may potentially decrease related complications, and personal and economic costs of the disease. Most important is that knowledge exists about who is at risk for diabetes by weight, family history of diabetes, ethnicity, and history of gestational diabetes that allows for the development and implementation of diabetes primary prevention programs. Multiple national health surveys and databases provide important information for health care providers, systems of care, and communities that can be used to guide such prevention, early screening, and disease detection and intervention programs aimed at decreasing the burden of diabetes.

The increasing prevalence of diabetes and prediabetes makes the cost of diabetes care a pressing concern. Nurses in all settings play a critical role in helping to reduce the cost of diabetes not only for individual patients but ultimately for the health care system. This article focuses on four main issues related to the economic impact of diabetes for patients and health systems: (1) overall estimates of the direct and indirect costs of diabetes and its associated complications, (2) the impact of cost on diabetes care and health outcomes, (3) the ways in which federal- and state-mandated

insurance for persons with diabetes is being used to promote more cost-effective and high-quality diabetes care, and (4) the use of cost-effectiveness analysis to evaluate interventions designed to prevent diabetes or diabetes-related complications.

Type 1 diabetes is a tremendously challenging and complex disease for children and families to manage. Advances in research are constantly bringing about changes in therapies and treatments with the hope of improving the quality of life for youth with type 1 diabetes and their families. Accurate diagnosis, education, treatment, and referral to a certified diabetes educator, endocrinologist, dietitian, social worker, and psychologist are needed to provide the child with the skills necessary to manage diabetes over a lifetime. Nurses and nurse practitioners must be informed of the most current treatments and research available for their patients so that they can encourage their patients to live full and healthy lives.

Type 2 diabetes mellitus (T2DM) is a heterogeneous group of metabolic diseases resulting from defects in insulin secretion, insulin action, or both. It comprises most diagnosed cases of diabetes and disproportionately affects minorities. This article describes the classification of diabetes mellitus; defines the metabolic syndrome; and discusses the diagnosis, risk factors, and screening criteria for T2DM. The pathophysiology of T2DM, its acute and chronic complications, and signs and symptoms are presented, along with a brief overview of treatment.

Women with diabetes face unique health challenges throughout their life cycle. Health concerns begin at puberty and continue throughout the reproductive years and later stages of life. Diabetes can have a significant impact on puberty, menstruation, reproduction, and cardiovascular and bone health. All women with diabetes require an individualized reproductive health plan that addresses contraception, the importance of planning pregnancies, and lifestyle changes. Anticipatory guidance and education in each phase of development can help the woman with diabetes avoid health care problems, reduce her risk of complications, and achieve a healthy outcome.

than 30 years ago. Appreciation of the multiple risk factors and complex pathophysiologic process responsible for cardiovascular disease in individuals with both type 1 and type 2 diabetes is critical for the prevention, early detection, and management of cardiovascular disease in this population. The focus of this article is on the acute and chronic manifestations of coronary heart disease.

FORTHCOMING ISSUES

RECENT ISSUES

THE CLINICS ARE NOW AVAILABLE ONLINE!

Access your subscription at:
http://www.theclinics.com

NURSING
CLINICS
OF NORTH AMERICA

Nurs Clin N Am 41 (2006) xi–xii

Preface

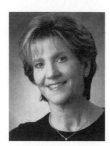

Gail D'Eramo Melkus, EdD, C-NP, CDE, FAAN
Guest Editor

The burgeoning of diabetes science and technology during the past decade has led to new knowledge that reconfigured diabetes health care delivery. Innovations in insulin therapy, blood glucose monitoring, early detection and treatment of complications, prevention efforts, and self-management interventions are just a few examples. The dissemination and translation of such advances and innovations are evident in established diabetes standards of care and education, reimbursement policies, and certification of diabetes educators and programs of diabetes care by national accrediting agencies. Despite these advances in science, technology, practice, and policy, however, there are continued increases in the incidence and prevalence of diabetes, particularly type 2 diabetes, and related complications, with elderly, ethnic minority, and rural populations experiencing the greatest burden.

This issue is a compilation of the current best practices and latest advances in the care of diabetes and diabetes-related complications. The reader will note that the number of persons affected by diabetes in the United States has increased to an estimated 21 million, accounting for more than $130 billion dollars in related health care costs. This care involves medical visits, emergency visits, hospitalizations, medical nutrition therapy, medications, self-management education, behavioral and psychologic counseling, and physical activity training. Multidisciplinary health care teams devoted to the delivery of quality diabetes care have been effective in improving health outcomes, but much more needs to be accomplished to decrease rates of diabetes morbidity and mortality and the health disparities for vulnerable populations. Numerous studies have shown that diabetes patient education

doi:10.1016/j.cnur.2006.08.002   *nursing.theclinics.com*

is an important prerequisite for behavioral change. Behavioral counseling and intervention strategies that facilitate and assist with maintenance of life-style modifications are necessary to sustain optimal daily diabetes self-management. Nurses dedicated to diabetes education and care have played a central and effective role within the diabetes health care delivery team. Like many of you, the authors of this issue are such nurses. They are leaders in diabetes care who have given generously of their time and expertise in their previous contributions to diabetes care, education, practice, policy, and research and to this issue of *Nursing Clinics of North America*. It is my hope that nurses and other health care professionals will find this issue informative and that the patients they care for will be the beneficiaries of what is derived.

Gail D'Eramo Melkus, EdD, C-NP, CDE, FAAN
Yale University School of Nursing
100 Church Street South
New Haven, CT 06536, USA

E-mail address: gail.melkus@yale.edu

ELSEVIER
SAUNDERS

Nurs Clin N Am 41 (2006) 487–498

NURSING
CLINICS
OF NORTH AMERICA

Epidemiologic Perspectives of Risk for Developing Diabetes and Diabetes Complications

Diane Berry, PhD, CANP[a],*,
Gail D'Eramo Melkus, EdD, C-NP, CDE, FAAN[b]

[a]School of Nursing, University of North Carolina at Chapel Hill, Carrington Hall,
Campus Box 7460, Chapel Hill, NC 27599–7460, USA
[b]Yale University School of Nursing, 100 Church Street South, PO Box 9740, New Haven,
CT 06536–0741, USA

Diabetes is a chronic metabolic condition in which the body fails to produce adequate insulin [1]. The classification of diabetes includes four clinical classes: (1) type 1 diabetes mellitus, which results from beta-cell destruction and leads to insulin deficiency; (2) type 2 diabetes mellitus (T2DM), which results from an insulin secretory defect; (3) other specific types, caused by genetic defects of beta-cell function or insulin action, diseases of the pancreas, or are drug or chemical induced; and (4) gestational diabetes mellitus [1]. T2DM accounts for 95% of individuals diagnosed with diabetes [1,2]. Prediabetes includes impaired fasting glucose (IFG) and impaired glucose tolerance (IGT) [1]. Both IFG and IGT are risk factors for the development of T2DM and cardiovascular disease (CVD). Diagnostic criteria for the diagnosis of IFG, IGT, and T2DM are as follows. IFG is diagnosed when fasting plasma glucose is between 100 mg/dL (5.6 mmol/L) and 125 mg/dL (6.9 mmol/L) [1]. IGT is diagnosed when during an oral glucose tolerance test the 2-hour plasma glucose is from 140 mg/dL (7.8 mmol/L) to 199 mg/dL (11 mmol/L) [1]. Diabetes is diagnosed if the patient has either the symptoms of diabetes (polydipsia, polyphagia, polyuria, unexplained weight loss) and a random glucose 200 mg/dL (11.1 mmol/L); fasting plasma glucose 126 mg/dL; or 2-hour plasma glucose 200 mg/dL (11.1 mmol/L during an oral glucose tolerance test using a glucose load containing the equivalent of 75-g anhydrous glucose dissolved in water [1].

* Corresponding author.
E-mail address: dberry@email.unc.edu (D. Berry).

Prevalence

The prevalence of diabetes globally has increased dramatically over the last several decades. A total of 18.2 million or 6.3% of the United States population have diabetes [3]. Of those 18.2 million people, 13 million are diagnosed and 5.2 million are undiagnosed [3]. Globally, diabetes is estimated to affect 151 million individuals with a projected increase by 2025 to 324 million [4]. The prevalence of diabetes varies by age, gender, and race and ethnicity. Approximately 0.26% (210,000) people under the age of 20 have diabetes with 1 in every 400 to 500 children and adolescents having type 1 diabetes [3]. In those people aged 20 years or older, 8.7% (18 million) have diabetes compared with 18.3% (8.6 million) of people aged 60 and older [3]. Over 8.7% of men (8.7 million) and 8.7% women (9.3 million) aged 20 years or older have diabetes [3]. If a male is diagnosed at age 40 with diabetes, his life expectancy decreases by approximately 11 years [5].

In those individuals born in the United States in 2000, the lifetime risk of developing diabetes is 39% for females and 33% for males, with Hispanic females the highest at 53% [5]. Hispanics, blacks, and American Indians are affected two to four times more than whites [2]. Within the past 10 years children and adolescents are diagnosed with T2DM more commonly than type 1 diabetes [6].

Etiology

The risk factors for developing T2DM include having a genetic predisposition, minority group, low birth weight, maternal diabetes, overweight and obesity, prediabetes, and certain environmental factors. The physiologic and molecular relationships between obesity and the development of T2DM continue to be an area of intense research [7].

The development of T2DM has been associated with a genetic predisposition. The thrifty genotype coupled with insulin resistance and beta-cell insufficiency has been found to contribute to the development of T2DM [8,9]. During the feast or famine times of hunter-gathers, survival was ensured with the ability to store energy as fat [2]. When famine is not an issue and individuals reduce energy expenditure, overweight and obesity develops.

Siblings of individuals with T2DM were found to have 3.5 times the risk of developing T2DM when compared with the general population [10]. In twins, monozygotic twins have an 80% to 100% chance of developing T2DM when compared with dizygotic twins [10]. Most T2DM in adults is polygenic [2,11].

Ethnic minority groups, such as Hispanics, blacks, American Indians, Pacific Islanders, and Asians, have a higher incidence of T2DM compared with whites [1]. Blacks are 1.4 to 2.2 times more likely to have diabetes compared with whites [1,3,5]. Hispanics have a higher prevalence of T2DM compared with whites, with Puerto Ricans and Hispanics living in the Southwest

having a higher incidence compared with Cubans [12,13]. American Indians are 2.8 times more likely to develop T2DM compared with whites. Asian and Pacific Islander communities (Japanese Americans, Chinese Americans, Filipino Americans, and Korean Americans) have a higher prevalence of T2DM when compared with whites [1,12,13].

Low birth weight is another risk factor that has been associated with the development of T2DM. Studies have demonstrated that impaired growth in utero caused by maternal malnutrition resulting in low birth weight has been associated with an increased incidence of glucose intolerance, insulin resistance, and T2DM in adults [14]. In addition, some fetal genetic factors determining insulin sensitivity might be linked to a reduction in fetal growth and the later development of diabetes [15]. Low birth weight has been found to be a risk factor for diabetes and increased rates of mortality. In one study, observed diabetes deaths were found to be greater than expected in the general population with 70% of excess deaths occurring among individuals who were low-birth-weight infants ($P < .001$) and to a lesser degree high-birth-weight infants ($P < .03$) compared with normal-weight infants [16].

Maternal diabetes has been found to be an important risk factor for the development of T2DM later in life. In one study, maternal gestational diabetes was associated with adiposity and higher glucose and insulin concentrations in female offspring at 5 years [17]. The absence of similar associations in offspring of diabetic fathers suggests a programming effect in the intrauterine environment of mothers with diabetes [17]. Further research confirms that alterations of the fetal and neonatal environment in offspring of mothers with diabetes who are low birth weight seem to program a predisposition to develop overweight, obesity, and T2DM later in life [18]. Another study confirmed that exposure to maternal obesity increased the risk of children developing the metabolic syndrome, which suggests that overweight or obese mothers who do not fulfill the clinical criteria of gestational diabetes mellitus may still have metabolic factors that affect fetal growth and postnatal outcomes [19]. Given the increased rates of overweight and obesity in the United States, these findings have implications for perpetuating the cycle of obesity, insulin resistance, and their consequences in future generations.

The increased incidence of diabetes has mirrored the obesity epidemic in the United States. Overweight and obesity is a multifaceted chronic disease involving genetic, environmental, physiologic, metabolic, behavioral, and psychologic components. The relationship between obesity and diabetes is mediated by nutritional and lifestyle factors [20,21]. Overweight and obesity is defined by body mass index, which is calculated by using the formula kilograms divided by meters squared (kg/m^2) [22]. In adults age 20 years and older, overweight is defined as a body mass index between 25 and 29.9 and obesity is defined as a body mass index ≥ 30 [23]. Currently, 64.5% (127 million) adults age 20 years and older in the United States are either

overweight or obese compared with 46% from 1976 to 1980 (Fig. 1) [13,22,24–26]. Overweight has increased steadily with age for both men and women with approximately 50% of all age groups being overweight and 20% being obese [13,22,24]. The age group with the highest prevalence of overweight and obesity, however, among men is 65 to 74 years and among women 55 to 64 years [13,22,27]. The risk for developing diabetes increases for women having a body mass index > 23 for 16 years and increases 20-fold for those women with a body mass index > 30 [28].

As overweight and obesity increases so does IGT and IFG, which establishes a foundation for the development of T2DM [1]. IFG is defined as having a glucose level between 110 and 125 mg/dL and IGT is defined as having a 2-hour postprandial blood glucose level between 140 and 199 mg/dL [1]. Individuals who are diagnosed with IFG and IGT have prediabetes. It has been reported that approximately 9.1 million overweight adults have IGT, 5.8 million have IFG, 11.9 million have prediabetes, and 3 million have IGT and IFG based on data from the Third National Health and Nutrition Examination Survey (1988–1994) [29].

The changing environment over the past several decades provides further understanding of the increase in T2DM in the United States and around the world. Over the past 30 years there has been an increasing positive energy balance because of increased food consumption and decreased physical activity. More meals are consumed in fast food restaurants than at home and those meals are higher in fat and calorie dense [29]. A decrease in physical activity and increase in sedentary activity is also an important factor in the development of obesity with several studies demonstrating that overweight subjects were less physically active when compared with leaner subjects [30,31].

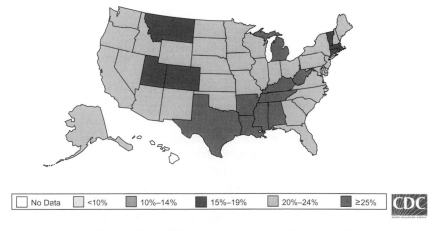

Fig. 1. Obesity trends among United States adults. Behavioral Risk Factor Surveillance System 2004. Body mass index ≥ 30 or approximately 30 lb overweight for a 5-ft 4-in person.

Cardiovascular risk

Diabetes has reached epidemic proportions globally and is likely to be one of the most important public health concerns and threat to health in the twenty-first century secondary to complications. Complications of diabetes can be classified as either microvascular or macrovascular. Microvascular complications include neuropathy, nephropathy, and retinopathy [1,32,33]. Macrovascular complications include CVD; stroke; and peripheral vascular disease, which can lead to ulcers, gangrene, and amputation [1]. Other complications of diabetes include infections and autonomic neuropathy [1]. This article concentrates on cardiovascular risk and the development of hypertension and dyslipidemia.

Hypertension

One in four adults in the United States has hypertension and hypertension is twice as common in individuals with diabetes compared with individuals without diabetes [34]. Hypertension contributes to microvascular and macrovascular complications and is a major contributor to the development of CVD [1]. Approximately 80% of early mortality in those patients with diabetes is related to CVD compared with 40% of those patients without diabetes [35,36].

Overweight and obesity contributes to the increased prevalence of T2DM and hypertension [36–38]. Over 50% of those patients diagnosed with T2DM have hypertension at diagnosis [36]. Overweight and obesity may be a common link between hypertension and diabetes, but insulin resistance and autonomic dysfunction may also be involved [1,34,39,40]. Central adiposity has been found to be a risk factor in the development of insulin resistance, T2DM, hypertension, dyslipidemia, and premature CVD [4,38,41,42]. This association is believed to be predisposed by a patient's amount of visceral fat [43]. Body mass index is believed to be a determinant of hypertension; however, visceral fat distribution seems to be an even more important risk factor for the development of hypertension [44,45]. In those individuals with central adiposity and increased visceral fat, fasting hyperinsulinemia [45] and elevated apolipoprotein B [46] have been found to be strong risk factors for the development of hypertension and CVD.

Approximately 25% of individuals with hypertension have adequate control of their blood pressure [34]. Reduction in blood pressure can decrease the risk of complications in those individuals with diabetes [1,34,39,40]. Hypertension is defined as follows: prehypertension is diagnosed when blood pressure is 120/80 to 139/89, stage I hypertension ranges from 140/90 to 159/99, and stage II hypertension is defined as a blood pressure $\geq 160/100$ on three occasions [47,48]. Patients with diabetes who have hypertension, however, should receive treatment to maintain a systolic blood pressure <130 mm Hg and a diastolic blood pressure <80 mm Hg [1].

Research studies have demonstrated the benefit of decreasing systolic blood pressure <140 mm Hg and diastolic blood pressure <80 mm Hg in decreasing cardiovascular events, stroke, and nephropathy [49–51]. Other studies have shown, however, that patients who have diabetes and a blood pressure >115/75 mm Hg have increased cardiovascular events and mortality [49,52,53]. The blood pressure goal <130/80 mm Hg is considered safe and reasonable [1].

Dyslipidemia

Diabetes has been defined as a CVD risk factor [54]. CVD is the leading cause of death for both men and women in the United States. CVD is caused by a narrowing of the coronary arteries that supply blood to the heart, and often results in a heart attack [54]. CVD caused 508,189 deaths in the United States in 2001 [54]. Men and women with diabetes with one or two risk factors had a 10-year cumulative incidence of CVD that was only 1.4 times higher than that of individuals without diabetes (14%) [55]. The 10-year incidence of CVD in subjects with diabetes and multiple risk factors increased to >40% with a higher incidence of fatal CVD compared with subjects without diabetes and previous CVD [55].

Dyslipidemia is defined as follows: a fasting total cholesterol ≥200 mg/dL; a low-density lipoprotein ≥100 mg/dL; a high-density lipoprotein ≤45 mg/dL; and triglycerides ≥150 mg/dL [56]. Elevated low-density lipoprotein is the primary contributing factor to the development and progression of coronary heart disease [57]. A major component of increased atherosclerotic plaques is related to excessive levels of low-density lipoprotein in the blood, which is deposited in the blood vessel wall [48,56]. Patients with diabetes should have a lipid profile drawn annually [1]. Patients with diabetes who have a low-density lipoprotein <100 mg/dL, high-density lipoprotein >50 mg/dL, and triglycerides <150 mg/dL can have a lipid profile every 2 years [1].

The Heart Protection Study demonstrated that in subjects with diabetes, when low-density lipoprotein was reduced approximately 30% from baseline with a statin, there was a 25% reduction in major first CVD events, independent of glycemic control, type of diabetes, years of diabetes, preexisting vascular disease, or baseline lipoprotein [58]. In another study, patients with T2DM were randomized to atorvastatin or placebo and those who received the atorvastatin had a significant decrease in CVD events [59]. Recent studies in high-risk patients have demonstrated that high doses of statins to achieve a low-density lipoprotein <70 mg/dL led to a significant reduction of future CVD events [60–62].

Diabetes Surveillance System

The Diabetes Surveillance System through the Centers for Disease Control and Prevention provides information on the prevalence and incidence,

mortality, hospitalizations, health care provider contacts, outpatient and emergency room visits, incidence of end-stage renal disease, disability, population statistics, and preventative care practices [63]. The incidence and prevalence of diabetes in the United States are determined by using data from the National Health Interview Survey (NHIS) of the National Center for Health Statistics (NCHS) conducted by the Centers for Disease Control and Prevention [64]. The NHIS has conducted an annual household survey since 1957 of approximately 120,000 residents. Each year, a subsample (one sixth) is asked whether in the last year any family member has had diabetes. Prevalence is defined as the total number of individuals with diabetes regardless of onset, and incidence is defined as individuals diagnosed with diabetes in the last year. The precision of prevalence and incidence estimates were improved by using 3-year moving averages. Then these estimates were applied to estimates of the United States population to determine the number of individuals diagnosed with diabetes [64].

The Behavioral Risk Factor Surveillance System (BRFSS) is used to estimate state-specific prevalence of diabetes [64]. The BRFSS is a monthly, state-based telephone survey of adults that is used to gather information on preventative health practices and behavioral risk factors. One question in the survey asks "Has a doctor every told you that you have diabetes"? If the individual answers "yes," then they are considered to have diabetes [64]. Both the NHIS and the BRFSS underestimate the prevalence of diabetes, however, because approximately one third of individuals do not know they have diabetes [65].

The NCHS at the Centers for Disease Control and Prevention collects and analyzes data annually on age, race, sex, state of residence, underlying cause of death, and multiple cause of death. These data are used to compile information on deaths associated with diabetes and examine emerging trends [66,67]. The most common cause of death in which diabetes was listed as a cause included diabetic ketoacidosis, stroke, ischemic heart disease, and major CVD [66,67]. Diabetes is underreported on death certificates. Among individuals with diabetes, only 40% have diabetes reported as a cause of death and only 10% have diabetes reported as an underlying cause of death [66,67]. Death certificate data cannot be used to examine overall mortality among individuals with diabetes.

The NCHS's National Hospital Discharge Data are used to estimate diabetes-related hospital discharges. Data are collected on age, race, sex, and length of stay. Hospital discharges with diabetes as a primary diagnosis include diabetic ketoacidosis, stroke, ischemic heart disease, major CVD, and nontraumatic lower-extremity amputation [68,69]. Hospitalizations caused by diabetes may be underestimated by 40% because of exclusion of long-term and federal hospitals from the data and a substantial proportion of discharges are missing racial classification [69].

The NHIS, National Ambulatory Care Survey, and National Hospital Ambulatory Medical Care Survey are collected by NCHS, Centers for

Disease Control and Prevention, and provide data on the use of health care services among individuals with diabetes. The NHIS is used to estimate the number and rate of health care provider contacts and visits among individuals with diabetes. These estimates include all contacts and visits regardless of reason, however, and reflect health care use among individuals with diabetes [63]. The National Ambulatory Care Survey is a national cross-sectional annual survey that provides data on office visits. Data are collected by health care providers and include practice characteristics, patient and visit characteristics, and health care provider's diagnoses [70]. The National Hospital Ambulatory Medical Care Survey is also a national cross-sectional annual survey that provides data on visits made to emergency departments and outpatient departments. Data are collected on patient and visit characteristics and the health care provider's diagnoses [71]. All three surveys underestimate the use of health care services by individuals with diabetes [65].

The US Renal Data System is a surveillance system for end-stage renal disease. The US Renal Data System is funded by the National Institute of Diabetes and Digestive and Kidney Diseases and the Health Care Financing Administration provides most of the data. The US Renal Data System data are used to examine the incidence and prevalence of end-stage renal disease attributed to diabetes. End-stage renal disease attributed to diabetes is defined as patients starting dialysis or kidney transplantation and having diabetes listed as their primary diagnosis. Those patients dying before receiving treatment or those patients not being included are limitations to data collection [72,73].

The NHIS provides indicators of disability among persons with diabetes. The two major indicators include activity limitation and activity restriction. Activity limitation reflects a long-term decrease in activity secondary to chronic disease. A decrease in activity is measured in terms of normal activities for each age group. For example, persons 18 to 69 years of age are measured by their ability to work or keep house and independence in basic life activities. Activity restriction is defined as a reduction of activity caused by either short- or long-term conditions. Estimates of disability by the NHIS underestimate the total amount of disability associated with diabetes.

The prevalence of state-specific diabetes preventative care is determined by using data from the BRFSS. Persons who responded "yes" to having diabetes are then asked how many times over the last year that they had their hemoglobin A_{1c} tested and had an eye and foot examination. Self-report of hemoglobin A_{1c} measurement has been shown to have high sensitivity and low specificity [74]. Further examination of the reliability and validity of self-report for eye and foot examinations is needed.

Summary

The incidence and prevalence of diabetes, particularly T2DM, is increasing both in the United States and worldwide. Identified risk factors, such as glucose intolerance, hypertension, and hyperlipidemia, often precede and

accompany the diagnosis of T2DM. Further, all are associated physiologic alterations of obesity. Obesity that has grown in epidemic proportion, because of overconsumption of calories in the presence of decreased physical activity, affects greater numbers of persons including children and adolescents. National recommendations for screening and diagnosis of diabetes, hypertension, and dyslipidemia provide a basis for early detection, treatment, and intervention that may potentially decrease related complications, and personal and economic costs of the disease. Most important is that knowledge exists about who is at risk for diabetes by weight, family history of diabetes, ethnicity, and history of gestational diabetes that allows for the development and implementation of diabetes primary prevention programs. Multiple national health surveys and databases provide important information for health care providers, systems of care, and communities that can be used to guide such prevention, early screening, and disease detection and intervention programs aimed at decreasing the burden of diabetes.

References

[1] American Diabetes Association. Clinical practice recommendations 2006. Diabetes Care 2006;29:S1–80.

[2] Permutt MA, Wasson J, Cox N. Genetic epidemiology of diabetes. J Clin Invest 2005;115: 1431–6.

[3] American Diabetes Association. National diabetes fact sheet. Chicago: American Diabetes Association; 2002.

[4] Zimmet PZ, Shaw JE, Albert KG. Preventing type 2 diabetes and the dysmetabolic syndrome in the real world: a realistic view. Diabet Med 2003;20:693–702.

[5] Narayan KM, et al. Life-time risk for diabetes mellitus in the United States. JAMA 2003;290: 1884–90.

[6] Alberti G, et al. Type 2 diabetes in the young: the evolving epidemic. The international diabetes federation consensus workshop. Diabetes Care 2004;27:1798–811.

[7] Speakman JR. Obesity: the integrated roles of environment and genetics. J Nutr 2004;134 (8 Suppl):2090S–105S.

[8] Neel JV. Diabetes mellitus: a "thrifty" genotype rendered detrimental by "progress"? Am J Hum Genet 1962;14:353–62.

[9] Lev-Ran A. Thrifty genotype: how applicable is it to obesity and type 2 diabetes? Diabetes Reviews 1999;7:1–22.

[10] Lindgren CM, Hirschhorn JN. The genetics of type 2 diabetes. Endocrinologist 2001;11: 178–87.

[11] American Diabetes Association. Consensus Development Conference On Insulin Resistance: 5–6 November 1997. Diabetes Care 1998;21:310–4.

[12] Liao Y, et al. REACH 2010 Surveillance for Health Status in Minority Communities, United States, 2001–2002. MMWR Morb Mortal Wkly Rep 2004;53:1–36.

[13] Mokdad AH, et al. The spread of the obesity epidemic in the United States, 1991–1998. JAMA 1999;282:1519–22.

[14] Ende N, Redd AS. Administration of human umbilical cord blood to low birth weight infants may prevent the subsequent development of type 2 diabetes. Med Hypotheses 2006;66:1157–60, Epub 2006 Feb 14.

[15] Igaki N, Tanaka M, Goto T. Low birth weight and insulin resistance associated with lean body adiposity in an adolescent onset diabetic patient. Internal Medicine 2006;45:5–9, Epub 2006 Feb 1.

[16] Leibson CL, et al. Relative risk of mortality associated with diabetes as a function of birth weight. Diabetes Care 2005;28:2839–43.

[17] Krishnaveni GV, et al. Anthropometry, glucose tolerance, and insulin concentrations in Indian children: relationships to maternal glucose and insulin concentrations during pregnancy. Diabetes Care 2005;28 2919–25.

[18] Plagemann A. Perinatal programming and functional teratogenesis: impact on body weight regulation and obesity. Physiol Behav 2005;86:661–8.

[19] Boney CM, et al. Metabolic syndrome in childhood: association with birth weight, maternal obesity, and gestational diabetes mellitus. Pediatrics 2005;115:290–6.

[20] Zimmet PZ. Diabetes epidemiology as a tool to trigger diabetes research and care. Diabetologia 1999;42:499–518.

[21] Hu FB, et al. Diet, lifestyle, and the risk of type 2 diabetes mellitus in women. N Engl J Med 2001;345:790–7.

[22] Centers for Disease Control and Prevention. What is BMI? United States Department of Health and Human Services. 2004. Available at: http://www.cdc.gov/nccdphp/dnpa/bmi/bmi-adult.htm. Accessed 2/15/2006.

[23] Hedley AA, et al. Overweight and obesity among US children and adolescents, and adults, 1999–2002. JAMA 2004;291:2847–50.

[24] Centers for Disease Control and Prevention. National Center for Health Statistics: overweight among US children and adolescents. National Health and Nutrition Examination Survey. 1999. Available at: http://www.CDC.gov/NCHS/NHANES.htm. Accessed 2/15/2006.

[25] National Health Center for Statistics. Centers for Disease Control and Prevention, and Health-E-Stats. Prevalence of overweight among children and adolescents: United States, 1999. 2001. Available at: http://www.cdc.gov/nchs/releases/01news/overweight99.htm. Accessed 2/15/2006.

[26] Flegal KM, et al. Prevalence and trends in obesity among US adults, 1999–2000. JAMA 2002;291:2847–50.

[27] Centers for Disease Control and Prevention. National Health and Nutrition Examination Survey. Atlanta: National Center for Health Statistics; 2002.

[28] Motala AA, Omar MA, Pirie FJ. Diabetes in Africa: epidemiology of type 1 and type 2 diabetes in Africa. J Cardiovasc Risk 2003;10:77–83.

[29] Troiano RP, et al. Overweight prevalence and trends for children and adolescents. The National Health and Nutrition Examination Surveys, 1963 to 1991. Arch Pediatr Adolesc Med 1995;149:1085–91.

[30] Davies PSW, Gregory J, White A. Physical activity and body fatness in pre-school children. Int J Obes Relat Metab Disord 1995;19:6–10.

[31] Moore LL, et al. Preschool physical activity level and change in body fatness in young children: the Framingham Children's Study. Am J Epidemiol 1995;142:982–8.

[32] Diabetes Control and Complications Trial (DCCT) Research Group. Effect of intensive insulin treatment on the development and progression of long-term complications in adolescents with insulin-dependent diabetes mellitus. Diabetes Control and Complications Trial. J Pediatr 1994;125:177–88.

[33] Engelgau MM, et al. The evolving diabetes burden in the United States. Ann Intern Med 2004;140:945–51.

[34] Konzem SL, Devore VS, Bauer DW. Controlling hypertension in patients with diabetes. Am Fam Physician 2002;66:1209–14.

[35] Leahy JL, Clark NG, Cefalu WT. Medical management of diabetes mellitus. New York: Marcel Dekker; 2000.

[36] Sowers JR, Raman B. Hypertension and diabetes. In: Leahy JL, Clark NG, Cefalu WT, editors. Medical management of diabetes. New York: Marcel Dekker; 2000. p. 573–82.

[37] Kirpichnikov D, Sowers JR. Diabetes mellitus and diabetes-associated vascular disease. Trends Endocrinol Metab 2001;12:225–30.

[38] Manrique C, et al. Hypertension and the cardiometabolic syndrome. J Clin Hypertens 2005; 7:471–6.

[39] American Diabetes Association. The treatment of hypertension in adult patients with diabetes. Diabetes Care 2002;25:134–47.

[40] American Diabetes Association. Hypertension management in adults with diabetes. Diabetes Care 2004;27:S65–7.

[41] Hu FB. Overweight and obesity in women: health risks and consequences. J Womens Health (Larchmt) 2003;12:163–72.

[42] Haffner SM. Metabolic syndrome, diabetes and coronary artery disease. Int J Clin Pract 2002;132:31–7.

[43] Caprio S. Relationship between abdominal fat visceral fat and metabolic risk factors in obese adolescents. Am J Human Biol 2001;11:259–66.

[44] Matsuzawa Y. Therapy Insight: adipocytokines in metabolic syndrome and related cardiovascular disease. Nature Clinical Practice Cardiovascular Medicine 2006;3:35–42.

[45] Reaven G. All obese individuals are not created equal: insulin resistance is the major determinant of cardiovascular disease in overweight/obese individuals. Diabetes and Vascular Disease Research 2005;2:105–12.

[46] Miller WM, et al. Obesity and lipids. Curr Cardiol Rep 2005;7:465–70.

[47] National High Blood Pressure Education Program. JNC 7 Express: the Seventh Report of the Joint National Committee on Prevention, Detection, Evaluation, and Treatment of High Blood Pressure. NIH Publication No. 03–5233. Washington: United States Department of Health and Human Services, National Institutes of Health, National Heart, Lung, and Blood Institute; 2003.

[48] US Department of Health and Human Services. Third Report of the National Cholesterol Education Program expert panel on the detection, evaluation, and treatment of high blood cholesterol in adults (Adult Treatment Panel III). NIH Publication No. 01–3670. Washington: United States Department of Health and Human Services; 2002.

[49] Chobanian AV, et al. The seventh report of the Joint National Committee on Prevention, Detection, Evaluation, and Treatment of High Blood Pressure: the JNC 7 Report. JAMA 2003;289:2560–72.

[50] United Kingdom Prospective Diabetes Study Group. Tight blood pressure control and risk of macrovascular and microvascular complications in type 2 diabetes. BMJ 1998;317: 703–13.

[51] Hansson L, et al. HOT Study Group: effects of intensive blood pressure lowering and low-dose aspirin in patients with hypertension. Principal results of the Hypertension Optimal Treatment (HOT) randomised trial. Lancet 1998;351:1755–62.

[52] Lewington S, et al. Age-specific relevance of usual blood pressure to vascular mortality: a meta-analysis of individual data for one million adults in 61 prospective studies. Lancet 2002;360:1903–13.

[53] Stamler J, et al. Diabetes, other risk factors, and 12-year cardiovascular mortality for men screened in the Multiple Risk Factor Intervention Trial. Diabetes Care 1993;16:434–44.

[54] American Heart Association. Heart and stroke statistics 2005 update. Dallas (TX): American Heart Association; 2005.

[55] Howard BV, et al. Coronary heart disease risk equivalence in diabetes depends on concomitant risk factors. Diabetes Care 2006;29:391–7.

[56] Grundy SM, et al. Implications of recent clinical trials for the National Cholesterol Education Program Adult Treatment Panel III Guidelines. Circulation 2004;110:227–39.

[57] Schaefer EJ, Seman LJ. The diagnosis and management of lipoprotein disorders. In: Leahy JL, Clark NG, Cefalu WT, editors. Medical management of diabetes mellitus. New York: Marcel Dekker; 2000. p. 499–526.

[58] Heart Protection Study Collaborative Group. MRC/BHF Heart Protection Study of cholesterol-lowering with simvastatin in 5963 people with diabetes: a randomised placebo-controlled trial. Lancet 2003;361:2005–16.

[59] Colhoun HM, et al. Primary prevention of cardiovascular disease with atorvastatin in type 2 diabetes in the Collaborative Atorvastatin Diabetes Study (CARDS): multicentre randomized placebo-controlled trial. Lancet 2004;364:685–6.

[60] Cannon CP, et al. Intensive versus moderate lipid lowering with statins after acute coronary syndromes. N Engl J Med 2004;350:1495–504.

[61] de Lemos JA, et al. Early intensive vs a delayed conservative simvastatin strategy in patients with acute coronary syndromes: phase Z of the A to Z trial. JAMA 2004;292:1307–16.

[62] Nissen SE, et al. Effect of intensive compared with moderate lipid-lowering therapy on progression of coronary atherosclerosis: a randomized controlled trial. JAMA 2004;291: 1071–80.

[63] Centers for Disease Control and Prevention (CDC). Data and trends of the Diabetes Surveillance System. Atlanta: National Center for Chronic Disease Prevention and Health Promotion; 2006.

[64] Massey JT, et al. Design and estimation for the National Health Interview Survey, 1985–94. Vital Health Stat 2 1989;110:1–40.

[65] Harris MI, et al. Prevalence of diabetes, impaired fasting glucose, and impaired glucose tolerance in US adults. The Third National Health and Nutrition Examination Survey, 1988–1994. Diabetes Care 1998;21:518–24.

[66] Bild DE, Stevenson JM. Frequency of recording of diabetes on US death certificates: analysis of the 1986 National Mortality Followback Survey. J Clin Epidemiol 1992;45:275–81.

[67] Ochi JW, et al. A population-based study of diabetes mortality. Diabetes Care 1985;8:224–9.

[68] Graves EJ. National Hospital Discharge Survey: annual summary, 1990. Vital Health Stat 13 1992;112:1–110.

[69] Ford ES, Wetterhall SF. The validity of diabetes on hospital discharge. Diabetes 1991; 40(Suppl 1):449A.

[70] Tenney JB, White KL, Williamson JW. National Ambulatory Medical Care Survey: background and methodology. Vital Health Stat 2 1974;34:1–85.

[71] McCaig LF, McLemore T. Plan and operation of the National Hospital Ambulatory Medical Survey Vital Health Stat 1 1994;34:1–226.

[72] US Renal Data System. USRDS 1999 annual data report. Bethesda: National Institutes of Health, National Institute of Diabetes and Digestive and Kidney Diseases; 1999.

[73] Centers for Disease Control and Prevention. Diabetes surveillance. Atlanta: US Department of Health and Human Services Public Health Service; 1992.

[74] Briggs-Fowels J, et al. The validity of self-reported diabetes quality of care measures. Int J Qual Health Care 1999;11:407–12.

ELSEVIER
SAUNDERS

NURSING
CLINICS
OF NORTH AMERICA

Nurs Clin N Am 41 (2006) 499–511

Economics of Diabetes Mellitus

Sarah L. Krein, PhD, RN[a,b,c,*],
Martha M. Funnell, MS, RN, CDE[c],
John D. Piette, PhD[a,b,c]

[a]VA Ann Arbor Healthcare System, Center for Practice Management and Outcomes
Research, 2215 Fuller Road, Ann Arbor, MI 48105, USA
[b]Department of Internal Medicine, University of Michigan Medical School,
300 North Ingalls, Suite 7C27, Ann Arbor, MI 48109, USA
[c]Michigan Diabetes Research and Training Center, University of Michigan, 1331 East Ann,
Box 0580, Room 5111, Ann Arbor, MI 48109, USA

There are over 20 million persons with diabetes in the United States (7% of the population) and projections suggest that the number of individuals diagnosed with diabetes could be as high as 39 million by the year 2050 [1–3]. In addition, an estimated 41 million adults have prediabetes (impaired fasting glucose or impaired glucose tolerance), a condition that raises the risk of developing type 2 diabetes substantially [2]. The increasing prevalence of diabetes, prediabetes, and diabetes risk factors, such as obesity, pose many challenges for the United States health care system in general and for the nursing profession in particular. Moreover, despite numerous treatment advances [4–11], diabetes remains a leading cause of blindness, end-stage renal disease, and amputation. In 2002, diabetes was the sixth leading cause of death in the United States [2,12] with most deaths and hospitalizations caused by macrovascular complications, such as heart attack and stroke [1,9,13].

Given the burden of diabetes on health systems, and on individual patients, the cost of diabetes care is a pressing concern. This article focuses on four main issues related to the economic impact of diabetes for patients and health systems: (1) overall estimates of the direct and indirect costs of

This work was supported in part by grant number NIH5P60 DK20572, 1 R18 0K062323 from the National Institute of Diabetes and Digestive and Kidney Diseases of the National Institutes of Health and DIB 98-001 from the Department of Veterans Affairs, Health Services Research and Development Service.

* Corresponding author. VA Ann Arbor Healthcare System, Center for Practice Management and Outcomes Research, 2215 Fuller Road, Ann Arbor, MI 48105.

E-mail address: skrein@umich.edu (S.L. Krein).

doi:10.1016/j.cnur.2006.07.003

nursing.theclinics.com

diabetes and its associated complications, (2) the impact of cost on diabetes care and health outcomes, (3) the ways in which federal and state mandated insurance for persons with diabetes are being used to promote more cost-effective and high-quality diabetes care, and (4) the use of cost-effectiveness analysis to evaluate interventions designed to prevent diabetes or diabetes-related complications.

The costs of diabetes and its complications

During the past decade, diabetes was ranked eighth among the 15 most costly medical conditions treated in the United States [14]. In 2002, diabetes costs in the United States were approximately $130 billion [15], which adjusted for inflation translates to approximately $149 billion in 2005. Diabetes costs include both the direct costs of medical care provided for patients and their diabetes-related complications, and the indirect costs associated with lost productivity and premature mortality. Given the current prevalence of diabetes in the United States, the total economic cost (ie, including both direct and indirect financial impacts) of diabetes could reach $192 billion by 2020 [15]. Considering the projected increasing rates of obesity and diabetes in many parts of the country, however, along with rising health care costs, the actual economic burden is likely to be significantly higher [1].

The direct cost of diabetes

Because diabetes has such pervasive effects on patients' medical needs, estimating direct medical costs requires data on a wide variety of inpatient and outpatient health services. Obtaining this information on a national basis can be challenging as described by Hogan and coworkers [15], who used data from several sources to produce a comprehensive assessment of diabetes-related costs in 2002. For example, estimates of the size of the population with diabetes were derived using data from the Census Bureau and the National Health Interview Survey, which identifies people with diabetes based on self-report and may underestimate the actual number of affected individuals. The fraction of patients' health care use attributable to their diabetes was estimated by compiling a number of different data sources (eg, National Inpatient Sample, National Ambulatory Medical Care Survey) to assess diabetes-related health care use across a spectrum of services including institutional care, outpatient care, medications, and supplies. Identifying the proportion of services used that are associated with diabetes is an important step because people with diabetes may also have health care needs not related to diabetes and the costs of these services should be excluded when measuring the resource intensity of diabetes care. Price estimates per unit of service were obtained primarily from the Medical Expenditure Panel Survey.

The analysis by Hogan and coworkers [15] showed that in 2002 health care spending for people with diabetes was $92 billion, including $23 billion

for health care events with a primary diagnosis of uncomplicated diabetes, and nearly $25 billion for treatment of diabetes-related cardiovascular disease. Other studies have also demonstrated the high cost burden of diabetes-related complications [16–18]. Although glycemic control is an important element of effective diabetes care, the management of macrovascular complications, such as heart attacks and strokes, represents the largest driver of medical service use and related costs, accounting for over 50% of expenditures [17].

As with many chronic illnesses, the most costly component of care for diabetes-related services are those provided as part of acute inpatient stays addressing either disease complications or (more rarely) acute episodes of severe glucose dysregulation [15]. Some estimates suggest that with appropriate nursing care management and other primary care services, many hospitalizations for diabetes complications could be prevented leading to over $2 billion in hospital costs averted and substantial savings for public health insurance programs, such as Medicare and Medicaid [19]. Nonetheless, in 2002, diabetes-related inpatient stays cost more than $40 billion; expenditures for nursing home care for diabetes patients cost almost $14 billion; diabetes medication (insulin and oral agents) and supply costs were $12 billion; and expenditures for office-based physician visits were $10 billion (Table 1) [15]. When all of these components are considered jointly, more than $1 in $10 spent on these types of health services in the United States was attributable to diabetes.

The indirect cost of diabetes

Even when their illness does not require medical intervention, diabetes can limit individuals' productivity, employability, and functioning while at

Table 1
Total economic cost of diabetes in the United States in 2002

Type of cost	Cost of diabetes: all ages ($ in millions)	Proportion of total cost (%)
Direct medical costs	91,860	
Institutional care	54,216	41
Outpatient care	20,129	15
Outpatient medication and supplies	17,515	13
Indirect costs	39,811	
Morbidity	18,253	14
Mortality	21,558	16
Total	131,671	100

Numbers do not add up to 100 because of rounding.
From Zhang P, Engelgau MM, Norris SL, et al. Application of economic analysis to diabetes and diabetes care. Ann Intern Med 2004;140:972–7; with permission.

work. Furthermore, diabetes is associated with premature mortality and these lost years of productive work life must also be taken into account when estimating the indirect cost of diabetes. In 2002, the cost of lost productivity because of diabetes was approximately $40 billion [15]. A more recent study based on a national household sample of Americans estimated that costs associated with diabetes-related mortality, disability, early retirement, and work absenteeism was more than $133 billion over the lifetime of the study cohort [20]. Large employer groups often must pay for the direct medical care of diabetes patients and the indirect costs associated with absenteeism. As a consequence many large employer groups have become interested in supporting novel workplace services designed to prevent diabetes by addressing risk factors, such as obesity, and to keep their employees healthy and on the job [21–23].

Predicting diabetes-related costs

Diabetes patients vary substantially in their patterns of health service use and costs. Risk factors for higher-than-average diabetes-related medical costs include insulin use, cardiovascular disease, depression, and higher hemoglobin A_{1c} levels, all of which are usually related to poorer outcomes, such as heart attacks and renal disease [24,25]. Indicators of patients' metabolic control (eg, blood pressure, lipid levels, and hemoglobin A_{1c}) also predict their risk of both macrovascular and microvascular complications [4–6,9]. Consequently, appropriate treatment and assisting patients in reaching metabolic targets is important to minimize morbidity and costly service use. As with most chronic conditions, however, diabetes requires a high level of self-management and outcomes are ultimately determined by patients' ability to self-monitor, adhere to treatment plans, and maintain critical lifestyle behavior changes. As such, the affect of cost on patients' ability to manage their condition is also an important issue to consider.

Impact of cost on diabetes patients' service use and health outcomes

Third-party health care payers increasingly face growing financial burdens and as a result are sharing an increasing proportion of these costs with health care consumers, including people with diabetes. Many patients pay at least some costs out-of-pocket for diabetes-related examinations and laboratory tests, blood glucose self-monitoring supplies, medical nutrition therapy, and diabetes self-management training [26,27]. A number of studies have examined the impact of this cost sharing on patients' use of essential treatments [26–30]. These studies consistently show that diabetes patients are sensitive to out-of-pocket medication costs and may decrease their use of important medications, including diabetes medications, because of cost pressures [27,28]. People with diabetes frequently take multiple medications

daily, both for their diabetes-related illnesses and to manage comorbidities, and even relatively small copayments can add up to a significant financial burden, especially for patients with limited financial resources.

Cost-related medication underuse has been linked to adverse health events among people with diabetes and other chronic health problems [31–33]. One study of diabetes patients found that those who reduced their use of hypoglycemic medications because of cost problems had poorer glycemic control. Patients who reported cutting back on medications because of the cost reported more diabetes-related symptoms, and poorer physical and mental functioning [32]. Additionally, third-party payers' efforts to control their costs by increasing patients' cost-sharing could actually lead to higher overall medical costs down the road because of the increased burden of treatment for preventable complications. For example, angiotensin-converting enzyme inhibitors slow the progression of renal disease and reduce cardiac morbidity and mortality among patients with diabetes and for many patients are critical components of their management plan. Rosen and coworkers [34] demonstrated that eliminating out-of-pocket costs for angiotensin-converting enzyme inhibitors among Medicare beneficiaries with diabetes could increase angiotensin-converting enzyme inhibitor use; prevent complications, such as myocardial infarction, stroke, and renal disease; and thereby reduce future Medicare expenditures. As a result, both public and private providers of prescription coverage are considering the ways in which "benefit-based copayment" strategies could improve both diabetes outcomes and their own bottom line [34,35].

Even if costs cannot be completely controlled, there are opportunities to address diabetes patients' cost-related medication adherence problems through interventions that assist patients in identifying programs to pay for their drugs and educating them about the importance of medication adherence. Unfortunately, diabetes patients frequently do not tell their providers when they are cutting back on medications because of cost pressures, and many patients with cost problems report that they have not received information or assistance from their health care providers to help them deal with cost pressures [27]. Piette and colleagues [27] found that 37% of older patients with diabetes who cut back on medications because of cost-pressures reported never talking with clinicians about medication costs. The most commonly cited reason for not discussing medication-related cost problems was because the clinician never asked [27].

These findings highlight an important gap in care for patients with diabetes where nurses could play a key role by identifying patients with cost-related concerns and by assisting them in accessing programs to help relieve cost barriers. Identifying potential cost-related problems can be as simple as asking a patient: Do you have problems paying for your medications? Do you ever miss or skip taking your medications because you do not have money to buy them? Have you talked with your insurer, care provider, or pharmacist about the cost of your medications? Nurses can help patients

identify how much they are currently spending out-of-pocket for medications and discuss the importance of using their medication as prescribed. Nurses also are ideally situated to assist patients who have potential cost-related adherence problems in talking with their prescribing provider about less expensive alternatives; which medications are the most important for them to take; and whether any medications could be eliminated, substituted, or taken at a lower dose [36].

In addition to medications, higher out-of-pocket costs have also been associated with decreased use of other recommended diabetes services [26,29,30]. One study found that among diabetes patients enrolled in 10 managed care health plans, those paying the full cost for services were less likely to have dilated eye examinations, attend health education classes, and, if on insulin, perform daily self-monitoring of blood glucose compared with enrollees with no copayment [26]. Another study found that patients with type 2 diabetes were more cost-sensitive in some areas of their care than others. In particular, patients reported they were less likely to follow their diet than take prescribed medications, with cost being one of the most frequently cited barriers to following dietary recommendations [30].

Structuring insurance benefits to promote more effective diabetes care

Because diabetes care is so costly, diabetes management has been singled out through mandated benefit and insurance coverage initiatives at both the state and federal levels. At the federal level, the Balanced Budget Act of 1997 explicitly acknowledged the value of diabetes self-management training (DSMT) and the provision of diabetes supplies. In addition, the Centers for Medicare and Medicaid Services (CMS) has specified a list of diabetes services and supplies as part of Medicare Part B coverage. These benefits were expanded as part of the Medicare Modernization Act of 2003 and as of January 1, 2005 [37], Medicare Part B coverage for eligible seniors included the services shown in Table 2.

For clinicians, including nurse practitioners and registered dietitians, who bill for providing services, CMS provides guidelines for the use of evaluation and management codes (which are used in conjunction with a specific diabetes diagnosis code) and the required documentation for appropriate billing [38]. Understanding how to use these codes is important to ensure proper reimbursement for time spent providing counseling or care coordination [38], activities that are often delivered by nurses and for which obtaining proper reimbursement has been problematic under the traditional fee-for-service system. In addition, reimbursement is more widely available for DSMT provided through a formal education program. To be eligible for Medicare reimbursement, DSMT programs must document that they meet the National Standards for Diabetes Self-Management Education and be recognized by the American Diabetes Association or Indian Health

Table 2
Medicare coverage of diabetes preventive services as of January 1, 2005

Services for which coverage is provided	Who or what is covered	Frequency
Diabetes screening tests	Medicare beneficiaries with certain risk factors for diabetes or diagnosed with prediabetes.	Two screening tests per year for those with prediabetes. One screening per year for those never tested or not diagnosed with prediabetes.
Diabetes self-management training	Medicare beneficiaries at risk for complications from diabetes or recently diagnosed with diabetes. Diabetes self-management training programs must be recognized by the American Diabetes Association or other approving body.	Requires written plan of care specifying number of sessions, frequency, and duration.
Medical nutrition therapy	Medicare beneficiaries diagnosed with diabetes or a renal disease.	First year, 3 hours of one-on-one counseling and 2 hours in subsequent years.
Diabetes supplies Blood glucose self-testing Therapeutic shoes Insulin pumps Diabetes-related durable Medical equipment	Blood glucose self-testing includes equipment and supplies; therapeutic shoes includes one pair of depth-inlay shoes and three pairs of inserts, or one pair of custom-molded shoes if the beneficiary cannot wear depth-inlay shoes because of a foot deformity, and two additional pairs of inserts within the calendar year; insulin pumps includes the pump and insulin used in the pumps.	Supplies may be limited based on treatment program.
Other services Foot care Hemoglobin A_{1c} tests Glaucoma screening Influenza and pneumococcal Polysaccharide vaccinations	Glaucoma screening is for beneficiaries with diabetes mellitus, family history of glaucoma, or African Americans age 50 and over. Vaccinations are available to all beneficiaries.	Glaucoma screening: annually for beneficiaries in one of the high-risk groups. Influenza vaccine: once per flu season. Pneumococcal vaccine: once in a lifetime.

Data from Medicare Learning Network (May 2005) Expanded Benefits Brochure. Centers for Medicare and Medicaid Services.

Service. Patients must also meet established referral criteria and obtain a physician prescription [39]. Benefits provided as part of the Medicaid program, which is a joint federal and state program, are generally determined at the state level.

In addition to these federal initiatives, most states have legislation requiring diabetes health insurance coverage by state-regulated insurers [40,41]. In 1987, Wisconsin enacted legislation requiring comprehensive coverage of diabetes services by insurers and other states have since followed suit. As of 2004, 46 states plus the District of Columbia had some type of required diabetes coverage [40–42]. In general, these coverage requirements relate to the provision of blood glucose monitors, test strips, and DSMT.

State-mandated coverage plays an important role in removing patients' cost barriers for certain services, such as testing supplies and self-management education. In addition, state-mandated coverage provides some degree of standardization for health care providers and may remove some of the difficulties associated with trying to determine what services are covered for a particular patient given their type of insurance coverage. Although these policies are encouraging, analysis by the Centers for Disease Control and Prevention showed that the content of the legislation varies from state to state and only 26% to 41% of the insured United States population with diabetes is covered by state-regulated plans [42]. Consequently, similar patients with different insurance benefits can have very different cost pressures, and clinicians often face a confusing array of insurance benefits within their panel of patients.

Another problem with state-mandated coverage is that such regulations are not generally focused on improving the quality of care for patients with diabetes [40]. Recent concepts in designing health care payment structures have emphasized the link between payment for health services and the quality of care received by patients [43]. Under these "pay-for-performance" initiatives, provider payment is no longer based solely on the process of care or the specific services and procedures provided to patients, but includes payments that in theory provide incentives to meet quality targets and improve patient outcomes.

CMS, along with a number of partnering agencies, is developing and implementing a set of pay-for-performance initiatives to support quality improvement in the care of Medicare beneficiaries, including those with diabetes, and reduce health care costs. CMS is motivated to improve the effectiveness of diabetes care, given that approximately 18% of Medicare beneficiaries have diabetes and these patients account for almost one third of Medicare spending [44]. Many of the demonstration programs currently being tested use existing disease management concepts and programs, which suggests that nurses are likely to play an integral part considering the prominent role of nursing in providing disease management services [45].

Medicare Health Support (Medicare Modernization Act section 721) includes a CMS pilot program designed to test a population-based model of disease management, whereby participating organizations are paid a monthly per beneficiary fee for managing a population of chronically ill patients with complex diabetes or advanced congestive heart failure. These

organizations, which include disease management vendors and insurance companies, must guarantee CMS a savings of at least 5% plus the cost of the monthly fees compared with a similar population of beneficiaries. Payment of fees is also contingent on performance on quality measures and satisfaction of both beneficiaries and providers. Nine sites have been selected for the 2-year pilot phase. Pending successful interim results, this pilot may be expanded nationwide.

Another initiative, the Disease Management Demonstration for Severely Chronically Ill Medicare Beneficiaries (Benefits Improvement and Protection Act 2000), is designed to test whether applying disease management and prescription drug coverage in a fee-for-service environment can improve outcomes and reduce costs for Medicare beneficiaries with diabetes and other chronic conditions. The three participating disease management organizations receive a monthly payment for every beneficiary they enroll to provide disease management services and a comprehensive drug benefit. In return, the organization must guarantee a net reduction in Medicare expenditures, and submit data on relevant clinical measures to permit evaluation of the demonstration's impact on quality.

Use of cost-effectiveness analysis to evaluate interventions designed to prevent diabetes or its complications

This section examines another way in which cost data are used to influence diabetes care and diabetes-related policies and programs. Cost-effectiveness studies are designed to assess the costs of a treatment or intervention relative to the health outcomes obtained. Such analyses are especially important in a time of rising health costs because they help inform decisions about which strategy for achieving the same outcome represents the "best buy" from the perspective of payers or society in general. Differing types of cost-effectiveness studies are distinguished by how they value the outcome of interest (eg, in monetary terms versus other units, such as quality-adjusted life years [QALY]). The outcome or effectiveness measure recommended by the Panel on Cost-Effectiveness [46] is the QALY, which takes into account not only changes in length of life associated with a particular intervention but the quality of any potential life years gained. One benefit of using QALYs, rather than other health outcome measures, as the standard for cost-effectiveness analyses is that QALYs allow for comparisons among interventions designed to produce different health effects (eg, glycemic control versus blood pressure control) and across interventions focusing on different health conditions (eg, diabetes versus cancer).

Much of the focus of diabetes care for both patients and providers is on preventing complications that may take many years to develop. As such, intervention studies generally focus on intermediate outcomes (eg, hemoglobin A_{1c}) that lead to these adverse outcomes rather than measuring the

effects on those outcomes directly. In contrast, diabetes cost-effectiveness studies often use modeling techniques that translate these shorter-term changes in key parameters (eg, hemoglobin A_{1c}) into longer-term outcomes (eg, rates of diabetes-related eye or kidney disease), which are subsequently used to generate QALYs. For example, the Centers for Disease Control and Prevention Diabetes Cost-effectiveness Group [47] used a statistical modeling approach to compare three important diabetes treatments for patients with type 2 diabetes age 25 years and older: (1) intensive glycemic control, (2) intensified hypertension control, and (3) reducing serum cholesterol levels. This analysis produced an incremental cost-effectiveness ratio (in 1997 United States dollars) of $41,384 per QALY for intensive glycemic control, $51,889 per QALY for serum cholesterol level reduction, and minus $1959 per QALY for intensified blood pressure control (ie, the intervention was both more effective than usual care while actually saving money) [47]. The investigators also found, however, that the cost-effectiveness ratios for both intensive glycemic control and serum cholesterol level varied by patient age. Specifically, intensive glycemic control costs were significantly lower for younger patients, whereas those for reducing cholesterol levels were lower for patients 45 to 85 years of age. A similar study using the United Kingdom Prospective Diabetes Study outcomes model also demonstrated a very favorable cost-effectiveness ratio (369 British pounds or approximately $644 per QALY) for intensive blood pressure control, although in this case it was not cost saving [48]. The cost-effectiveness ratio (6028 pounds or approximately $10,500 per QALY) for intensive blood glucose control was somewhat higher but still economically favorable compared with many other types of interventions [48].

More recently, cost-effectiveness analyses have been used to evaluate interventions that delay or prevent the development of type 2 diabetes among high-risk adults [49,50]. Herman and colleagues [49] conducted a cost-effectiveness analysis of the lifestyle modification and metformin interventions implemented as part of the Diabetes Prevention Program [51]. They estimated health system costs per QALY of approximately $1100 for lifestyle interventions and $31,300 for interventions using metformin. Although the lifestyle intervention was considered cost-effective for all age groups, the metformin intervention was over $100,000 per QALY for those over age 65 years. Whereas there is some debate about what cost per QALY represents a reasonable investment of public health dollars, most policy-makers agree that interventions with a ratio above $100,000 are likely not the best of use of resources [52]. Another study suggested that the cost of implementing the lifestyle modification program used in the Diabetes Prevention Program might be higher than previously found and possibly more than most insurers are willing to cover [50]. All of these studies demonstrate the ways in which cost-effectiveness analysis and modeling can be useful tools for evaluating diabetes interventions and for assisting health plans and payers in allocating scarce resources.

Summary

Diabetes care represents a significant economic cost in the United States and without a concerted effort both to prevent diabetes-associated complications and the number of individuals who develop diabetes, these costs are likely to continue to rise. Health insurers are straining under the burden of diabetes-related expenditures, and increasingly are sharing these costs with their covered patients. As a consequence, some diabetes patients forgo needed treatment because of cost problems and many fail to address this issue with their clinicians. There are many initiatives to improve the management of diabetes both by health care providers and patients, including specified coverage for certain diabetes services and programs that target high-risk and high-cost patients. It is also important, however, to recognize the many ways in which nurses can help reduce the economic impact of diabetes, such as assisting patients with cost-related self-management problems, helping ensure that proper reimbursement is maintained to sustain critical diabetes services, and being an active participant in programs designed to provide better quality and more cost-effective care for individuals with diabetes or prediabetes. In these ways and many others nurses play a critical role in helping to reduce the cost of diabetes not only for individual patients but ultimately for the health care system and society as a whole.

References

[1] Engelgau MM, Geiss LS, Saaddine JB, et al. The evolving diabetes burden in the United States. Ann Intern Med 2004;140:945–50.

[2] Centers for Disease Control and Prevention. National diabetes fact sheet: general information and national estimates on diabetes in the United States, 2005. Atlanta (GA): US Department of Health and Human Services, Centers for Disease Control and Prevention; 2005.

[3] Honeycutt AA, Boyle JP, Broglio KR, et al. A dynamic Markov model for forecasting diabetes prevalence in the United States through 2050. Health Care Manag Sci 2003;6: 155–64.

[4] UK Prospective Diabetes Study Group (UKPDS). Tight blood pressure control and risk of macrovascular and microvascular complications in type 2 diabetes (UKPDS 38). BMJ 1998; 317:703–13.

[5] The Diabetes Control and Complications Trial Research Group. The effect of intensive treatment of diabetes on the development and progression of long-term complications in insulin-dependent diabetes mellitus. N Engl J Med 1993;329:977–86.

[6] UK Prospective Diabetes Study Group (UKPDS). Intensive blood-glucose control with sulphonylureas or insulin compared with conventional treatment and risk of complications in patients with type 2 diabetes (UKPDS 33). Lancet 1998;352:837–53.

[7] Vijan S, Stevens DL, Herman WH, et al. Screening, prevention, counseling, and treatment for the complications of type II diabetes mellitus: putting evidence into practice. J Gen Intern Med 1997;12:567–80.

[8] The Early Treatment of Diabetic Retinopathy Study Research Group. Early photocoagulation for diabetic retinopathy. ETDRS Report Number 9. Ophthalmology 1991;98:766–85.

[9] Vijan S, Hayward RA. Treatment of hypertension in type 2 diabetes mellitus: blood pressure goals, choice of agents, and setting priorities in diabetes care. Ann Intern Med 2003;138: 593–602.

[10] Vijan S, Hayward RA. Pharmacologic lipid-lowering therapy in type 2 diabetes mellitus: background paper for the American College of Physicians. Ann Intern Med 2004;140:650–8.

[11] Singh N, Armstrong DG, Lipsky BA. Preventing foot ulcers in patients with diabetes. JAMA 2005;293:217–28.

[12] Anderson RN, Minino AM, Hoyert DL, et al. Comparability of cause of death between ICD-9 and ICD-10: preliminary estimates. Natl Vital Stat Rep 2001;49:1–32.

[13] Snow V, Weiss KB, Mottur-Pilson C. The evidence base for tight blood pressure control in the management of type 2 diabetes mellitus. Ann Intern Med 2003;138:587–92.

[14] Druss BG, Marcus SC, Olfson M, et al. The most expensive medical conditions in America. Health Aff (Millwood) 2002;21:105–11.

[15] Hogan P, Dall T, Nikolov P. Economic costs of diabetes in the US in 2002. Diabetes Care 2003;26:917–32.

[16] O'Brien JA, Patrick AR, Caro J. Estimates of direct medical costs for microvascular and macrovascular complications resulting from type 2 diabetes mellitus in the United States in 2000. Clin Ther 2003;25:1017–38.

[17] Caro JJ, Ward AJ, O'Brien JA. Lifetime costs of complications resulting from type 2 diabetes in the US. Diabetes Care 2002;25:476–81.

[18] Killilea T. Long-term consequences of type 2 diabetes mellitus: economic impact on society and managed care. Am J Manag Care 2002;8(16 Suppl):S441–9.

[19] Economic and health costs of diabetes. Agency for Healthcare Research and Quality (AHRQ) HCUP Highlights. Pub. No. 04–0034. Rockville (MD): US Department of Health and Human Services, Agency for Healthcare Research and Quality; 2005.

[20] Vijan S, Hayward RA, Langa KM. The impact of diabetes on workforce participation: results from a national household sample. Health Serv Res 2004;39(6 Pt 1):1653–69.

[21] Chapman LS. Reducing obesity in work organizations. Am J Health Promot 2004;19:1–8 [discussion: 12].

[22] Yancey AK, McCarthy WJ, Taylor WC, et al. The Los Angeles Lift Off: a sociocultural environmental change intervention to integrate physical activity into the workplace. Prev Med 2004;38:848–56.

[23] Katz DL, O'Connell M, Yeh MC, et al. Public health strategies for preventing and controlling overweight and obesity in school and worksite settings: a report on recommendations of the Task Force on Community Preventive Services. MMWR Recomm Rep 2005;54(RR-10); 1–12.

[24] Gilmer TP, O'Connor PJ, Rush WA, et al. Predictors of health care costs in adults with diabetes. Diabetes Care 2005;28:59–64.

[25] Brandle M, Zhou H, Smith BR, et al. The direct medical cost of type 2 diabetes. Diabetes Care 2003;26:2300–4.

[26] Karter AJ, Stevens MR, Herman WH, et al. Out-of-pocket costs and diabetes preventive services: the Translating Research Into Action for Diabetes (TRIAD) study. Diabetes Care 2003;26:2294–9.

[27] Piette JD, Heisler M, Wagner TH. Problems paying out-of-pocket medication costs among older adults with diabetes. Diabetes Care 2004;27:384–91.

[28] Roblin DW, Platt R, Goodman MJ, et al. Effect of increased cost-sharing on oral hypoglycemic use in five managed care organizations: how much is too much? Med Care 2005;43: 951–9.

[29] Soumerai SB, Mah C, Zhang F, et al. Effects of health maintenance organization coverage of self-monitoring devices on diabetes self-care and glycemic control. Arch Intern Med 2004; 164:645–52.

[30] Vijan S, Stuart NS, Fitzgerald JT, et al. Barriers to following dietary recommendations in type 2 diabetes. Diabet Med 2005;22:32–8.

[31] Heisler M, Langa KM, Eby EL, et al. The health effects of restricting prescription medication use because of cost. Med Care 2004;42:626–34.

[32] Piette JD, Wagner TH, Potter MB, et al. Health insurance status, cost-related medication underuse, and outcomes among diabetes patients in three systems of care. Med Care 2004; 42:102–9.

[33] Tamblyn R, Laprise R, Hanley JA, et al. Adverse events associated with prescription drug cost-sharing among poor and elderly persons. JAMA 2001;285:421–9.

[34] Rosen AB, Hamel MB, Weinstein MC, et al. Cost-effectiveness of full Medicare coverage of angiotensin-converting enzyme inhibitors for beneficiaries with diabetes. Ann Intern Med 2005;143:89–99.

[35] Fendrick AM, Smith DG, Chernew ME, et al. A benefit-based copay for prescription drugs: patient contribution based on total benefits, not drug acquisition cost. Am J Manag Care 2001;7:861–7.

[36] Piette JD. Medication cost-sharing: helping chronically ill patients cope. Med Care 2005;43: 947–50.

[37] Merin M. New Medicare benefits for people with diabetes. The new year brings new Medicare benefits and services for people with diabetes. Diabetes Forecast 2005;58:77.

[38] Bartol T. Coding and billing for patients with diabetes. Nurse Pract 2005;30:47–53.

[39] American Diabetes Association. Third-party reimbursement for diabetes care, self-management education, and supplies. Diabetes Care 2006;29(Suppl 1):S68–9.

[40] Guglielmo WJ. Does mandated diabetes coverage boost compliance? Med Econ 2001;78: 61–2, 65.

[41] National Conference of State Legislatures. State Laws Mandating Diabetes Health coverage. Available at: www.ncsl.org/programs/health/diabetes.htm. Accessed January 27, 2006.

[42] Hartsfield D, Vinicor F. The role of law in health services delivery: diabetes and state-mandated benefits. J Law Med Ethics 2003;31(4 Suppl):51.

[43] Conrad DA, Christianson JB. Penetrating the black box: financial incentives for enhancing the quality of physician services. Med Care Res Rev 2004;61(3 Suppl):37S–68S.

[44] Centers for Medicare and Medicaid Services. Medicare awards for programs to improve care of beneficiaries with chronic illnesses. Medicare Fact Sheet. Washington: Department of Health & Human Services, Centers for Medicare & Medicaid Services; 2004.

[45] Norris SL, Nichols PJ, Caspersen CJ, et al. The effectiveness of disease and case management for people with diabetes: a systematic review. Am J Prev Med 2002;22(4 Suppl): 15–38.

[46] Gold MR, Siegel JE, Russell LB, et al, editors. Cost-effectiveness in health and medicine. New York: Oxford University Press; 1996.

[47] CDC Diabetes Cost-effectiveness Group. Cost-effectiveness of intensive glycemic control, intensified hypertension control, and serum cholesterol level reduction for type 2 diabetes. JAMA 2002;287:2542–51.

[48] Clarke PM, Gray AM, Briggs A, et al. Cost-utility analyses of intensive blood glucose and tight blood pressure control in type 2 diabetes (UKPDS 72). Diabetologia 2005; 48:868–77.

[49] Herman WH, Hoerger TJ, Brandle M, et al. The cost-effectiveness of lifestyle modification or metformin in preventing type 2 diabetes in adults with impaired glucose tolerance. Ann Intern Med 2005;142:323–32.

[50] Eddy DM, Schlessinger L, Kahn R. Clinical outcomes and cost-effectiveness of strategies for managing people at high risk for diabetes. Ann Intern Med 2005;143:251–64.

[51] Knowler WC, Barrett-Connor E, Fowler SE, et al. Reduction in the incidence of type 2 diabetes with lifestyle intervention or metformin. N Engl J Med 2002;346:393–403.

[52] Laupacis A, Feeny D, Detsky AS, et al. How attractive does a new technology have to be to warrant adoption and utilization? Tentative guidelines for using clinical and economic evaluations. CMAJ 1992;146:473–81.

ELSEVIER
SAUNDERS

Nurs Clin N Am 41 (2006) 513–530

NURSING
CLINICS
OF NORTH AMERICA

Type 1 Diabetes

Andrea Dann Urban, MSN, APRN, CDE[a,b,*],
Margaret Grey, DrPH, FAAN, CPNP[a]

[a]Yale University School of Nursing, 100 Church Street South, PO Box 9740,
New Haven, CT 06536–0740, USA
[b]Yale Pediatric Diabetes Clinic, New Haven, CT, USA

One in every 400 to 600 children in the United States has type 1 diabetes (T1D) [1]. In the United States the risk of developing T1D is higher than almost all other chronic illnesses of childhood [1]. With T1D having such a high prevalence, nurses and advanced practice nurses interface with children and young adults living with this disease in many health care settings. Health care professionals need to be knowledgeable about pathophysiology, diagnosis, and management of the child and young adult living with T1D. The treatment of T1D in children changes so rapidly that these youth should be managed by a diabetes care team consisting of a nurse, diabetes educator, pediatric endocrinologist, dietitian, social worker, psychologist, and exercise physiologist. These professionals are constantly seeking cutting edge treatments for the child with diabetes while guiding them through the many challenges they face as they grow and develop.

Epidemiology

The incidence of T1D varies tremendously throughout the world. Scandinavia has the highest incidence of the disease, with about 30 new cases annually per 100,000 populations [2]. A child in Finland is 40 times more likely to develop T1D than a child in Japan and 100 times more likely than a child in China. The rate of increase of the disease has been the highest in the infant and toddler age group (ages 0–4 years), but there are a large number of adolescents who present in early puberty [2,3]. One third of the cases of T1D are diagnosed in adulthood, but diagnosis is rare after age 45. Males and females are equally affected [2].

* Corresponding author.
E-mail address: andrea.urban@yale.edu (A.D. Urban).

0029-6465/06/$ - see front matter © 2006 Elsevier Inc. All rights reserved.
doi:10.1016/j.cnur.2006.07.013
nursing.theclinics.com

Genetics

T1D is a genetic disease of the immune system where the genes responsible for the disease are carried on the DQ band of the short arm of chromosome 6. These genes controlling the immune system are part of the major histocompatibility complex. If these genes malfunction, they can impair the immune system's ability to recognize itself [4,5]. It is not genes alone, however, that cause T1D to develop. Rather, it is thought to be the interplay between genetic susceptibility and environmental factors that provide the elements for the disease to occur [3]. Environmental factors that have been suspected to be triggers of T1D include viruses, foods, and toxins [6]. To date, there have been no scientific studies proving the relationship between any of these environmental factors and the disease itself.

Currently, it is believed that the susceptibility for T1D is inherited and the individual experiences a triggering event that begins the misdirected inflammatory response against the pancreatic islet cells. Islet cells are the insulin-producing cells. This inflammatory response against the islet cells is accompanied by the production of serum antibodies, which contribute to the inflammatory process. Islet cell antibodies are present in the serum of about 80% of individuals at the time of diagnosis. The most prevalent autoantibody is GAD65, which is directed against the enzyme glutamic acid decarboxylase [2]. These antibodies alone are not sufficient or necessary in making the diagnosis of T1D. Rather, they can be helpful in clinical situations where it is unclear whether the individual has type 1 or type 2 diabetes [6].

Pathophysiology

Insulin is produced by the β cells of the islet of Langerhans of the pancreas. It is a protein hormone secreted by the β cells, which is then deposited into intracellular space [4]. Insulin is an anabolic hormone that regulates the manner in which the body stores glucose and uses those glucose stores. Insulin is stimulated by a rise in blood glucose and is necessary for the transport of glucose into muscle cells to be used for fuel or storage by the cell [2,4]. In the liver, insulin stimulates glycogen synthesis, while inhibiting gluconeogenesis and glycogenolysis [2].

The absence of insulin creates a starvation state within the body despite the fact that the body is being nourished [4]. Glucose transporters in the peripheral tissues depend on insulin to be able to use the glucose by the tissues. When glucose is unavailable, the tissues essentially starve. The liver further stimulates glycogenolysis and gluconeogenesis and hyperglycemia worsens. Osmotic diuresis begins to occur, which leads to urinary losses of fluid and electrolytes. Glucose production continues along with decreased peripheral glucose uptake and fluid losses, which leads to a progressive dehydration and hyperosmolality [2].

Diabetic ketoacidosis (DKA) is a life-threatening complication of T1D. DKA is actually defined as a blood sugar level of >240 mg/dL, ketonemia or ketonuria, and a pH level less than 7.3 [2]. DKA is the result of absolute or relative insulin deficiency along with increased levels of catecholamines, glucagon, cortisol, and growth hormone. When peripheral glucose uptake is disrupted and hyperglycemia and hyperosmolality ensue, fat tissue is used for energy by the body by the process of lipolysis. Increased lipolysis and ketogenesis cause ketonemia and if left untreated, metabolic acidosis [7].

Diagnosis of type 1 diabetes

The diagnosis of T1D is made by looking at the clinical signs and symptoms of polyuria, polydipsia, and polyphagia. The diagnosis must be made carefully because there is a wide differential diagnosis associated with these signs and symptoms. Intercurrent illnesses, typically viral infections, are sometimes present at time of diagnosis and can mask the diagnosis of diabetes. Hyperglycemia and the hyperosmolar state cause osmotic diuresis and the increased thirst, urination, and hunger that are associated with the diagnosis. The length of time between the onset of symptoms and the diagnosis of diabetes can vary greatly from child to child, but is typically only a few weeks in duration [2].

Children typically have some amount of weight loss and experience fatigue as insulin deficiency continues and protein and fat stores are lost [2]. As counterregulatory hormones increase and ketosis worsens, a situation of acute illness develops that typically includes nausea, abdominal pain, and vomiting. If this condition is untreated, it continues to progress to a more serious level of acidosis and dehydration and can include, lethargy, confusion, stupor, and coma [2]. Approximately 15% to 67% of those newly diagnosed with T1D in Europe and North America present in DKA. In addition, DKA accounts for 65% of all hospital admissions of children with T1D under age 19 years [6].

A careful history and review of systems should be completed at the time of suspected diagnosis of T1D and should include a family history of endocrine-related disorders. The physical examination should focus first and foremost on the level of hydration and include a careful assessment of heart rate, blood pressure, mucous membranes, pulses, capillary refill, and skin temperature. An estimation of dehydration status is helpful in facilitating rehydration in the emergency room and hospital. Careful examination and documentation of neurologic status is critical and should be done at the place of diagnosis in the event that there is a change in this status en route to the hospital. In addition, the physical examination must include respiratory and abdominal examinations, and endocrine examinations. Kussmaul respirations are the body's way of compensating for the metabolic acidosis and are characterized by deep, sighing respirations. DKA is at times accompanied by a "fruity" odor to the breath, but this cannot be used as

a diagnostic tool. It is most important that the child be examined for signs and symptoms of adrenal or thyroid disorders that are also associated with autoimmunity [2].

Elevated blood glucose must be documented to confirm the diagnosis of diabetes. In the asymptomatic child or adolescent criteria for diagnosis include a fasting plasma glucose of >126 mg/dL, or random glucose >200 mg/dL, which should be repeated on another day to confirm the diagnosis. The child or adolescent who is symptomatic and has a random plasma glucose of >200 mg/dL does not require repeat testing to make the diagnosis. Glucose tolerance testing is typically not necessary except in cases that are difficult to diagnose (eg, where there are many normal, plasma glucose readings). Regardless of the severity at the time that the diagnosis is made, children and adolescents require immediate medical treatment and education about how to manage the disease [8].

Medical and nursing management

It is the recommendation of the American Diabetes Association (ADA) that a specialized team consisting of a pediatric endocrinologist, diabetes nurse educator, dietitian, mental health professional, and an exercise physiologist manage the care of the child or adolescent with T1D [9]. These professionals provide the patients with the most up-to-date treatment, education, and support, which is critical in a specialty that changes very rapidly. These providers understand the issues that arise as a child and adolescent grows and develops and how this can affect their diabetes treatment. In addition, it is imperative that the diabetes team be well versed in the differences in treatment of type 1 versus type 2 diabetes [9].

Whether the education and initial treatment of the youth with T1D is delivered in the hospital or the home, the plan should include education in the use of insulin, meal planning, training in blood glucose monitoring, urine ketone testing, hypoglycemia and hyperglycemia management, and emotional support of the child and family [6]. The initial training that the family receives in diabetes management should be viewed as an important investment in their future and affords them the skills they need to manage the disease for a lifetime. The initial education is reviewed at subsequent visits to the care provider; as they become ready to learn it, more advanced education is presented to the child and family [6,10–12].

Current goals for therapy of children and adolescents with T1D are to achieve near normal glycemia, minimize the risk of severe hypoglycemia, limit excess weight gain while encouraging normal growth and development, prevent vascular complications, and improve the quality of life for patients and their families [13]. In 1993, the Diabetes Control and Complications Trial (DCCT) recommended that tight control of blood glucose be the standard of care for most patients with T1D. DCCT research found that

patients who were intensively managed and had tight blood glucose control had a significant decrease in the risk of microvascular complications of the eyes, kidneys, and nerves [14]. The DCCT study included youth between the ages of 13 and 17 years. As a result of the DCCT, intensive management has become the standard of care for most children and adolescents with T1D [15].

Glycemic goals have traditionally been based on the age of the child because of physiologic and developmental factors (Table 1). The standard of care published by the ADA recommends that children below the age of 6 years have a hemoglobin A_{1c} between 7.5% and 8.5%. The reason for this is the relationship between hypoglycemia and the potential for neuro-psychologic impairment. The concern is that the developing brain of a young child is more susceptible to the detrimental effects of hypoglycemia than that of an older child or adolescent. There have been no studies to date that have documented these findings in a longitudinal, prospective clinical trial [9]. Management of diabetes in the 6- to 12-year-old age range requires close communication between the parents, the child, the school personnel, and the diabetes care team. Many children in this age group can make decisions around food choices and insulin amounts, but they still need the close super-vision of an adult who is trained in diabetes management. The ADA has recommended a hemoglobin A_{1c} level of <8% for this age group. A hemoglobin A_{1c} level of <7.5% is suggested for ages 13 to 19 years, although some teenagers safely keep their hemoglobin A_{1c} at a lower level than 7.5% [9].

Insulin therapy

The goal of insulin therapy is to approximate the requirements of the body for basal insulin and food coverage with the use of subcutaneous in-jections. There are many types of insulin preparations available, with

Table 1
Plasma blood glucose and hemoglobin A_{1c} goals for type 1 diabetes by age group

Plasma blood glucose goal, range (mg/dL)				
Values by age	Before meals	Bedtime or overnight	Hemoglobin A_{1c}	Rationale
Toddlers and preschoolers (<6 y)	100–180	110–200	<8.5% (but >7.5%)	Vulnerability to hypoglycemia
School age (6–12 y)	90–180	100–180	<8%	Risk of hypoglycemia
Adolescents and young adults	90–130	90–150	<7.5%	Risk of hypoglycemia and psychologic issues

Adapted from Silverstein J, Klingensmith G, Copeland K, et al. Care of children and ado-lescents with type 1 diabetes. A statement of the American Diabetes Association. Diabetes Care 2005;28:186–212; with permission. © 2005 American Diabetes Association.

different onset, peak, and duration [2]. Insulins generally used in children are the rapid-acting insulin analogues and intermediate-acting insulin. Occasionally, long-acting insulin is used in the adolescent [9].

Insulin requirements for children are typically based on weight, age, and pubertal status. Children with newly diagnosed T1D usually require between 0.5 and 1 units/kg of insulin per day divided into two or three doses. Younger children, who are prepubertal, usually require lower doses than children who are in puberty or who have been in acidosis at the time of diagnosis. Infants and toddlers may require amounts smaller than 0.5 units of insulin; the insulin must be diluted with a special diluent available through the manufacturer [9].

The honeymoon period begins for most children and adolescents several weeks after the initiation of insulin therapy. During the honeymoon phase, the pancreas produces small amounts of insulin, which help to keep the blood glucoses at near normal levels. Insulin requirements typically decrease during this period of insulin production and insulin doses may decrease to a few units of intermediate-acting insulin per day. Unfortunately, the β-cell destruction within the pancreas continues. Youth who have been in severe DKA may not experience a honeymoon, because they have depleted the functioning β cells. Insulin requirements during growth and puberty increase to counteract the effect of the increased growth hormone and sex hormone secretion [9].

Most children on insulin injections receive three injections per day. Traditional insulin regimens for children consist of two thirds of the daily insulin dose given in the morning before breakfast and one third in the evening. The morning injection typically consists of rapid-acting and intermediate-acting insulin, which covers breakfast, lunch, and the afternoon. The dinner injection consists of rapid-acting insulin to cover the evening and the bedtime injection of intermediate-acting insulin to cover hormone surges during the sleeping hours. The rapid-acting insulins are termed "insulin analogues." They arise from the biochemical alteration of the human insulin molecule and are available on the market as Humalog and NovoLog [6]. These insulin analogues have an onset from 15 to 30 minutes, a peak of approximately 1 hour, and duration of 3 to 5 hours. NPH is a commonly used intermediate-acting insulin and has an onset of 2 to 4 hours, a peak of 4 to 10 hours, and a duration of 12 to 24 hours. Lente had been used in the pediatric population until recently, when it was discontinued by insulin manufacturers [2]. Premixed insulin is popular among adults for its ease of administration, but is not commonly used in children and adolescents unless all other insulin programs have failed. Usually, use of premixed insulin is considered when youth have difficulty in managing more complex regimens. These mixtures contain a set amount of short-acting with a larger amount of intermediate-acting insulin.

Glargine (Lantus) is a long-acting insulin analogue. It is meant to function as basal insulin and is not meant to cover meals or snacks. It is thought to be

a peakless insulin and has a duration of about 24 hours or longer. The most common method of using glargine is to deliver it in one injection per day and use a rapid-acting insulin analogue for meals and large snacks. This insulin must be injected alone and not mixed with another type of insulin in the syringe. Glargine has not been approved for use in children <6 years old [6].

Insulin pumps became available in the mid 1970s along with the introduction of self-monitoring of blood glucose, hemoglobin A_{1c} tests, and more aggressive treatment of T1D [12]. It was thought that the improvement of metabolic control from these intensive therapies might delay the development or progression of complications of diabetes caused by hyperglycemia [15]. This issue was resolved in 1993 with the release of the results of the DCCT, where intensive control was found to reduce significantly the onset and progression of retinopathy and microalbuminuria in adolescents [13,16].

Continuous subcutaneous insulin infusion or insulin pump therapy was used in few children until recently because of the large size of the earlier pumps and the cost associated with this therapy [12]. Insulin pumps that are in use today are compact, comfortable, and covered by most insurance companies. They are becoming extremely popular with all age groups including infants and toddlers with T1D. Insulin pump therapy has some clear advantages over insulin injection therapy. Most importantly, pump treatment allows for more physiologic insulin delivery than injections. From the patient's and family's point of view the biggest advantage is the ability to be flexible with meal and snack times. The child is no longer forced to eat based on the peak of intermediate- or long-acting insulin, because insulin pumps deliver rapid-acting insulin alone. A second large advantage is that the number of injections is decreased from several per day to one injection for pump catheter insertion every second or third day. Most children and adolescents find this to be a huge benefit. Lastly, blood glucose control is as evidenced by hemoglobin A_{1C} levels is improved on pump therapy over injection therapy [12]. Parents have reported less stress and worry about hypoglycemia, meal times, and diabetes care overall on pump therapy. They enjoy more freedom and flexibility in all aspects of their lives [17].

It is critical to the success of continuous subcutaneous insulin infusion to have a team of highly trained clinicians, including certified diabetes educators, who are expert in managing children on pumps, and patients and families who are able to carry out the intensive program that goes along with pump therapy [13]. Individuals on the insulin pump must be willing to monitor their blood glucose five to six times per day and follow the carbohydrate counting meal plan. The insulin pump uses rapid-acting insulin alone. Small amounts of insulin are delivered every few minutes as a basal rate and additional insulin is delivered through the pump to cover carbohydrate ingestion and correct hyperglycemia as a bolus. Basal rates can be programmed to change every 30 minutes and temporary basal rates can be set at lower or higher amounts to cover exercise, illness, and menstrual cycles [12].

Blood glucose monitoring

Self-monitoring of blood glucose allows individuals living with diabetes to measure blood glucose levels in an accurate and convenient manner. It is a necessary part of attaining optimal glycemic control because research has shown a positive relationship between the frequency of glucose testing and glycemic control [9,18]. Insulin doses, whether they are with a syringe or continuous subcutaneous insulin infusion, should always be based on the interpretation of blood glucose levels. Blood glucose levels also are a key piece in planning insulin and food coverage of exercise and sick day management. Blood glucose readings should be closely observed for trends of hypoglycemia or hyperglycemia and insulin adjusted accordingly. It is the recommendation of the ADA that all children with T1D test their blood glucose a minimum of four times per day. Young children who are unable to feel the symptoms of hypoglycemia should have their glucose tested even more frequently [9]. New blood glucose meters are constantly being developed. The current meters use a small amount of blood and are approved for use in alternate sites, such as the forearm and the palm of the hand.

Nutrition for type 1 diabetes

Nutrient recommendations for children with T1D are the same as for children and adolescents without a chronic illness [19]. Healthy eating habits should be adopted by all youth to ensure adequate intake of essential vitamins and minerals [20]. Youth with T1D should have a consultation with a registered dietitian who has experience in diabetes. The meal plan should be individualized to take into account food preferences, cultural influences, exercise patterns, and daily schedules [9]. The carbohydrate counting meal plan, where total carbohydrate content of all meals and snacks is counted, is currently used for children and adolescents. Youth on injection therapy are encouraged to follow a set carbohydrate range for meals and snacks. Youth on continuous subcutaneous insulin infusion therapy are afforded more flexibility because they dose their insulin based on the amount of carbohydrate ingested and the level of blood glucose. Growth, weight gain, and body mass index should be measured at follow-up visits (every 3 months) and plotted on the growth curve. All children with T1D should have access to a dietitian at least annually [9].

Physical activity and exercise

Maintaining an active lifestyle should be a goal for all children, but especially those with diabetes. Exercise can benefit insulin sensitivity, glucose use, and cardiovascular health [2,21]. Clinically, this can translate to lower insulin requirements in general. Physical activity is also associated with a higher self-esteem and improved motivation to manage diabetes [2].

Massin and colleagues [21] found that most children and adolescents with T1D in their study did meet the pediatric guidelines for physical activity and exercised as much as their healthy peers.

The effects of exercise must be carefully reviewed with children and their families at the time of diagnosis [2]. Moderate and vigorous activity can predispose the child to hypoglycemia either during or after the exercise is completed. Overnight hypoglycemia after exercise is common in children with T1D and points to the necessity of modifying diabetes management to reduce the risk of hypoglycemia [22]. Blood glucose should be monitored before, during, and after moderate and vigorous exercise. Youth on an insulin injection program should decrease the evening intermediate-acting insulin and those youth on continuous subcutaneous insulin infusion should implement a temporary basal rate at a decreased rate for several hours through the night. It is wise to test the blood glucose during the night following afternoon or evening exercise.

Appropriate self-management and family involvement by age (Table 2)

Infants and toddlers

The diagnosis of T1D in the infant and toddler places the parents in a position where they must learn many new skills to care for their child [23]. The awesome amount of responsibility for their child and the fear of hypoglycemia can be extremely stressful for the parents [24]. Infants and toddlers are unable to recognize the symptoms of hypoglycemia; the risk of moderate or severe hypoglycemia is the highest in these two age groups [25]. Toddlers typically present a challenge with food because their appetites are typically erratic. This eating pattern may cause the family to become very anxious about the increased chances of hypoglycemia with poor appetite. Parents and caregivers of infants and toddlers must have adequate training by a dietitian to learn to manage their child's food intake and how it relates to insulin administration [9]. Insulin pumps are becoming increasingly popular among this age group because doses of rapid-acting insulin can be more efficiently titrated to the needs of the small child. Discipline of the toddler should be reviewed at the time of diagnosis because temper tantrums are quite common in this age group. Parents should be instructed to test their child's blood glucose first, and if the reading is low, then the glucose should be treated accordingly. Parents and caregivers of this age group need much emotional support and assistance from the diabetes care team and from family and friends.

Preschool and early school-aged children (3–7 years)

Preschool and early school-aged children are gaining confidence in their ability to master tasks, but do not have the coordination and cognitive development needed to perform most diabetes tasks. Children of this age

Table 2
Major developmental issues and their effect on diabetes in children and adolescents

Developmental stage	Normal developmental tasks	Diabetes management priorities	Family issues with diabetes
Infancy and toddlerhood (0–36 mo)	Developing a trusting relationship with caregiver Developing sense of mastery and autonomy	Preventing and treating hypoglycemia Managing irregular food intake	Coping with stress Sharing the care with others to avoid parent burnout Establishing a schedule Setting limits on the child
Preschool (3–7 y)	Developing initiative in activities and self-confidence	Preventing and treating hypoglycemia Unpredictable appetite and food intake Positive reinforcement for cooperation with regimen	Reassuring child that diabetes is not their fault Educating other caregivers about diabetes
School-age (8–11 y)	Developing skills in athletic, cognitive, artistic, and social area Developing self-esteem within peer group	Making diabetes regimen flexible to allow for participation in school-sports-peer activities	Maintaining parental involvement while allowing for child to perform some diabetes tasks Continue to educate school and other caregivers

| Early adolescence (12–15 y) | Managing physiologic changes Developing strong sense of self-identity | Managing increased insulin requirements during puberty Weight and body image concerns | Negotiation of parent and teenager's roles, in diabetes management Learning coping skills to enhance ability to self-manage Preventing and intervening with diabetes-related family conflict Monitoring for signs of depression, psychiatric illnesses, and risky behaviors |
| Later adolescence (16–19 y) | Establishing sense of identity after | Integrating diabetes into new lifestyle | Supporting the transition to independence Learning coping skills to enhance ability to self-manage Preventing and intervening with diabetes-related family conflict Monitoring for signs of depression, psychiatric illnesses, and risky behaviors |

Adapted from Silverstein J, Klingensmith G, Copeland K, et al. Care of children and adolescents with type 1 diabetes. A statement of the American Diabetes Association. Diabetes Care 2005;28:186–212; with permission.

usually take great pride in being able to set up the blood glucose test and may even be able to do the test with supervision. As they learn how to read, many children enjoy reading food labels and participating in carbohydrate counting and meal planning. Childcare providers, school nurses, and babysitters are becoming involved in the care of this age group. To be effective, parents need to work with these other providers to ensure that they can manage diabetes, and this requires significant training on the part of the parents. It is often difficult for the parents to hand over the diabetes care to other caregivers because of fear of what happens to their child when they are not in their care [24]. The diabetes care team can play a role in training of school nurses and child care providers by performing in-services and education, providing clear guidelines for when the diabetes team and parents should be contacted, and being available by telephone for questions on a daily basis. Undetected hypoglycemia is still a concern for caregivers of children of this age group [9].

School-aged children (8–11 years)

School-aged children are often interested in performing many of the tasks associated with their diabetes care, with adult supervision. They typically perform all blood glucose tests, and participate in carbohydrate counting and insulin injections or pump catheter insertion. Several studies have shown that children need much adult supervision and support with their diabetes care. It has been shown that metabolic control suffers when families allow children to exert total independence over diabetes tasks and the responsibilities should be shared [9,26,27]. Conflict between the child with diabetes and their parent has been found to begin before the adolescent period because some of the increased demands and responsibilities of diabetes treatment that can lead to parent-child conflict [28]. Davis and colleagues [29], however, found through their research that greater parental warmth and caring in children might improve adherence through reduced family conflict, and an increase in family cohesion. It is important to encourage children with T1D to participate in school activities and sports to facilitate the development of normal peer relationships [30].

Adolescents

Teenagers experience rapid biologic change during adolescence, which is accompanied by increased physical, emotional, and cognitive maturity. They are struggling to become their own person with their own thoughts and feelings, apart from their families [9]. This adolescent struggle can present difficulties when parent and teenager differ in their views of how diabetes should be managed. The parent may have been the main decision maker in the diabetes care up until this point, when the teenager wants to take on more of the responsibility. A certain amount of conflict is to be expected

between teenagers and their parents, however, and teenagers with T1D have been found to have the same amount of conflict with their parents as their nonaffected peers [31]. Parents should continue to stay involved in their teenager's diabetes care. Anderson and colleagues [32] found that diabetes-specific conflict and adherence to blood glucose monitoring was strongly linked to the teenager's glycemic control. It is for these reasons that interventions to build positive family involvement and interaction around diabetes care are provided, so that negative behaviors are not established. Parents and caregivers of adolescents with T1D need to be cognizant of the teenager's emotional state because this age group has been found to have higher levels of depression and lower satisfaction with life than their peers without diabetes [33].

Acute and chronic complications

Hypoglycemia is the most common acute complication of diabetes and is a direct result of insulin therapy. The occurrence of mild hypoglycemia is to be expected when trying to achieve good control of blood glucose. Symptoms typically associated with mild hypoglycemia are diaphoresis, tremor, headache, abdominal pain, and mood change. These signs and symptoms should be promptly treated with juice, glucose tablets, or another source of quick-acting carbohydrate. Severe hypoglycemia may lead to severe alterations in consciousness, seizures, coma, and the possibility of death if the glucose level is left untreated. Moderate and severe hypoglycemia should be treated with glucose gel and glucagon if necessary. In children, the chronic effects of moderate or severe hypoglycemia on cognitive development are worrisome and somewhat limit the extent to which the goals of intensive therapy can be applied [2]. In adolescents and young adults, moderate and severe hypoglycemia is particularly worrisome when the individual is operating an automobile. It is the responsibility of the diabetes care provider to train young adults to test their blood glucose immediately before driving and to have treatment for hypoglycemia available in the automobile.

Adolescents and young adults should also be counseled on the risk of hypoglycemia with alcohol consumption. Alcohol inhibits gluconeogenesis and glycogenolysis and if ingested without simultaneous food consumption, hypoglycemia may occur. Carbohydrates should be eaten along with any alcohol [34]. Individuals with diabetes should space a serving of an alcoholic beverage over 1 hour and should limit their total intake to three beverages.

DKA is also known to occur in children with known T1D. It is most commonly caused by the omission of insulin, intercurrent illness, malfunctioning of insulin pump or pump catheter, and trauma [35]. Children being treated for DKA are at a higher risk of cerebral edema during acute treatment. DKA accounts for 20% of all deaths in children with diabetes less than 20 years old and can be avoided in most cases by prompt treatment

with insulin, fluids, and increased testing of blood glucose and urine ketone levels [36]. Emotional stress and a lack of parental supervision can contribute to insulin omission and should be addressed by the diabetes provider, social worker, and psychologist [9].

The association of T1D and autoimmune thyroid disease is well established. In many patients, autoimmune thyroid disease is subclinical and is detected by routine screening of thyroid-stimulating hormone and thyroid autoantibody levels [37]. The prevalence of thyroid autoantibodies and thyroid dysfunction has been found to increase with age and duration of diabetes. In children with T1D, studies have shown the prevalence of thyroid antibodies between 10% and 22% and subsequent thyroid dysfunction rates to be 3% to 7% [37–44]. Youth found to have abnormal thyroid function studies should be evaluated and treated by a pediatric endocrinologist.

The prevalence of celiac disease, a gluten-sensitive enteropathy, in the general population is estimated at 1:122 to 1:300 [45–47]. The disease is thought to be underdiagnosed in the population at large. The association between celiac disease and T1D is thought to occur with a frequency of up to 20% [48]. In celiac disease, gluten peptides trigger an immune response with inflammation in the small intestine. The inflamed intestines release tissue transglutaminase, which is a highly specific endomysial autoantigen that can be readily detected in the blood [2]. Children who have elevated tissue transglutaminase levels may or may not experience abdominal discomfort, including, cramping, bloating, and diarrhea. Elevated tissue transglutaminase levels warrant referral to a pediatric gastroenterologist, who performs a small intestinal biopsy to confirm the diagnosis. If the diagnosis of celiac disease is made, the child or adolescent must follow a meal plan that is free of gluten-containing products.

Diabetic nephropathy is the leading cause of end-stage renal disease in developed countries. Twenty-five percent of patients with T1D go on to develop diabetic nephropathy at some point in their lives. At the time of diagnosis with diabetes, glomerular filtration rate, urinary albumin excretion, and kidney size are increased; however, they return to normal with treatment of the hyperglycemia. Even with standard diabetes care, however, glomerular filtration rate and kidney size remain mildly elevated over the next 10 years. This is termed the "silent phase" of diabetic renal disease, where structural changes may be occurring within the kidney without any signs and symptoms [49]. Microalbuminuria (urinary albumin excretion rate) is defined as 30 to 300 mg per 24 hours or 20 to 200 µg/min [2,49]. The next phase, termed "incipient nephropathy," is characterized by subtle blood pressure changes, microalbuminuria, and possible decreased creatinine clearance [49]. In studies with children and adolescents, the presence of microalbuminuria is much greater in patients who are over 12 to 15 years old, indicating a relationship with the onset of puberty [50,51]. Studies have shown that it is possible for patients to reverse the progression of microalbuminuria to normal urinary albumin excretion by lowering hemoglobin

A_{1c} levels, lowering blood pressures, and lowering lipid levels [52,53]. Patients with urinary microalbuminuria should be aggressively treated by improving metabolic control, lowering blood pressure with the use of angiotensin-converting enzyme inhibitors, using lipid-lowering agents, and frequent follow-up with the diabetes care team [49]. All youth with T1D should have urinary microalbumin levels performed on an annual basis.

Diabetic retinopathy is the most common microvascular complication of diabetes and is the leading cause of blindness in the United States. The earliest lesion detected is nonproliferative retinopathy, which consists of microaneurysms. More severe forms include exudates and venous beading of the retina. Proliferative retinopathy causes fibrous proliferation, new blood vessel formation, and macular edema and is associated with a progressive loss of vision. Proliferative retinopathy occurs in 50% of diabetics after a 20-year duration of diabetes, but is rarely seen in children before the age of 15 years [2]. Children and adolescents with T1D should have an initial dilated eye examination by an ophthalmologist within 3 to 5 years after the onset of diabetes and annually thereafter [8].

Children and adolescents with T1D are known to be at risk for developing psychiatric problems. This increased risk has been attributed to the stress of the chronic illness, the demanding nature of diabetes care, the threat of future complications, and possibly the pathophysiology of T1D [54–57]. The comorbidity of diabetes and depression in children and adolescents is a serious issue, which affects up to 20% of youth with diabetes compared with less than 7% of youth without diabetes [58]. Studies have also shown that anxiety disorders and eating disorders have an increased prevalence in youth with diabetes [54,59,60]. The ADA recommends that all individuals over the age of 8 years with T1D be screened annually for depression using a reliable and valid depression screening tool. Diabetes providers are given the opportunity to monitor the patient's psychosocial and psychiatric status at the time of diagnosis and at follow-up appointments and make the appropriate referrals for mental health providers [8]. Family adjustment and support are correlates of depression in youth with diabetes, suggesting that family approaches, such as coping skills training and behavioral therapy for families, may be effective in preventing or treating depression in these youth [58].

Summary

T1D is a tremendously challenging and complex disease for children and families to manage. Advances in research are constantly bringing about changes in therapies and treatments with the hope of improving the quality of life for youth with T1D and their families. Accurate diagnosis, education, treatment, and referral to a certified diabetes educator, endocrinologist, dietitian, social worker, and psychologist are needed to provide the child with

the skills necessary to manage diabetes over a lifetime. Nurses and nurse practitioners must be informed of the most current treatments and research available for their patients so that they can encourage their patients to live full and healthy lives.

References

[1] American Diabetes Association. The dangerous toll of diabetes. ADA Website, 2006.
[2] Weinzimer S, Magge S. Type 1 diabetes mellitus in children. In: Bell LM, Pasquariello PS, editors. Pediatric endocrinology: the requisites in pediatrics. Philadelphia: Elsevier Mosby; 2005. p. 3–18.
[3] Devendra D, Liu E, Eisenbarth G. Type 1 diabetes: recent developments. BMJ 2004;328: 750–5.
[4] Guthrie R, Guthrie D. Pathophysiology of diabetes mellitus. Crit Care Nurs Q 2004;27: 113–25.
[5] Morwessel NJ. The genetic basis of diabetes mellitus. AACN Clin Issues Adv Pract Crit Care 1998;9:609–14.
[6] Laffel L, Pasquarello C, Lawlor M. Treatment of the child and adolescent with diabetes. In: Kahn C, King G, Moses A, et al, editors. Joslin's diabetes mellitus. 14th edition. New York: Lippincott Williams and Wilkins; 2005. p. 711–36.
[7] Agus M, Wolfsdorf MB. Diabetic ketoacidosis in children. Pediatr Clin North Am 2005;52: 1147–63.
[8] American Diabetes Association. Clinical practice recommendations 2006. Diabetes Care 2006;29(Suppl 1):S4–42.
[9] Silverstein J, Klingensmith G, Copeland K, et al. Care of children and adolescents with type 1 diabetes. A statement of the American Diabetes Association. Diabetes Care 2005;28: 186–212.
[10] Mensing C, Boucher J, Cypress M, et al. National standards for diabetes self-management education: task force to review and revise the national standards for diabetes self-management education programs. Diabetes Care 2000;23:682–9.
[11] Etzwiler DD. Education of the patient with diabetes. Med Clin North Am 1978;62:857–66.
[12] Tamborlane T, Fredrickson L, Ahern J. Insulin pump therapy in childhood diabetes mellitus. Treat Endocrinol 2003;2:11–21.
[13] The Diabetes Control and Complications Research Group. The effect of intensive treatment of diabetes on the development and progression of long-term complications in insulin-dependent diabetes mellitus. N Engl J Med 1993;329:977–86.
[14] Rapaport R, Sills IN. Implications of the DCCT for children and adolescents with IDDM. N J Med 1994;91:227–8.
[15] Tamborlane WV, Sherwin RS, Genel M, et al. Reduction to normal of plasma glucose in juvenile diabetes by subcutaneous administration of insulin with a portable infusion pump. N Engl J Med 1979;300:573–8.
[16] The Diabetes Control and Complications Trial Research Group. The effect of intensive diabetes treatment on the development of long-term complications in adolescents with insulin-dependent diabetes mellitus. J Pediatr 1994;125:177–88.
[17] Sullivan-Bolyai S, Knafl K, Tamborlane WV, et al. Parent's reflections on managing their children's diabetes with insulin pumps. J Nurs Scholarsh 2004;36:316–23.
[18] Anderson B, Ho J, Brackett J, et al. Parental involvement in diabetes management tasks: relationships to blood glucose monitoring adherence and metabolic control in young adolescents with insulin-dependent diabetes mellitus. J Pediatr 1997;130:257–65.
[19] Institute of Medicine. Dietary reference intakes: energy, carbohydrate, fiber, fat, fatty acids, cholesterol, protein, and amino acids. Washington: National Academics Press; 2002.

[20] American Dietetic Association. Position of the American Dietetic Association: dietary guidance for healthy children ages 2 to 11 years. J Am Diet Assoc 2004;104:660–77.

[21] Massin MM, Lebrethon MC, Rocour D, et al. Patterns of physical activity determined by heart rate monitoring among diabetic children. Arch Dis Child 2005;90:1215–7.

[22] Tsalikian E, Mauras N, Beck RW, et al. Impact of exercise on overnight glycemic control in children with type 1 diabetes mellitus. J Pediatr 2005;147:528–34.

[23] Martin R, Kupsis B, Novak P, et al. The infant with diabetes mellitus: a case study. Pediatr Nurs 1994;20:27–34.

[24] Banion CR, Miles MS, Carter MC. Problems of mothers in management of children with diabetes. Diabetes Care 1983;6:548–51.

[25] Ryan CM, Becker DJ. Hypoglycemia in children with type 1 mellitus: risk factors, cognitive function, and management. Endocrinol Metab Clin North Am 1999;28:883–900.

[26] Fonagy P, Moran GS, Lindsay MK, et al. Psychological adjustment and diabetic control. Arch Dis Child 1987;62:1009–13.

[27] Follansbee DS. Assuming responsibility for diabetes management: what age? what price? Diabetes Educ 1989;15:347–53.

[28] Anderson B. Family conflict and diabetes management in youth: clinical lessons from child development and diabetes research. Diabetes Spectrum 2004;17:22–5.

[29] Davis CL, Delamater AM, Shaw KH, et al. Parenting styles, regimen adherence, and glycemic control in 4–10 year-old children with diabetes. J Pediatr Psychol 2001;26:123–9.

[30] Pond JS, Peters ML, Pannell DL, et al. Psychosocial challenges for children with insulin-dependent diabetes mellitus. Diabetes Educ 1995;21:297–9.

[31] Viikinsalo MK, Crawford DM, Kimbrel H, et al. Conflicts between young adolescents with type 1 diabetes and their parents. JSPN 2005;10:69–79.

[32] Anderson BJ, Vangsness A, Connell D, et al. Family conflict, adherence, and glycemic control in youth with short duration type 1 diabetes. Diabet Med 2002;19:635–42.

[33] Faulkner MS. Quality of life for adolescents with type 1 diabetes: parental and youth perspectives. Pediatr Nurs 2003;29:362–8.

[34] van de Wiel A. Diabetes mellitus and alcohol. Diabetes Metab Res Rev 2004;20:263–7.

[35] Harris GD, Fiordalisi I, Harris WL, et al. Minimizing the risk of brain herniation during treatment of diabetic ketoacidemia: a retrospective and prospective study. J Pediatr 1990; 117:22–31.

[36] Finberg L. Fluid management of diabetic ketoacidosis. Pediatr Rev 1996;17:46–52.

[37] Hansen D, Bennedbaek FN, Hoier-Madsen M, et al. A prospective study of thyroid dysfunction, morphology and an auto-immunity in young patients with type 1 diabetes. Eur J Endocrinol 2003;148:245–51.

[38] McKenna MJ, Herskowitz R, Wolfsdorf JI. Screening for thyroid disease in children with IDDM. Diabetes Care 1990;13:801–3.

[39] Darendeliler FF, Kadioglu A, Bas F, et al. Thyroid ultrasound in IDDM. J Endocrinol 1994; 7:33–7.

[40] Lorini R, d'Annunzio G, Vitali L, et al. IDDM and autoimmune thyroid disease in the pediatric age group. J Pediatr Endocrinol Metab 1996;9:89–94.

[41] Roldan MB, Alonso M, Barrio R. Thyroid autoimmunity in children and adolescents with type 1 diabetes mellitus. Diabetes Nutr Metab 1999;12:27–31.

[42] Holl RW, Bohm B, Loos U, et al. Thyroid autoimmunity in children and adolescents with type 1 diabetes mellitus. Horm Res 1999;52:113–8.

[43] Kordonouri O, Deiss D, Danne T, et al. Predictivity of thyroid antibodies for the development of thyroid disorders in children and adolescents with type 1 diabetes. Diabet Med 2002; 19:518–21.

[44] Prina-Cerai LM, Weber G, Meschi F, et al. Prevalence of thyroid autoantibodies and thyroid autoimmune disease in diabetic children and adolescents. Diabetes Care 1994;17:782–3.

[45] Spiekerkoetter U, Seissler J, Wendel U. General screening for celiac disease is advisable in children with type 1 diabetes. Horm Metab Res 2002;34:192–5.

[46] Johnston SD, Watson RG, McMillan SA, et al. Prevalence of celiac disease in Northern Ireland. Lancet 1997;350:1370.
[47] Pruessner HT. Detecting celiac disease in your patients. Am Fam Physician 1998;57: 1034–41.
[48] Boudraa G, Hachelaf W, Benbouabdellah M, et al. Prevalence of celiac disease in diabetic children and their first-degree relatives in west Algeria. screening with serological markers. Acta Paediatr Suppl 1996;412:58–60.
[49] Ellis E. Diabetes mellitus and the kidney in adolescents. Adolesc Med 2005;16:173–84.
[50] Mathiesen ER, Saurbrey N, Hommel E. Prevalence of microalbuminuia in children with type 1 diabetes mellitus. Diabetologia 1986;29:640–3.
[51] Quattrin T, Waz WR, Duffy LC. Microalbuminuria in an adolescent cohort with insulin dependent diabetes mellitus. Clin Pediatr 1995;34:12–7.
[52] Gorman D, Sockett E, Daneman D. The natural history of microalbuminuria in adolescents with type 1 diabetes. J Pediatr 1999;134:333–7.
[53] Rudberg S, Dahlquist G. Determinants of progress of microalbuminuria in adolescents with IDDM. Diabetes Care 1996;19:369–71.
[54] Kovacs M, Goldston D, Obrosky D, et al. Psychiatric disorders in youths with IDDM: rates and risk factors. Diabetes Care 1997;20:36–44.
[55] Johnson SB. Psychosocial factors in juvenile diabetes: a review. J Behav Med 1980;3:95–116.
[56] Johnson SB. Diabetes mellitus in childhood. In: Routh DK, editor. Handbook of pediatric psychology. New York: Guilford Press; 1988. p. 9–31.
[57] Drash AL, Becker DJ. Behavioral issues in patients with diabetes mellitus, with special emphasis on the child and adolescent. In: Rifkin H, Porte D, editors. Ellenberg and Rifkin's diabetes mellitus. theory and practice. 4th edition. New York: Elsevier; 1990. p. 922–34.
[58] Grey M, Whittemore R, Tamborlane WV. Depression in type 1 diabetes in children: natural history and correlates. J Psychosom Res 2002;53:907–11.
[59] Gavard JA, Lustman PJ, Clouse RE. Prevalence of depression in adults with diabetes: an epidemiological evaluation. Diabetes Care 1993;16:1167–78.
[60] Lustman PJ, Amado H, Wetzel RD. Depression in diabetics: a critical appraisal. Compr Psychiatry 1983;24:65–74.

ELSEVIER
SAUNDERS

NURSING
CLINICS
OF NORTH AMERICA

Nurs Clin N Am 41 (2006) 531–547

Type 2 Diabetes Mellitus

Anne H. Skelly, PhD, RN, CS, FAANP

School of Nursing, The University of North Carolina at Chapel Hill,
Carrington Hall, CB# 7460, Chapel Hill, NC 27599, USA

Diabetes mellitus is a heterogeneous group of metabolic diseases resulting from defects in insulin secretion, insulin action, or both, resulting in hyperglycemia [1]. The major categories or classifications of diabetes are type 1 (T1DM), type 2 (T2DM), gestational diabetes, other specific types, and prediabetes. T2DM is the most common form of diabetes affecting 17 million Americans or over 6.5% of the population [2]. The incidence of T2DM is reaching epidemic proportions worldwide paralleling increases in obesity and more sedentary lifestyles. The World Health Organization estimates that by the year 2025, over 300 million individuals may have diabetes [3].

T2DM disproportionately affects members of minority groups including African Americans, Native Americans, Latinos, Asian Americans, and Pacific Islanders. Although T2DM is usually diagnosed in individuals after the age of 30, increasing numbers of children and adolescents are now being diagnosed with the disease, especially among minority populations. T2DM is a chronic disorder characterized by progressive β-cell dysfunction and varying degrees of insulin resistance. In some individuals this may progress to an absolute deficiency of insulin secretion [3]. T2DM formerly was referred to as "non–insulin-dependent diabetes mellitus," "maturity-onset diabetes," or "adult-onset diabetes." This terminology often created confusion with individuals who have T1DM.

Although the precise etiology of T2DM is not known, genetics and environment seem to play major roles. A 75% concordance rate has been found in studies of identical twins with T2DM, but the exact genes involved have not been identified. Islet cells antibodies found in T1DM are not present in T2DM. Obesity seems to be the most important factor in the pathogenesis of T2DM, with greater than 80% of individuals obese, or having a history of obesity, at the time of diagnosis [3]. Sedentary lifestyle has also been linked to the development of T2DM. Other important risk factors for the

E-mail address: askelly@email.unc.edu

0029-6465/06/$ - see front matter © 2006 Elsevier Inc. All rights reserved.
doi:10.1016/j.cnur.2006.07.011
nursing.theclinics.com

development of T2DM are age, ethnicity, insulin resistance, impaired fasting glucose, impaired glucose tolerance, and previous gestational diabetes.

Persons with T2DM may or may not present with the classic symptoms of diabetes: polydipsia, polyphagia, polyuria, and weight loss. They frequently present with symptoms of microvascular, macrovascular, and neuropathic complications, however, such as numbness and tingling in the extremities and lipid abnormalities, because of the extended length of time (up to 4–7 years) between the onset of hyperglycemia and the diagnosis of T2DM [3,4]. Children may present with ketoacidosis; however, β-cell destruction is usually not found, nor evidence of active autoimmunity.

The Diabetes Prevention Program demonstrated the ability to delay or prevent the development of T2DM through lifestyle changes, particularly weight loss and increased physical activity [5]. These findings provide an opportunity for nurses and other health care professionals to intervene with at-risk families and individuals to prevent proactively the development of T2DM. This article sets out to

1. Describe the classification of diabetes mellitus
2. Define the metabolic syndrome, the different criteria used for diagnosis, and its relationship to T2DM
3. Present criteria for the diagnosis of diabetes
4. Discuss the risk factors and screening criteria for T2DM
5. Discuss the pathophysiology of T2DM and of acute and chronic complications
6. Discuss the signs of symptoms of persons presenting with T2DM
7. Briefly present an overview of the treatment of T2DM

Classification of diabetes mellitus

In 2003, the American Diabetes Association revised the diagnostic and classification criteria for diabetes to reflect new understanding of the pathogenesis and, in certain cases, the causes of the various categories. The five major categories are T2DM, T2DM, gestational diabetes, other specific types, and prediabetes (Box 1) [6].

Type 1 diabetes

T1DM results from cell-mediated autoimmune destruction of the pancreatic β cells that ultimately leads to an absolute deficiency of insulin. Patients with T1DM usually have an onset of symptoms before the age of 30, have severe insulinopenia, and are prone to ketoacidosis [7]. T1DM was previously known as "insulin-dependent diabetes mellitus" or "juvenile-onset diabetes."

A form of T1DM can also present later in life. Latent autoimmune diabetes of aging is a slow, progressive form of hyperglycemia with β-cell

---

**Box 1. Categories of diabetes mellitus and other classes
of abnormal glucose metabolism**

Type 1: Immune-medicated absolute deficiency of insulin
Type 2: Insulin resistance with relative insulin deficiency
Gestational diabetes: Diabetes first diagnosed during pregnancy
Other types
Genetic defects in insulin action
Genetic defects in β-cell function
Endocrine disorders
Diseases of the exocrine pancreas, infections
Drug or chemical-induced diabetes
Prediabetes
Individuals with plasma glucose higher than normal but not
    diagnostic for diabetes mellitus
Impaired fasting glucose
Impaired glucose tolerance

Adapted from Burant CF. Medical management of type 2 diabetes. 5th edition.
Alexandria (VA): American Diabetes Association; 2004. p. 4, 11.

---

destruction caused by autoimmune processes, which may not require insulin for years. In adults, anti-glutamic acid decarboxylase autoantibodies are positive in approximately two of three cases and may be useful in the diagnosis. Because of the slow development of symptomatology, individuals with latent autoimmune diabetes of aging may be misclassified as having T2DM [3].

Type 2 diabetes

T2DM is a heterogenetic disorder characterized by a combination of varying degrees of progressive β-cell dysfunction and insulin resistance that typically lead to a relative (rather than an absolute) deficiency of insulin [7]. Although the specific causes of T2DM are not known, autoimmune destruction of the pancreas does not occur and individuals do not have any of the other known causes of diabetes shown in Box 1. Persons diagnosed with T2DM usually are diagnosed after the age of 30 years, are obese, and have a family history of T2DM.

Type 2 in youth

Concurrent with the increase in obesity, T2DM in children and adolescents is becoming more common, particularly in minority populations. The incidence of T2DM is surpassing that of T1DM in children and may be provoked by the onset of puberty. The pathophysiology of T2DM in

young individuals is likely very similar to that seen in adults. Obesity and physical inactivity seem to be the primary factors involved related to increased consumption of high caloric foods, decreased leisure time physical activity, and increased time spent viewing television. In the adolescent, T2DM can be differentiated from T1DM by the absence of islet cell antibodies, normal or elevated C-peptide levels, the presence of obesity, a significant family history of T2DM, and the presence of acanthosis nigricans. Youths presenting with T2DM may present with ketonuria, or even ketoacidosis, but not weight loss [3].

Other specific types of diabetes

Disorders in this category include a range of genetic disorders and maturity-onset diabetes of the young. Among the genetic disorders that result in diabetes are disorders of β-cell function; genetic defects in insulin action; diseases of the exocrine pancreas; endocrinopathies (eg, Cushing's syndrome, pheochromocytoma, acromegaly, hyperthyroidism); drug- or chemical-induced diabetes; infections; uncommon forms of immune-mediated diabetes (eg, stiff-man syndrome); and other genetic syndromes sometimes associated with diabetes. Although this category represents a small subset of persons with diabetes, identification is important because the treatment often differs.

Maturity-onset diabetes of the young

Maturity-onset diabetes of the young is characterized by an onset of hyperglycemia at an early age, usually before the age of 25. Maturity-onset diabetes of the young is seen in families and is inherited as an autosomal-dominant pattern. In maturity-onset diabetes of the young, insulin secretion is impaired. Unlike T2DM, however, minimal or no defects in insulin action are seen [3,7]. Maturity-onset diabetes of the young was considered a subset of T2DM but now is listed under the category "other specific types."

Gestational diabetes

This is glucose intolerance first identified during pregnancy. Scrupulous glycemic control is necessary to prevent fetal macrosomia. Approximately 50% of women diagnosed with gestational diabetes develop T2DM [3].

Prediabetes

Individuals in this category have plasma glucose levels higher than normal but not diagnostic for diabetes mellitus. This category includes impaired fasting glucose with values between 100 and 125 mg/dL (6.1–6.9 mmol/L) and impaired glucose tolerance with values between 140 and 199 mg/dL (7.8–11 mmol/L) in the 2-hour sample after a 75-g oral glucose tolerance test (OGTT). Individuals in this category are at risk for the development of diabetes and cardiovascular disease and benefit from education and lifestyle modifications.

The metabolic syndrome and insulin resistance

The metabolic syndrome is a constellation of risk factors, mostly metabolic in origin, that tend to coexist and complicate and exacerbate each other (Fig. 1) [8]. Individuals with the metabolic syndrome are at increased risk of developing both cardiovascular disease and T2DM. T2DM and prediabetes are manifestations of the metabolic syndrome and closely linked to insulin resistance [3]. The metabolic syndrome is commonly defined by the markers of insulin resistance (see Fig. 1). Insulin resistance is present in more than 90% of patients with T2DM and is also prevalent in obese individuals, particularly those with visceral or abdominal obesity [9].

Insulin resistance is the failure of insulin, at relatively normal concentrations, to exert its normal effects. As the concentration of glucose in the blood increases, insulin is released in greater quantities from the pancreas. In obese persons, insulin concentrations in the plasma are actually greater than normal. Some people can maintain this increased insulin secretion and carry on as obese, nondiabetic individuals. In genetically predisposed others, however, the ability of the β cells to sustain these higher rates of insulin begins to fail resulting in impaired glucose tolerance and progression to clinical diabetes mellitus (Fig. 2).

Questions have been expressed about whether the metabolic syndrome actually comprises a syndrome or whether the different components may have disparate pathologies [10]. The criteria for metabolic syndrome or insulin resistance syndrome have been variably defined by the World Health Organization [11], the National Cholesterol Education Program Adult Treatment Panel III [12], the International Diabetes Federation [13], and the American Association of Clinical Endocrinology [14]. Although there are no commonly accepted criteria for the metabolic syndrome, the most widely accepted definition in the United States is that of the National Cholesterol Education Program Adult Treatment Panel III (Table 1). Although

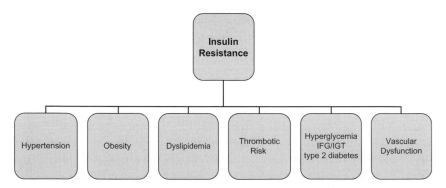

Fig. 1. Clinical components in type 2 diabetes and the metabolic syndrome. Insulin resistance is proposed to play a central role in the development of many of the associated features. IFG, impaired fasting glucose; IGT, impaired glucose tolerance.

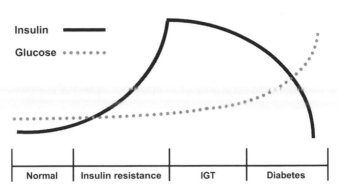

Fig. 2. Glucose and insulin changes in the progression to type 2 diabetes mellitus. IGT, impaired glucose tolerance.

the definitions proposed by the World Health Organization and the American Association of Clinical Endocrinology include a measure of insulin resistance, the National Cholesterol Education Program Adult Treatment Panel III criteria do not, avoiding the implication that insulin resistance is the primary or the only cause of the associated risk factors [15]. Revised guidelines for the definition and diagnosis of metabolic syndrome are currently under review by the American Heart Association/National Heart, Lung, and Blood Institute and the International Diabetes Federation. It is hoped that these new criteria provide a consistent approach to the identification of individuals with metabolic syndrome to facilitate early interventions.

The incidence of metabolic syndrome varies in different ethnic populations, perhaps because of the differing criteria for diagnosis, and its prevalence increases with age. It is now estimated that up to 8% to 45% of new cases of diabetes among children and adolescents are T2DM. An even larger proportion of obese youth are developing the metabolic syndrome or prediabetes. This is alarming given the length of time these individuals are exposed to risk factors for diabetes-related complications and underscores the need for appropriate and timely interventions [16].

Diagnostic criteria for diabetes

The criteria for the diagnosis of diabetes, impaired fasting glucose and impaired glucose tolerance, are shown in Fig. 3. The diagnosis of diabetes can be made using a random plasma glucose plus signs and symptoms of diabetes, a fasting plasma glucose, or an OGTT. In the absence of unequivocal hyperglycemia with acute metabolic decompensation, test results should be confirmed on a different day. The fasting plasma glucose remains the test of choice because of its accuracy and convenience. The OGTT is useful if the patients adhere to a diet adequate in carbohydrates (150 g/day for 3 days);

Table 1
Current criteria for the diagnosis of the metabolic syndrome

	WHO	NCEP ATP III	AACE
Hypertension	Current antihypertensive therapy or BP >160/90	BP >130/85	Hypertension
Dyslipidemia	Plasma triglycerides >1.7 mmol/L or HDL cholesterol	Plasma triglycerides >150 mg/dL, HDL cholesterol <40 mg/dL in men and <50 mg/dL in women	Dyslipidemia (HDL cholesterol <45 mg/dL in women, <35 mg/dL in men, or triglycerides >150 mg/dL)
Obesity	BMI >30 or waist/ hip ratio >0.90 in males, >0.85 in females	Waist circumference >40 cm in males and >50 cm in females	Waist circumference >102 cm for men and >88 cm for women
Glucose	Type 2 diabetes or IGT	Fasting blood glucose >110 mg/dL	Impaired fasting blood glucose or type 2 diabetes
Other	Microalbuminuria = over-night urinary albumin excretion rate >20 μg/min		Insulin resistance (denoted by hyperinsulinemia relative to glucose levels or acanthosis nigricans)
Requirements for diagnosis	Requires diagnosis of type 2 diabetes or IGT and any *two* of the previous criteria; if normal glucose tolerance, must demonstrate three other disorders	Requires any *three* of the previous disorders	Minor criteria including hypercoagulability, PCOS, vascular or endothelial dysfunction, microalbuminuria, and coronary heart disease

Abbreviations: AACE, American Association of Clinical Endocrinology; BMI, body mass index; BP, blood pressure; HDL, high-density lipoprotein; IGT, impaired glucose tolerance; NCEP ATP III, National Cholesterol Education Program—Adult Treatment Panel III; PCOS, polycystic ovary syndrome; WHO, World Health Organization.

From Harmel A, Mathur R, editors. Davidson's diabetes mellitus. 5th edition. Philadelphia: WB Saunders, 2004; with permission.

have no underlying illnesses; or interfering drugs [3]. The OGTT should not be performed if the fasting plasma glucose is ≥126 mg/dL. The OGTT is performed in nonpregnant adults using a 75-g oral glucose load with examination of the 2-hour plasma glucose value [3].

Risk factors and screening recommendations for diabetes

Diabetes screening is recommended for all at-risk individuals. The present recommendations for screening to detect diabetes and prediabetes are

Diagnosis of Diabetes

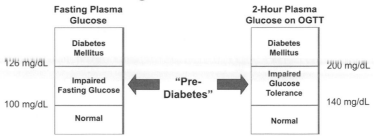

Fig. 3. Diagnosis of diabetes. OGTT, oral glucose tolerance test. (*Adapted from* the American Diabetes Association. Diagnosis and Classification of Diabetes Mellitus. Diabetes Care 2004; 27:S5–10.)

to test all individuals ≥45 years of age, particularly those with a body mass index ≥25 kg/m^2 (this may not be correct for all ethnic groups). If the results are normal, testing should be repeated at 3-year intervals [17].

Testing should be considered at a younger age (starting at 10 years of age) and conducted more frequently in individuals who are overweight and demonstrate one or more of the following risk factors [17]:

- Are physically inactive
- Have a first-degree relative with diabetes
- Are of African America, Latino, Native American, Asian American, or Pacific Islander ethnicity
- Delivered a baby weighing ≥9 lb
- Have been previously diagnosed with gestational diabetes
- Diagnosed with polycystic ovary syndrome
- Are hypertensive (≥140/90 mm Hg)
- Have a high-density lipoprotein cholesterol level <35 μm/dL or a triglyceride level >250 μm/dL
- Have a history of impaired fasting glucose or impaired glucose tolerance
- Have a history of vascular diseases
- Have other clinical conditions associated with insulin resistance (eg, acanthosis nigricans, polycystic ovary syndrome)

A fasting plasma glucose test is recommended initially for screening in nonpregnant adults because of its convenience, cost, and ease of administration. The 2-hour OGTT should be considered in patients who present with impaired fasting glucose to define better their risk of diabetes.

Screening pregnant women for gestational diabetes should occur at the first prenatal visit by assessing for risk factors and, if appropriate, an OGTT. Important risk factors include marked obesity, history of gestational diabetes, and family history of diabetes. Women at high-risk, not found to have gestational diabetes at the initial screening, and average-risk

women should be tested between 24 and 28 weeks of gestation using the OGTT. Women who are <25 years, have a normal body weight, no first-degree relatives with diabetes, and are white with a low risk of gestational diabetes need not be screened [3].

Only children and youth at increased risk for the development of T2DM should be screened. The American Academy of Pediatrics and the American Diabetes Association recommend screening at age >10 or the onset of puberty in children who have any of the following risk factors [18]:

Body mass index >85th percentile
First- or second-degree relative with diabetes
Member of an at-risk ethnic group
Signs of insulin resistance (eg, polycystic ovary syndrome, dyslipidemia, hypertension, acanthosis nigricans)

To screen, either a fasting plasma glucose test or a 2-hour OGTT may be used. Follow-up testing is recommended at 2-year intervals for at-risk youths.

Pathophysiology of type 2 diabetes

The pathogenesis of T2DM involves both relative insulin deficiency and impairment of insulin action. Both are usually seen in affected individuals and are caused by a combination of both genetic and environmental factors. Epidemiologic studies indicate that T2DM seems to result from the interaction of multiple genes each of which confers a risk for the development of the disease [19]. Genetic factors are even more important than in T1DM. In first-degree relatives (and nonidentical twins) of individuals with T2DM the risk of developing diabetes is 20% to 40%, versus 5% to 7% in the population at large [20].

The two major metabolic defects that characterize T2DM are a derangement in β-cell secretion of insulin and a decreased response of the peripheral tissues to insulin (insulin resistance). Increased glucose production by the liver is also seen. Whether impaired insulin secretion or impaired insulin action is the primary pathogenic defect in the etiologic process of T2DM is still debated. Abnormalities in the uptake and metabolism of fatty acids in the peripheral tissues and β cells may be a primary event in the development of insulin resistance and β-cell failure [3].

Defects in β-cell secretion

In populations at risk for developing T2DM, a modest hyperinsulinemia may be observed related to hyperresponsiveness by the β cell to physiologic elevations in blood glucose. The pattern of insulin secretion changes with the development of overt disease. Early in the course of T2DM, insulin secretion seems to be normal and plasma insulin levels are not reduced.

The normal pattern of insulin secretion is lost, however, and the rapid first phase of insulin secretion triggered by glucose is blunted [20]. With reductions in this early phase of insulin secretion, the concentration of insulin in the portal vein remains low after food intake and hepatic glucose production is not suppressed. This continuing production of glucose by the liver in addition to the glucose entering the circulation from a meal leads to hyperglycemia. Reduced uptake of glucose by the skeletal muscle caused by reduced insulin secretion further contributes to hyperglycemia. Early in the course of diabetes, this reduced first-phase of insulin secretion is followed by a late phase of increased insulin secretion with the plasma glucose returning to a normal level. This late-phase insulin secretion diminishes as β cells continue to fail resulting in overt diabetes [3]. Collectively, these changes suggest derangements in β-cell responses to hyperglycemia early in T2DM, rather than deficiencies in insulin synthesis.

Later in the course of T2DM, a mild to moderate deficiency of insulin develops, which is less severe than seen in T1DM. The cause of the insulin deficiency is not entirely clear, but irreversible β-cell damage does seem to be present. Unlike T1DM, there is no evidence for viral or immune-mediated injury to the islet cells. The somatic cells of predisposed individuals, including the pancreatic β cells, may be more genetically vulnerable to injury, leading to accelerated cell turnover and premature aging, and ultimately to a modest reduction in β-cell mass [20].

Pathogenesis of insulin resistance

Although insulin deficiency is present late in the course of T2DM, it is not of sufficient magnitude to explain the metabolic disturbances seen. Rather, a major factor in the development of T2DM is the reduced responsiveness of peripheral tissues (insulin resistance). Skeletal muscle, liver, and adipose tissue are primary sites of insulin resistance.

Insulin resistance is a complex phenomenon that is not restricted to diabetes. In both obesity and pregnancy, insulin sensitivity of target tissues decreases (even in the absence of diabetes), and insulin levels may be elevated. Insulin resistance in the main insulin target organs (liver and skeletal muscle) may initially be compensated for by the increased production of insulin (hyperinsulinemia), so that overt diabetes does not occur until there is β-cell failure (see Fig. 2) [3,20].

The molecular basis of insulin resistance is not clear. Postreceptor signaling by insulin is impaired and there may be a decrease in the number of insulin receptors. Binding of insulin to its receptors leads to translocation of glucose transporters (gluts) to the cell membrane, which in turn facilitates cellular uptake of glucose. It is suspected that reduced synthesis and translocation of gluts in muscle and fat cells underlie the insulin resistance found in obesity and T2DM. Other postreceptor signaling defects have also been described. From a physiologic standpoint, insulin resistance, regardless of

its mechanism, results in the inability of circulating insulin properly to dispose of glucose and other metabolic fuels, and more persistent hyperglycemia resulting in more persistent stimulation of the pancreatic β cell. Chronic hyperglycemia may exhaust the ability of the β cells to function as a consequence of persistent β-cell stimulation [20].

Obesity

Regardless of which initiating event is proposed for T2DM, obesity is an extremely important environmental influence. Insulin resistance is part of the metabolic syndrome and obesity is the most common acquired cause of insulin resistance. Approximately 80% of adults with T2DM are obese, with abdominal obesity having a greater metabolic impact. Intra-abdominal fat catabolism delivers free fatty acids to the liver, yet is relatively resistant to the modulating effects of insulin. Although abdominal obesity and insulin resistance could be expressions of a third unknown factor, the possibility that they are casually related should be considered [21]. Insulin resistance, frequently associated with obesity, produces excessive stress on the β cells, which may fail in the face of a sustained hyperinsulinemia.

Pathophysiology of chronic complications

Although the major types of diabetes have different pathogenic mechanisms, the long-term complications (macrovascular disease, microvascular disease, and neuropathy) are the same and are major causes of morbidity and death. The pathologic basis of these complications continues to be studied [22,23]. Clinical evidence, however, points to the role of chronic hyperglycemia in causing the metabolic derangements seen. This is supported by data from multicenter clinical trials that have demonstrated delays in the progression of microvascular complications with strict glycemic control [24].

Two metabolic events seem to be involved in the genesis of chronic complications of diabetes: nonenzymatic glycosylation and intracellular hyperglycemia with disturbances in the polyol pathway [20]. Nonenzymatic glycosylation is a process by which glucose chemically attaches to the amino group of proteins without the aid of enzymes. The degree of enzymatic glycosylation is directly related to the level of blood glucose. These products undergo a slow series of chemical changes to form advanced glycosylation end product accumulations in interstitial and blood vessel walls. These advanced glycosylation end products have a number of chemical and biologic characteristics that are potentially damaging [25]. Some structures in the body, such as the nerves, lens of the eye, kidneys, and blood vessels, do not require insulin to transport glucose into the cells. In these tissues, increases in intracellular glucose (hyperglycemia) are metabolized by aldose reductase to sorbitol (a polyol) and then to fructose. This change in metabolic pathways causes increased intracellular osmolarity and influx of water,

and eventually osmotic cell injury because of the accumulated levels of sorbitol and fructose. An example of this may be seen in the eye with swelling of the lens of the eye, injury to the Schwann cells and pericytes of the retinal capillaries, and retinal microaneurysms.

For an in depth discussion of these complications, their clinical manifestations, underlying pathophysiology, and treatment, the reader is referred to other articles in this issue.

Signs and symptoms

Most cases of T2DM are diagnosed after the age of 40, most typically in individuals who are obese or have a family history of diabetes. The risk for T2DM increases with age. Because of the presence of some circulating endogenous insulin in individuals with T2DM, ketoacidosis is uncommon but certain individuals may be at risk for hyperosmolar hypertonic nonketotic coma (HHNK). Severe hypoglycemia is rare in T2DM.

Individuals with T2DM may present with increased thirst (polydipsia) and increased urination (polyuria), but rarely weight loss. Other common symptoms include headache, weakness, fatigue, and blurred vision. On occasion, individuals with T2DM may present with signs and symptoms of peripheral neuropathy or cardiac complications including dyslipidemias (hypertriglyceridemia) resulting from undiagnosed diabetes over a period of time. In women with T2DM, chronic skin infections, reoccurring vulvovaginitis or pruritus, or urinary tract infections may be the initial presenting complaints. Especially in obese individuals, patients may be asymptomatic because of an insidious onset of hyperglycemia. These individuals may be first diagnosed during work up for another medical problem or as part of a routine physical examination.

An evaluation of the signs for T2DM should include assessment of the other clinical conditions associated with the metabolic syndrome including insulin resistance and visceral adiposity (see Fig. 1). Height, weight, and waist circumference should be measured and a body mass index calculated. The American Diabetes Association Clinical Practice Recommendations [17] present criteria for an initial, comprehensive physical examination including vital signs; sexual maturation staging (during the pubertal period); examination of the skin; funduscopic and oral examinations; palpation of the thyroid; examination of the heart, abdomen, and extremities (with special attention to the hands, fingers, and feet); palpation and auscultation of the pulses; and examination of the neurologic system. The presence of acanthosis nigricans should be assessed in children. Acanthosis nigricans is present in 90% of children with T2DM and is characterized by hyperpigmented, velvety patches most prominent in the intertriginous areas (eg, axilla or groin) or the back of the neck.

The recommended initial laboratory studies for T2DM include a fasting plasma glucose; hemoglobin A_{1c}; fasting lipid profile (total cholesterol,

triglycerides, and high- and low-density lipoprotein cholesterol); test for microalbuminuria (in all patients with T2DM on presentation); serum creatinine (may also include a calculated glomerular filtration rate); thyroid-stimulating hormone (if clinically indicated); and a urinanalysis for glucose, ketones, protein, and sediment. An electrocardiogram is indicated for adults over the age of 35 or with a significant medical history. In situations where the diagnosis of whether the patient is T1DM or T2DM (eg, an older patient with new-onset diabetes who is lean), a postprandial C-peptide test may be helpful. C-peptide is produced during the conversion of proinsulin to insulin and correlates with circulating endogenous insulin levels.

Based on this evaluation, the individual may be referred for an eye examination, for family planning, or for medical nutrition therapy consultations, or to a foot specialist, diabetes educator, or behavioral specialist.

Acute complications of type 2 diabetes mellitus

The two acute complications seen with T2DM are HHNK and hypoglycemia. HHNK coma evolves over time and is characterized by blood glucoses ≥ 600 mg/dL with minimal ketosis, serum osmolality >340 mOsm/L, and profound dehydration. Although HHNK results in no metabolic acidosis, the degree of hyperglycemia and dehydration is more severe than seen in diabetic ketoacidosis [26]. HHNK may be precipitated by hyperglycemic-inducing drugs, such as steroids or diuretics; dialysis; hyperalimentation; surgery; or acute stress. It is more prominent in institutionalized elderly, mentally impaired individuals, and those with an impaired thirst mechanism or an inability to express their need for water. HHNK is considered a life-threatening condition and requires immediate hospitalization.

Hypoglycemia occurs when glucose use by the body exceeds glucose intake or production resulting in low blood glucose levels (<60 mg/dL) and accompanying adrenergic and neuroglycopenic symptoms. Factors that contribute to hypoglycemia include decreased caloric intake or increased physical activity in patients using insulin or certain oral hypoglycemic agents; missed meals; and extra administration of insulin or certain oral hypoglycemic agents (eg, secretagogues). Although symptoms may vary with individuals, common adrenergic symptoms are diaphoresis, tremors, hunger, and palpitations. As hypoglycemia advances, persons may complain of headache and experience mood or behavioral changes, such as increased irritability (most prominent in children). If unrecognized or untreated, unconsciousness, seizures, and coma can develop because of neuroglycopenia.

The most effective treatment for HHNK and hypoglycemia is prevention. This involves patient, family, and health-care provider education about how to prevent these occurrences; what signs and symptoms to be alert for; and how to respond to them when they occur. Patients and families need to know how to treat hypoglycemia effectively and to recognize the life-threatening nature of HHNK and the need for immediate hospitalization.

Treatment of type 2 diabetes

Newer therapeutic products and techniques have provided the ability proactively to fine-tune glycemic control to achieve control 24 hours a day rather than simply correcting glucose excursions. Achieving greater glycemic control improves patient outcomes. For example, a statistical model that compared the lifetime risk of complications in patients with the difference in hemoglobin A_{1c} of 10% versus 7.2% equates to a projected reduction in lifetime risk of complications of 87% reduction for renal failure, 72% for blindness, 68% for symptomatic neuropathy, and 67% for lower-extremity amputation [27].

Current approaches to treatment recognize the progressive nature of T2DM. It is expected that individuals need changes in their treatment regimen as their disease progresses. The concept of treating to target is important in that it focuses on the goals of management, which include normalizing glycemic control and correction of other metabolic parameters incident to diabetes. Pharmacologic interventions are needed when lifestyle change is not enough. The availability of pharmacologic aids, however, does not justify inattention to lifestyle change. An understanding of the pathophysiology of T2DM helps to clarify the mechanisms of action of the variety of pharmacologic agents available to treat T2DM (Fig. 4).

The core components of management for T2DM include education for the person with T2DM and their family, medical nutrition therapy, regular

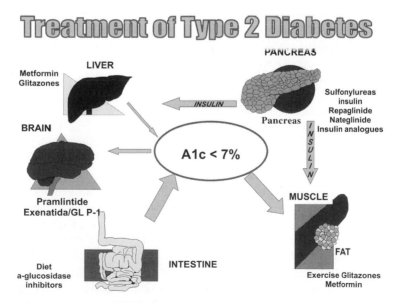

Fig. 4. Treatment of type 2 diabetes. (*Adapted from* Sonnenberg GE, Kotchen TA. New therapeutic approaches to reversing insulin resistance. Curr Opin Nephrol Hypertens 1998;7:551–5; with permission.)

physical activity, use of medications or insulin, and preventive care. Diabetes education remains the cornerstone of care whether it is provided by a certified diabetes educator or a nurse at the bedside. The American Association of Diabetes Educators has published curriculum guides for diabetes education [28] and the American Diabetes Association has national standards available for diabetes education programs [29]. The reader is referred to articles elsewhere in this issue for a detailed discussion of the use of medical nutrition therapy, physical activity, medications, and insulin in T2DM; and for a discussion of behavioral interventions for diabetes and diabetes self-management education.

Management of type 2 diabetes in youths

With the increasing prevalence of T2DM seen in youths over the past 10 years, researchers continue to search for evidence of the best treatment approaches to this problem [30]. At present, there is a lack of evidence-based guidelines specific to this population [31]. A major factor attributed to this rise in cases of T2DM is the increase in obesity caused by intake of high-caloric foods and an increasing sedentary lifestyle. Another factor is the increased demands placed on the body during puberty [32]. At present, the only oral diabetes agent approved for use in youths is metformin [33], although studies have been conducted using other agents and insulin with varying results. Treatment plans for this population should address the lifestyle and risk factors of the entire family to be effective, because family members often share the same risk factors and lifestyle habits [31,34]. The reader is referred to an article elsewhere in this issue for a discussion of families and diabetes.

Management of prediabetes

The most effective management of diabetes is prevention. Aggressive treatment is needed before and after the diagnosis of diabetes. Providers need to identify individuals with prediabetes (impaired fasting glucose and impaired glucose tolerance) and encourage them to make the needed lifestyle changes [35]. Although doing so may be difficult for both the individuals with prediabetes and their health care providers, studies have been able to demonstrate clearly a slowing in the progression to T2DM [5,36].

Summary

Diabetes is a progressive, chronic disorder that places great burdens on affected individuals and their families as they deal with an often complex, demanding self-care regimen. Nurses are in an excellent position to support families with diabetes through patient and family education regarding prevention and management of T2DM; advocacy on the individual,

community, and national levels; and through nursing research to develop culturally sensitive models of diabetes self-care leading to better outcomes.

Acknowledgment

The author thanks April C. M. Soward and Dr. Jenniefer Leeman for their thoughtful critiques of this manuscript, and R. Preston D. Soward, III, for his assistance with the artwork and graphic design.

References

[1] Report of the Expert Committee on the Diagnosis and Classification of Diabetes Mellitus. Diabetes Care 1997;20:1183.

[2] Mokdad AH, Ford ES, Bowman BA, et al. Diabetes trends in the US 1990–1998. Diabetes Care 2000;23:1278.

[3] Burant CF, editor. Diagnosis and classification. In: Medical management of type 2 diabetes. 5th edition. Alexandria (VA): American Diabetes Association; 2004. p. 6.

[4] Harris MI, Klein R, Welborn TA, et al. Onset of NIDDM occurs at least 4–7 yr before clinical diagnosis. Diabetes Care 1992;15:815.

[5] Diabetes Prevention Program Research Group. Reduction in the incidence of type 2 diabetes with lifestyle intervention or metformin. N Engl J Med 2002;346:393–403.

[6] American Diabetes Association. Diagnosis and classification of diabetes mellitus. Diabetes Care 2004;27(Suppl 1):S5–10.

[7] Harmel A, Mathur R, editors. Classification of diabetes mellitus. In: Davidson's diabetes mellitus. 5th edition. Philadelphia: WB Saunders; 2004. p. 10–7.

[8] Freeman S. The metabolic syndrome: diagnosis and management. Women's Health Care 2005;4:11 30.

[9] Frayn K. Diabetes mellitus. In: Malden MA, editor. Metabolic regulation: a human perspective. 2nd edition. Malden (MA): Blackwell Sciences; 2003. p. 284–5.

[10] Kahn R, Buse J, Ferrannini E, et al. The metabolic syndrome: time for a critical appraisal. Joint statement from the American Diabetes Association and the European Association for the Study of Diabetes. Diabetes Care 2005;28:2289–304.

[11] Alberti KGMM, Zimmet PZ, , for the WHO Consultation. Definition, diagnosis, and classification of diabetes mellitus and its complications. Part 1: diagnosis and classification of diabetes mellitus. Provisional report of a WHO consultation. Diabetes Med 1998;15:539–53.

[12] Executive Summary of the Third Report of the National Cholesterol Education Program (NCEP) Expert Panel on Detection, Evaluation, and Treatment of High Blood Cholesterol in Adults (Adult Treatment Panel III). JAMA 2001;285:2486.

[13] International Diabetes Federation. The IDF consensus worldwide definition of the metabolic syndrome. Available at: www.idf.org/webdata/docs/Metac_syndrome_def.pdf. Accessed 2/12/06.

[14] Einhorn D, Reaven GM, Cobin RH, et al. American College of Endocrinology position statement on the insulin resistance syndrome. Endocr Pract 2003;9:237–52.

[15] Grundy SM, Hansen B, Smith SC Jr, et al. Clinical management of the metabolic syndrome. Report of the American Heart Association/ National Heart, Lung, and Blood Institute/ American Diabetes Association conference on scientific issues related to management. Circulation 2004;109:551–6.

[16] Caprio S. Prediabetes and the metabolic syndrome in obese children. Cadre's Current Diabetes Practices 2005;3:7–8.

[17] American Diabetes Association. Standards of medical care in diabetes: 2006. Diabetes Care 2006;29(Suppl 1):S4–42.

[18] American Diabetes Association. Screening for type 2 diabetes (position statement). Diabetes Care 2004;27(Suppl 1):S11–4.

[19] Hattersley A. Genetic factors in the etiology of non-insulin-dependent diabetes. Front Horm Res 1997;22:157.

[20] Cotran R, Kumar V, Collins T. The endocrine pancreas. In: Robbins' pathologic basis of disease. 6th edition. Philadelphia: WB Saunders; 1999. p. 911–29.

[21] Boden G. Pathogenesis of type 2 diabetes: insulin resistance. Endocrinol Metab Clin North Am 2001;30:801–15.

[22] Semenkovich CF, Heinecke JW. The mystery of diabetes and atherosclerosis: time for a new plot. Diabetes 1997;46:327.

[23] Nathan DM. The pathophysiology of diabetes complications: how much does the glucose hypothesis explain? Ann Intern 1996;124:86.

[24] UK Prospective Diabetes Study (UKPDS) Group. Intensive blood glucose control with sulfonylureas or insulin compared with conventional treatment and risk of complications in patients with type 2 diabetes (UKPDS 33). Lancet 1998;352:837–53.

[25] Vlassara H. Recent progress in advanced glycation end products and diabetic complications. Diabetes 1997;46(Suppl 2):S19–25.

[26] Matz R. Hyperosmolar nonacidotic diabetes. In: Porte DJ, Sherwin RS, editors. Ellenberg & Rifkin's diabetes mellitus. 5th edition. Stamford (CT): Appleton & Lange; 1997. p. 845.

[27] Funnell M, Kruger D. Type 2 diabetes: treat to target. Nurse Pract 2004;29:11–5, 19–23.

[28] Franz M, editor. A core curriculum for diabetes education. 4th edition. Chicago: American Association of Diabetes Educators, 2001.

[29] Mensing C, Boucher J, Cypress M, et al. National standards for diabetes self-management education. Diabetes Care 2006;29:S78–85.

[30] Rizvi A. Type 2 diabetes: epidemiologic trends, evolving pathogenic concepts, and recent changes in therapeutic approach. South Med J 2004;97:1079–87.

[31] Pinhas-Hamiel O, Zeitler P. Barriers to the treatment of adolescent type 2 diabetes: a survey of provider perceptions. Pediatr Diabetes 2003;4:24–8.

[32] Motil K. Dietary history and recommended dietary intake in children. Available at: http://www.uptodate.com. Accessed April 13, 2005.

[33] Zuhri-Yafi M, Brosnan PG, Hardin DS. Treatment of type 2 diabetes in children and adolescents. J Pediatr Endocrinol Metab 2002;15:541–6.

[34] McKnight-Menci H, Sababu S, Kelly SD. The care of children and adolescents with type 2 diabetes. J Pediatr Nurs 2005;20:96–106.

[35] Kahn S. The case for aggressive treatment before and after diagnosis in type 2 diabetes. Cadre's Current Diabetes Practices 2004;3:1–2.

[36] Gaede P, Vedel P, Larsen N, et al. Multifactorial intervention and cardiovascular disease in patients with type 2 diabetes. N Engl J Med 2003;348:383–93.

NURSING
CLINICS
OF NORTH AMERICA

Nurs Clin N Am 41 (2006) 549–565

Women and Diabetes

Carol J. Homko, RN, PhD, CDE[a,b,c,*],
Kimberly Trout, PhD, RN[d]

[a]*Department of Obstetrics and Gynecology, Temple University School of Medicine,*
Philadelphia, PA, USA
[b]*Department of Medicine, Temple University School of Medicine, Philadelphia, PA, USA*
[c]*General Clinical Research Center, Temple University School of Medicine, Temple University*
Hospital, 3401 North Broad Street, 4 West, Philadelphia, PA 19140, USA
[d]*College of Nursing, Villanova University, Villanova, PA, USA*

Diabetes mellitus is a serious chronic illness affecting almost 20 million Americans, of which more than half are women. Diabetes is responsible for more deaths in women than either breast or ovarian cancer. Women with diabetes face unique health challenges throughout their life cycle. This article examines the available data concerning the impact of diabetes on women beginning with adolescence, continuing through their reproductive years, and culminating with its effects in later life on the risks for cardiovascular disease and osteoporosis. Also examined is how blood glucose levels may be affected by the hormonal changes associated with puberty, the menstrual cycle, pregnancy, and menopause.

Puberty

Adolescence is characterized by sexual maturation and increased circulating concentrations of sex steroids. Findings of the effect of diabetes on age at menarche have been inconsistent. Some clinical studies and retrospective analysis have found delays [1,2], whereas others have found normal ages at menarche [3–5]. The Wisconsin Diabetes Registry Project [6], which is a population-based incident cohort of individuals with type 1 diabetes, found that age of menarche was moderately delayed by approximately 3 months in young women with type 1 diabetes as compared with the overall United States population. Menstruation was delayed by 1.3 months for each 1% increase in hemoglobin A_{1c} in the 3 years

---

* Corresponding author.
E-mail address: homkoc@temple.edu (C.J. Homko).

before menarche. This study was also the first to identify hemoglobin A_{1c} levels as an important modification factor affecting menstruation.

Historically, the diagnosis of diabetes in an individual under 20 years of age was categorized as type 1 diabetes. The prevalence of type 2 diabetes mellitus is increasing in children and adolescents, however, reaching epidemic proportions in many western countries. In 1994, type 2 diabetes accounted for approximately a third of all cases of diabetes in teenagers and as many as half of all new cases of diabetes in certain populations [7]. The increasing prevalence of type 2 diabetes has closely paralleled the increase in childhood obesity noted across most of the Western world. Most recent studies indicate that the prevalence is even higher among ethnic minorities and that young adult women seem to be affected two to three times as often as their male counterparts [8,9].

The onset of puberty is also a culprit in the development of type 2 diabetes in adolescents. Increases in growth hormone secretion during midpuberty accentuate insulin resistance leading to type 2 diabetes in susceptible teenagers. Studies during adolescence have noted a 30% reduction in insulin-stimulated glucose disposal, with girls being more insulin resistant than boys [10]. Puberty creates an insulin-resistant state making glycemic control more challenging. Conversely, chronic suboptimal glycemic control seems to delay puberty.

Adolescent girls need to understand the effects of diabetes on their reproductive health, sexuality, and future pregnancies. Preconception counseling should begin in puberty and young women must be taught the importance of planning pregnancy and the meticulous use of contraception. Young women should also be instructed on the importance of taking multivitamins daily containing at least 400 µg of folic acid. This recommendation is particularly important for women with pregestational diabetes, because their offspring are at higher risk of developing neural tube defects, and folic acid supplementation in women of childbearing age has been shown to decrease the incidence of neural tube defects [11].

The reproductive years

Pregnancy

It is estimated that 150,000 pregnancies are complicated by diabetes each year in the United States. Gestational diabetes accounts for 135,000 of these pregnancies, type 2 diabetes for 12,000 pregnancies, and type 1 diabetes for 7000 pregnancies [12]. White's classification remains the most commonly accepted system for categorizing diabetes during pregnancy (Table 1). This system relates the onset of disease, disease duration, and the presence of vascular complications to the risk of adverse outcomes in pregnancy.

Table 1
Whites classification of diabetes in pregnancy

Class A	Gestational diabetes mellitus
Class B	Onset at age 20 or older and <10-y duration
Class C	Onset between 10 and 19 years of age or 10–19 years duration
Class D	Onset <10 y of age or >20 y duration
Class F	Diabetic nephropathy
Class R	Proliferative retinopathy
Class FR	Nephropathy and proliferative retinopathy
Class H	Heart disease
Class T	Renal transplantation

Fuel metabolism

Pregnancy is recognized as having a profound effect on maternal carbohydrate metabolism. These alterations in fuel metabolism are necessary to meet the demands of the developing fetus. Early pregnancy is characterized by a greater than normal insulin sensitivity. This produces a milieu that favors maternal fat accumulation in preparation for the increasing energy requirements of late gestation and lactation. Late pregnancy is characterized by accelerated growth of the fetus and placenta, elevated concentrations of several diabetogenic hormones including human placental lactogen and estrogens, and increasing insulin resistance. Studies have consistently demonstrated that insulin sensitivity is reduced by 33% to 50% by the third trimester of pregnancy [13,14]. Although the cause or causes are not entirely clear, the parallel decline in insulin sensitivity and increases in blood levels of human placental lactogen and other diabetogenic hormones, including cortisol, progesterone, and estrogens, suggest that these hormones are responsible for much of the observed insulin resistance. In healthy pregnant women insulin secretion must be increased by 200% to 300% in late gestation to overcome the resistance and maintain euglycemia. Women who are unable to increase their insulin secretion to compensate for the physiologic changes of advancing gestation go on to develop impaired glucose tolerance and gestational diabetes.

Diabetes-related congenital malformations

Congenital malformations continue to complicate between 6% and 10% of all diabetic pregnancies and are the major cause of mortality among these infants [15]. The malformations associated with diabetes can involve multiple organ systems but defects of the cardiovascular and nervous systems are most common. The defects most frequently associated with diabetes occur very early (before the seventh week of gestation) before most women realize they are pregnant. It is well accepted that diabetes-related congenital malformations are related to hyperglycemia during the period of organogenesis [15–18]. Numerous clinical trials in humans have demonstrated that strict glycemic control before and during early pregnancy can

reduce the rate of these defects in most cases to the background level [19,20]. These data highlight the importance of pregnancy planning and preconception care to optimize glycemic control.

Gestational diabetes mellitus

Gestational diabetes mellitus (GDM) is a common problem complicating approximately 5% of all pregnancies in the United States [21]. The likelihood of developing gestational diabetes is significantly increased in women with a positive family history of type 2 diabetes, advancing maternal age, obesity, and nonwhite ethnicity. Excess risks for both gestational diabetes and impaired glucose tolerance have been demonstrated in African American, Hispanic, and Native American women, and women from the Indian subcontinent and the Middle East [22].

The American College of Obstetricians and Gynecologists recommends that all pregnant patients should be screened for GDM at least by history, clinical risk factors, or a laboratory test [23]. There are certain groups of low-risk women in whom it may not be cost-effective to routinely do laboratory screening for GDM. This low-risk group includes women who are not members of the previously described ethnic groups, who have all of the following characteristics: age less than 25 years, normal body weight, no previous history of adverse obstetric outcomes usually associated with GDM, no personal history of abnormal glucose tolerance, and no family history of diabetes mellitus [23]. Universal laboratory screening is recommended for women in all high-risk groups. Laboratory screening should be performed between the 24th and 28th week of gestation (Box 1). Women who have significant risk factors or a previous history of gestational diabetes, however, should be screened earlier in pregnancy.

Management of the pregnancy complicated by diabetes

The main goal of management for pregnancies complicated by diabetes is to achieve or maintain strict glycemic control throughout gestation. The treatment approach requires a combination of medical nutrition therapy, exercise, pharmacologic therapy, and blood glucose monitoring. The goals of nutrition therapy are to provide adequate maternal and fetal nutrition, to achieve appropriate maternal weight gains, and to optimize glucose control. Consensus has not been reached regarding optimal nutrition recommendations for women with diabetes. The most current guidelines suggest that the composition of the diabetic diet be based on an individualized nutrition assessment [24].

Evidence regarding the risks or benefits of exercise in pregnant women with pregestational diabetes is limited. Mild exercise in the form of walking, however, is possible for most women and has been reported to improve lipid and blood glucose profiles [25]. Regular aerobic exercise has been shown to

---

Box 1. Gestational diabetes mellitus

Definition
Carbohydrate intolerance of variable severity with onset or first recognition during the current pregnancy

Screening
50-g 1-hour oral glucose challenge
Positive: plasma glucose ≥140 mg/dL

Diagnosis
100-g 3-hour oral glucose tolerance test
Positive if two or more values are met or exceeded
    Fasting blood sugar ≥95 mg/dL
    1 hour ≥180 mg/dL
    2 hour ≥155 mg/dL
    3 hour ≥140 mg/dL

Postpartum follow-up
75-g 2-hour oral glucose tolerance test

---

lower fasting and postprandial glucose concentrations in women with GDM. Several randomized controlled trials have demonstrated that upper-extremity exercise for 20 minutes three times a week can significantly improve blood glucose levels and reduce the need for insulin therapy [26,27]. In addition, these trials found no significant increase in adverse pregnancy outcomes.

The past several years have seen the addition of rapid-acting analogues and oral agents to the pharmacologic management of pregnancies complicated by diabetes. Traditionally, insulin was the only therapy recommended to treat diabetes during pregnancy. The goal of insulin therapy is to achieve blood glucose levels that are nearly identical to those observed in nondiabetic pregnant women. Human insulin is the least immunogenic of all insulins and is exclusively advised for use in pregnancy. There are multiple approaches to insulin administration; however, the superiority of one regimen over another has never been demonstrated. The new rapid-acting insulin analogues with peak hypoglycemic action 1 to 2 hours after injection offer the potential for improved postprandial glucose control. Most evidence at this time suggests that insulin lispro, the most widely studied of the analogues, does not cross the placenta and does not have adverse maternal or fetal effects [28–30]. Continuous subcutaneous insulin infusion pumps are another treatment option that has been used successfully during pregnancy [31].

The growing numbers of women with type 2 diabetes and GDM has led to increased interest in the use of oral agents during pregnancy. Historically, oral hypoglycemic agents have not been recommended for use during

pregnancy because of concerns regarding transplacental passage and the risk of fetal teratogenesis and prolonged neonatal hypoglycemia. To date, there has only been one randomized controlled trial [32] to test the effectiveness and safety of sulfonylurea therapy in the management of women with GDM. Women were randomized to receive glyburide, a second-generation sulfonylurea, or insulin according to an intensified treatment protocol. Both groups of women were able to achieve satisfactory glucose control and had similar perinatal outcomes. Glyburide was not detected in the cord serum of any infant in the glyburide group and only 4% of women failed to achieve glucose control with the maximal dose of glyburide. There is also a considerable wealth of evidence from retrospective studies and extensive clinical experience that have failed to demonstrate any adverse effects [33–35]. It seems that glyburide can be safely and effectively used in GDM.

Diabetes control is monitored through a combination of self blood glucose monitoring, ketone measurements, and hemoglobin A_{1c} concentrations. Although it is widely accepted that the level of metabolic control achieved in the pregnancy complicated by diabetes significantly affects perinatal outcome, what constitutes optimal control has yet to be established. Most experts recommend that plasma blood glucose levels not exceed 95 mg/dL in the fasted state and 120 mg/dL after meals in the antepartum period. Nocturnal glucose levels should not decrease below 60 mg/dL. Patients should be questioned regarding their awareness of hypoglycemic episodes and to make sure that they know how to respond to those episodes. Family members should also be instructed on what to do for hypoglycemia, and glucagon kits should be made available to all patients on insulin [11]. During labor and delivery, maternal blood glucose levels should be maintained at a level below 110 mg/dL with the use of an insulin-glucose infusion.

Complications

Women with diabetes are at greater risk for a number of pregnancy-related complications. These include preterm labor, infectious morbidities, hydramnios, hypertensive disorders, and operative delivery. Women with both type 1 and type 2 diabetes are also at increased risk for spontaneous abortions and their offspring are at increased risk for congenital malformations. Perinatal morbidity and mortality rates are also higher in pregnancies complicated by diabetes. Neonatal morbidities include neonatal hypoglycemia and other metabolic abnormalities, respiratory distress syndrome, and macrosomia [36,37]. It is well accepted that the risk for these complications increases as maternal glucose levels rise. Elevations in postprandial glucose levels have been specifically linked to an increased risk for macrosomia, the most common complication affecting the offspring of women with diabetes. The evidence does not support induction of labor for suspected fetal macrosomia, because this has not been shown to improve maternal or fetal outcomes. The American College of Obstetricians and Gynecologists states,

however, that elective cesarean delivery may be considered if the estimated fetal weight is greater than 4500 g [11].

Lactation

Breast-feeding should be encouraged in women with both pregestational and GDM. For women with diabetes in good metabolic control, the quality of breast milk is not substantially affected [38]. Increasing evidence suggests that breast-feeding may offer the offspring protection from type 2 diabetes and a decreased likelihood of developing obesity in childhood and young adulthood [39–41]. Lower glucose levels at the time of postpartum oral glucose tolerance testing and lower rates of diabetes also have been found in women with GDM who continued to breast-feed compared with those who did not continue [42]. Most recently, the Nurses Health study found that the duration of breast-feeding was inversely associated with the risk of type 2 diabetes in two large cohorts of women [43].

Postpartum

For women with type 1 and type 2 diabetes, the primary goal of the postpartum period is continued maintenance of strict glycemic control and for women with GDM it is the prevention of overt diabetes. An individualized reproductive health plan needs to be developed that addresses contraception, the importance of planning future pregnancies, and lifestyle changes aimed at preventing diabetes or its long-term complications.

The use of contraception in all women with diabetes or a history of GDM cannot be stressed strongly enough. A variety of family planning methods can be used. Natural family planning is a contraceptive method that requires women abstain from intercourse during the fertile phase of the menstrual cycle. Barrier methods of contraception, which create mechanical or chemical barriers to fertilization, include diaphragms, male condoms, spermicidal foam, jelly or foam, cervical caps, and female condoms. Although these methods pose no health risks to the woman with diabetes, they are user-dependent and consequently have a high failure rate particularly in the first year.

Oral contraceptives remain the most popular form of birth control despite the risk of potential side effects. The main reasons for their popularity are their low failure rate (generally $<1\%$) and ease of use. The lowest dose formulations should be used whenever possible. Oral contraceptives are not recommended for women with vascular complications or risk factors, such as smoking or a strong family history of cardiac disease [44,45]. Their effects on carbohydrate and lipid metabolism are minimal and in women with GDM, their long-term use has not been shown to increase the risk for overt diabetes [46]. Progestin only (mini-pill) oral contraceptives are an option for women with contraindications to the estrogen component, such as hypertension or thrombosis [44,45]. In women with GDM, however,

progestin-only oral contraceptives during breast-feeding increased their risk for diabetes almost threefold and this risk rose with increased duration of use [46].

An intrauterine device is the most effective of the nonhormonal devices. Cooper intrauterine devices have not been associated with an increased risk of pelvic inflammatory disease in women with either type 1 or type 2 diabetes and are considered the intrauterine device of choice [46]. Patient education should include the early signs of sexually transmitted diseases, such as increased and abnormal vaginal discharge; dyspareunia; heavy, painful menses; lower abdominal pain; and fever [44,45].

Depo-Provera is a long-acting progestin with a very low failure rate. Depo-Provera, which is administered intramuscularly every 3 months, works by inhibiting ovulation. Its effectiveness and prolonged action make it an attractive option for women with a history of poor medication compliance [44,45]. This long-acting progestin has not been studied, however, in women with diabetes. Deterioration of carbohydrate tolerance has been demonstrated in healthy women and it is not considered first-line therapy.

Permanent sterilization, including tubal ligation and vasectomy, may be considered by the patient or her partner when they desire no more children.

Other reproductive health issues

Effects of menstrual cycle on glucose control

Menstrual cycle–related alterations in blood glucose control have been reported in some women with type 1 diabetes. Most of these women describe deterioration in glycemic control around the time of menstruation, although some women have reported improvements [47]. An epidemiologic study found that women with the symptom complaints of premenstrual syndrome reported the need to make more frequent adjustments in insulin dosage because of premenstrual increases in blood glucose [48]. As early as 1942, both diabetic ketoacidosis and mild and severe hypoglycemia have been noted to occur more frequently in the perimenstrual period [49]. The exact mechanism of these changes in glucose homeostasis in women with diabetes is unknown but it is presumed to be related to changes in levels of estrogen, progesterone, and other reproductive hormones. Studies examining this phenomenon have yielded controversial results.

Some studies have demonstrated decreased insulin sensitivity during the luteal as compared with the follicular phase, whereas other studies have not found these differences [47,50,51]. Data from Widom and colleagues [52] suggest that there is a subgroup of women with type 1 diabetes who exhibit worsening premenstrual (luteal phase) hyperglycemia and a decline in insulin sensitivity. In these studies this deterioration in glucose use was associated with greater increments in estradiol levels from the follicular to the luteal phase. A study investigating insulin sensitivity by cycle phase

(follicular versus luteal) using minimal model analysis of the frequently sampled intravenous glucose tolerance test in five type 1 diabetic women found that there was a decline in insulin sensitivity in the luteal phase for three of the five women studied [53]. In this study, greater increments in estradiol levels in the luteal phase were not correlated with the decline in insulin sensitivity in those subjects, suggesting the role of another unidentified factor. There was a trend noted in this study of decreased insulin sensitivity (S_I) with increased plasma progesterone levels (R = −.50), although this was not statistically significant ($P = 0.14$) with this small group of subjects. Of note, the women in this study had been screened for premenstrual syndrome, although none of the women who completed the study actually had premenstrual syndrome.

Another study was performed where four women with type 1 diabetes were on continuous glucose monitoring through three complete menstrual cycles. Interestingly, analysis revealed that two of the four women had profiles with an increased frequency of hyperglycemia in the luteal phase. For the other two women in the study, no cycle-related pattern was identified [54]. The researchers concluded that the menstrual cycle has an effect on glucose control for a subset of women.

From a clinical perspective women with diabetes need to be counseled regarding the possibility of altered glucose control at various points in the menstrual cycle. They need to monitor blood glucose levels more frequently and adjust insulin dosages accordingly. In some women increases in food cravings for high-carbohydrate food during the premenstrual phase may further accentuate the loss of glucose control. Attention to dietary changes is also important.

Polycystic ovarian syndrome

Polycystic ovarian syndrome (PCOS) is an endocrine disorder that affects 4% to 6% of all women. There is no universally accepted definition of PCOS. The diagnosis is based on the presence of hyperandrogenism and ovulatory dysfunction, after all other known causes of androgen excess or ovulatory dysfunction have been excluded. The presence of polycystic ovaries on sonography is suggestive of PCOS but is not diagnostic because that can be present in women without PCOS. Most women with PCOS demonstrate frank elevations in circulating androgens, in particular free testosterone, and approximately 60% of these women are obese [55]. Although not part of the diagnostic criteria, many women with PCOS are also insulin resistant and exhibit secondary hyperinsulinemia.

Clinical PCOS tends to develop shortly after menarche and persists throughout most of the woman's reproductive life. The menstrual irregularities and hyperandrogenism seem to normalize as women approach the perimenopause. The associated metabolic abnormalities, in particular glucose intolerance, actually worsen with age. The inherent insulin

resistance present in PCOS, aggravated by the high prevalence of obesity, places these women at increased risk for impaired glucose tolerance. Approximately 40% of individuals with PCOS go on to develop either type 2 diabetes or impaired glucose tolerance [56]. PCOS has also been shown to confer an increased risk for cardiovascular disease and reproductive cancers.

PCOS is associated with reduced fertility and an increased rate of first-trimester pregnancy loss if pregnancy is achieved. GDM, preeclampsia, and premature delivery have all been reported to occur with an increased incidence in women with PCOS [57–59]. Lifestyle modifications, which include diet and exercise, are considered to be the first line of therapy. Modest weight loss increases the frequency of ovulation; improves conception; and reduces miscarriage, hyperlipidemia, hyperglycemia, and insulin resistance in women with PCOS. Other treatment approaches include insulin-sensitizing agents, such as the thiazolidinediones, and metformin. A recent meta-analysis [60] showed that metformin is effective in achieving ovulation in women with PCOS, with odds ratio of 3.88 (95% confidence interval 2.25–6.69) for metformin compared with placebo and 4.41 (2.37–8.22) for metformin and clomiphene compared with clomiphene alone.

Because of the increased risk for GDM, many women with PCOS are being treated with metformin throughout pregnancy. In one study, treatment of PCOS with metformin throughout pregnancy was associated with a 10-fold reduction in one study in the incidence of GDM [61]. Two subsequent non-randomized trials by the same group reported similar findings [62,63]. A recent randomized, double-blind, placebo-controlled trial, however, reported similar rates of GDM between women who continued metformin throughout gestation as women who discontinued it following conception [64]. At the present time the data are too limited to determine whether women should continue its use throughout pregnancy. Counseling for women with PCOS should emphasize the importance of lifestyle interventions to prevent diabetes.

Diabetes in older women

Menopause

Menopause marks an important transition into the last third of a woman's life. Women with type 1 diabetes are twice as likely as nondiabetic women to experience an early menopause. The mean age of menopause has been studied only in small numbers of women. Menopause occurred at a mean age of 41.6 years in 15 women with type 1 diabetes as compared with a mean age of 49.9 years in the nondiabetic sisters and a mean age of 48 in other nondiabetic women [4,65]. The role of glyucemia in relation to the age of onset of menopause is not clear but it has been speculated there may be a direct toxic effect of hyperglycemia on the viability of the oocyte [66].

Data are also limited for women with type 2 diabetes. A cross-sectional study of 51 women with type 2 diabetes found they had an earlier mean

age of 45.7 as compared with the nondiabetic controls of 48 years with similar degrees of obesity [67]. Earlier age at diagnosis of diabetes was associated with earlier age of menopause. In contrast, a larger study in 404 women with type 2 diabetes and regular menstrual cycles found that the mean age of menopause did not differ from nondiabetic controls [68].

Hormone replacement therapy

Hormone-replacement therapy is no longer recommended for the prevention of cardiovascular disease or fractures in women with or without diabetes. In 1998, the HERS trial [69] demonstrated that hormone-replacement therapy had an early adverse effect in women with pre-existing coronary disease. Several years later, the Woman's Health Initiative [70], which investigated the health risks and benefits of combined estrogen and progestin replacement therapy in healthy postmenopausal women, was discontinued early because it was discovered that the risk of breast cancer and increases in the risk of coronary heart disease, stroke, and pulmonary embolism outweighed any potential benefits. Data specific to hormone-replacement therapy in women with diabetes mellitus are scarce. The Third National Health and Nutrition Examination Survey [71] found that postmenopausal women with diabetes using hormone-replacement therapy had significantly better lipoprotein profiles and glycemic control than did women with diabetes who were never or previous users of hormone-replacement therapy. Hormone-replacement therapy may still be appropriate for short-term therapy for menopausal symptoms including vasomotor instability with hot flushes, sleep disturbance, night sweats, and mood lability.

Cardiovascular disease

Cardiovascular disease is the leading cause of death among women with diabetes, exceeding both breast and ovarian cancers [72]. Although women without diabetes are generally protected from heart disease before menopause, this protective effect is absent in women with diabetes. Studies have found that individuals with diabetes are at increased risk for cardiovascular disease as compared with individuals without diabetes and that the risk for women with diabetes actually surpasses that of men with diabetes. Lundberg and colleagues [73] found that the relative risk for cardiovascular disease was 2.9 in diabetic men but 5 in women with diabetes, in a population-based study of almost 2500 individuals. In addition, they reported that the mortality rate from myocardial infarction was four times higher in diabetic men and seven times higher in diabetic women. Both the Strong Heart Study [74] and Rancho Bernardo Study [75] reported similar increases in mortality. Not only are diabetic women at increased risk for cardiovascular disease compared with their nondiabetic female counterparts, they seem to fare worse in terms of morbidity and mortality compared with diabetic

men. The mechanisms postulated for this increased risk have included higher triglyceride levels, lower high-density lipoprotein cholesterol, and greater abdominal pattern obesity seen in women with type 2 diabetes [76]. Other differences have been found in presentation and treatment of coronary heart disease in women. Studies have found that women are more likely to have their initial manifestation as angina pectoris, are more likely to be referred for diagnostic tests at a more advanced stage of disease, and less likely than men to have corrective invasive procedures [77]. Because women with diabetes carry a disproportionate risk for the development of premature coronary heart disease, early and ongoing assessment of cardiovascular risk factors and intense intervention is needed for all women with diabetes (Box 2). Interventions should include counseling regarding weight management, regular physical activity, a diet low in saturated fats, smoking cessation, and interventions for dyslipidemia and control of blood pressure.

Box 2. Prevention of diabetes and its complications

Medical nutrition therapy
To normalize blood glucose levels
To achieve or maintain normal body weight
To reduce risk for cardiovascular disease and osteoporosis
    Reduce fat
    Increase dietary fiber
    Limit sodium chloride
    Maintain adequate intake of calcium

Routine physical activity
Engage in ≥30 minutes of moderate-intensity physical activity five to seven times per week
Smoking prevention and cessation

Control of lipids and blood pressure
Achieve and maintain blood pressure <140 mm Hg with optimal goal <120 /80 mm Hg
Achieve and maintain
    Total cholesterol <200
    High-density lipoprotein >45
    Low-density lipoprotein <100
    Triglycerides <150

Minimize stress

Osteoporosis

Osteoporosis is the most prevalent metabolic bone disease in the United States. Although more common in white women, it does affect both sexes and all ethnic groups. Whether there is an increase risk of osteoporosis in individuals with type 1 and 2 diabetes remains controversial. Most studies in women with type 1 diabetes have reported lower bone mineral density levels than in nondiabetic controls [78] but not all [79]. In addition, the risk of hip fracture seems to be substantially increased among individuals with type 1 diabetes. In contrast, studies of bone mineral density in type 2 diabetes have reported a broader range of results that do not suggest a pattern of lower bone mineral density. Despite normal bone mineral density levels, individuals with type 2 diabetes have an increased risk for fractures (both hip and foot fractures) like their counterparts with type 1 diabetes [80]. Why these differences occur is not well understood. The increase in risk is at least partially accounted for by a greater tendency to fall (secondary to poor balance, poor vision, and neuropathy) and fall prevention measures should be a consideration with older diabetic patients. All women with diabetes should be evaluated for the risk of osteoporosis and related fractures. Women with diabetes and osteoporosis should be provided treatment similar to those recommended for osteoporosis in general. There is at least some initial evidence that antiresorptive treatments known to preserve bone in nondiabetic women have a similar effect on bone mineral density among those with diabetes. In addition, they should be counseled regarding appropriate preventive measures, which include adequate dietary calcium intake, regular exercise, and avoidance of smoking and other potential risk factors.

Summary

In women with diabetes, health concerns begin at puberty and continue throughout the reproductive years and later stages of the life cycle. Anticipatory guidance and education in each phase of development can help the woman with diabetes avoid health care problems, reduce her risk of complications, and achieve a healthy outcome. Regardless of the stage of life, proper nutrition, increased physical activity, smoking prevention or cessation, and control of lipids, blood pressure, and glucose levels are the key.

References

[1] Kjaer K, Hagen C, Sando SH, et al. Epidemiology of menarche and menstrual disturbances in a group of women with insulin dependent diabetes mellitus compared to controls. J Clin Endocrinol Metab 1992;75:524–9.
[2] Tatersall RB, Pyke DA. Growth in diabetic children: studies in identical twins. Lancet 1973;2:1105–9.

[3] Salerno M, Argenziano A, DiMaio S, et al. Tenore maturation, and final height in children with IDDM: effects of age at onset and metcoli. Diabetes Care 1997;20:721–4.

[4] Strotmeyer ES, Strotmeyer ES, Steenkiste AR, et al. Menstrual cycle differences with type 1 diabetes and women without diabetes. Diabetes Care 2003;26:1016–21.

[5] Schriock EA, Winter RJ, Traisman HS. Diabetes mellitus and its effects on menarche. J Adolesc Health Care 1984;5:101–4.

[6] Danielson KK, Palta M, Allen C. Wisconsin Diabetes Registry Project. J Clin Endocrinol Metab 2005;90:6466–71.

[7] Pinhas-Hamiel O, Standiford D, Hamiel D, et al. The type 2 family: a setting for development and treatment of adolescent type 2 diabetes mellitus. Arch Pediatr Adolesc Med 1999;153:1063–7.

[8] Ludwig DS, Ebbeling CB. Type 2 diabetes mellitus in children: primary care and public health considerations. JAMA 2001;286:1427–30.

[9] Rosenbloom AL, Joe JR, Young RS, et al. Emerging epidemic of type 2 diabetes in youth. Diabetes Care 1999;22:345–54.

[10] Thrailkill KM. Diabetes care for adolescents. In: Reece EA, Coustan DR, Gabbe SG, editors. Diabetes in women: adolescence, pregnancy and menopause. 3rd edition. Philadelphia: Lippincott Williams & Wilkins; 2004. p. 37–56.

[11] ACOG Practice Bulletin #60: pregestational diabetes mellitus. Washington: American College of Obstetricians and Gynecologists; 2005.

[12] Engelgau NM, Herman WH, Smith PJ, et al. The epidemiology of diabetes and pregnancy in the US, 1988. Diabetes Care 1995;18:1029–33.

[13] Homko CJ, Sivan E, Reece EA, et al. Fuel metabolism during pregnancy. Semin Reprod Endocrinol 1999;17:119–25.

[14] Catalano PM, Tyzbir ED, Roman NM, et al. Longitudinal changes in insulin release and insulin resistance in nonobese pregnant women. Am J Obstet Gynecol 1991;165:1667–72.

[15] Reece EA, Homko CJ, Wu YK. Multifactorial basis of the syndrome of diabetic embryopathy. Teratology 1996;54:171–82.

[16] Eriksson UJ. Congenital malformations in diabetic animal models-a review. Diabetes Res 1984;1:57–61.

[17] Rose BI, Graff S, Spencer R, et al. Major congenital anomalies in infants and glycosylated hemoglobin levels in insulin-requiring diabetic mothers. J Perinat 1998;8:309–11.

[18] Ylinen K, Aula P, Stenman UH, et al. Risk of minor and major fetal malformations in diabetics with high hemoglobin A1c values in early pregnancy. BMJ 1984;289:345–6.

[19] Kitzmiller JL, Gavin LA, Gin GD, et al. Preconception care of diabetes: glycemic control prevents congenital anomalies. JAMA 1991;265:731–6.

[20] Kitzsmiller JL, Buchanan TA, Kjos S, et al. Pre-conception care of diabetes, congenital malformations, and spontaneous abortions. Diabetes Care 1996;19:514–41.

[21] Metzger BE, Coustan DR. Summary and recommendations of the Fourth International Workshop-Conference on gestational diabetes. Diabetes Care 1998;21(Suppl 2):B161–7.

[22] Marshall JA, Hamman RF, Baxter J, et al. Ethnic differences in risk factors associated with prevalence of non-insulin dependent diabetes mellitus. The San Luis Valley Diabetes Study. Am J Epidemiol 1993;137:706–18.

[23] ACOG Practice Bulletin #30: gestational diabetes. Washington: American College of Obstetricians and Gynecologists; 2001.

[24] Homko CJ. Woman and diabetes. In: Childs BP, Cypress M, Spollett G, editors. Complete nurse's guide to diabetes care. Alexandria: American Diabetes Association; 2005. p. 272–85.

[25] Hollingsworth DR, Moore TR. Postprandial walking exercise in pregnant insulin dependent (type I) diabetic women: reduction of plasma lipid levels but absence of a significant effect on glycemic control. Am J Obstet Gynecol 1987;157:1359–63.

[26] Jovanovic-Peterson L, Peterson CM. Exercise and the nutritional management of diabetes during pregnancy. Obstet Gynecol Clin North Am 1996;23:75–86.

[27] Bung P, Artal R, Khodiguian N, et al. Exercise in gestational diabetes: an optional therapeutic approach? Diabetes 1991;40(Suppl 2):182–5.

[28] Bhattacharyya A, Brown S, Hughes S, et al. Insulin lispro and regular insulin in pregnancy. QJM 2001;94:255–60.

[29] Jovanovic L, Ilic S, Pettitt DJ, et al. Metabolic and Immunologic effects of insulin lispro in gestational diabetes. Diabetes Care 1999;22:1422–7.

[30] Wyatt JW, Frias JL, Hoyme HE, et al. Congenital anomaly rate in offspring of mothers with diabetes treated with insulin lispro during pregnancy. Diabet Med 2004;22:803–7.

[31] Jornsay DL. Pregnancy and continuous insulin infusion therapy. Diabetes Spectrum 1998; 11:26–32.

[32] Langer O, Conway DL, Berkus M, et al. A comparison of glyburide and insulin in women with GDM. N Engl J Med 2000;343:1134–8.

[33] Kremer CJ, Duff P. Glyburide for the treatment of gestational diabetes. Am J Obstet Gynecol 2004;190:1438–9.

[34] Chmait R, Dinise T, Moore T. Prospective observational study to establish predictors of glyburide success in women with gestational diabetes mellitus. J Perinatol 2004;24:617–22.

[35] Jacobson GF, Ramos GA, Ching JY, et al. Comparison of glyburide and insulin for the management of gestational diabetes in a large managed care organization. Am J Obstet Gynecol 2005;193:118–24.

[36] Weintrob N, Karp M, Hod M. Short- and long-range complications in offspring of diabetic mothers. J Diabetes Complications 1996;10:294–301.

[37] Schwarz R, Teramo KA. Effects of diabetic pregnancy on the fetus and newborn. Semin Perinatal 2000;24:120–35.

[38] Van Geusekon CM, Annnet Zeegers T, Martini IA, et al. Milk of patients with tightly controlled insulin-dependent diabetes mellitus has normal macronutrient and fatty acid composition. Am J Clin Nutr 1993;57:938–43.

[39] von Kries R, Koletzko B, Sauerwald T, et al. Breast feeding and obesity: cross sectional study. BMJ 1999;319:47–150.

[40] Arstrong J, Reilly JJ. Breastfeeding and lowering the risk of childhood obesity. Lancet 2002; 359:2003–4.

[41] Pettitt DJ, Knowler WC. Long-term effects of the intrauterine environment, birth weight, and breast-feeding in Pima Indians. Diabetes Care 1998;21(Suppl 2):B138–41.

[42] Kjos SL, Henry O, Lee TM, et al. The effect of lactation on glucose and lipid metabolism in women with recent gestational diabetes. Obstet Gynecol 1993;82:451–5.

[43] Stuebe AM, Rich-Edwards JW, Willett WC, et al. Duration of lactation and incidence of type 2 diabetes. JAMA 2005;294:2601–10.

[44] Kjos SL. Contraception in women with diabetes mellitus. Diabetes Spectrum 1993;6:80–6.

[45] Kjos SL. Postpartum care of women with diabetes. Clin Obstet Gynecol 2000;43:46–55.

[46] Kjos SL, Peters RK, Xiang A, et al. Contraception and the risk of type 2 diabetes mellitus in Latina women with prior gestational diabetes mellitus. JAMA 1998;280:533–8.

[47] Case A, Reid RL. Effects of the menstrual cycle on medical disorders. Arch Intern Med 1998; 158:1405–12.

[48] Cawood EH, Bancroft J, Steel JM. Perimenstrual symptoms in women with diabetes mellitus and the relationship to diabetic control. Diabet Med 1993;10:444–8.

[49] Cramer HI. The influence of menstruation on carbohydrate tolerance in diabetes mellitus. Can Med Assoc J 1942;47:51–5.

[50] Jarrett RJ, Graver HJ. Changes in oral glucose tolerance during the menstrual cycle. BMJ 1968;2:528–9.

[51] Moberg E, Kollind M, Lins PE, et al. Day-to-day variation of insulin sensitivity in patients with type 1 diabetes: role of gender and menstrual cycle. Diabet Med 1995;12:224–8.

[52] Widom B, Diamond MP, Simonson DC. Alterations in glucose metabolism during menstrual cycle in women with IDDM. Diabetes Care 1992;15:213–20.

[53] Trout KK, Rickels M, Petrova M, et al. Menstrual cycle effects on insulin sensitivity in women with type 1 diabetes [abstract]. Diabetes 2005;54:A645.

[54] Goldner WS, Kraus VL, Sivitz WI, et al. Cyclic changes in glycemia assessed by continuous glucose monitoring system during multiple complete menstrual cycles in women with type 1 diabetes. Diabetes Technol Ther 2004;6:473–80.

[55] Legro RS, Azziz R. Androgen excess disorders. In: Scott JR, Gibbs RS, Kaplan BY, et al, editors. Danforth's obstetrics and gynecology. 9th edition. Philadelphia: Lippincott Williams & Wilkins; 2003. p. 669–72.

[56] Bloomgarden ZT. Diabetes issues in women and children. Diabetes Care 2003;26:2457–63.

[57] Bjercke S, Dale PO, Tanbo T, et al. Impact of insulin resistance on pregnancy complications and outcome in women with polycystic ovary syndrome. Gynecol Obstet Invest 2002;54: 94–8.

[58] Mikola M, Hilesmaa V, Haltunen M, et al. Obstetric outcome in women with polycystic ovarian syndrome. Hum Reprod 2001;16:226–9.

[59] Costello MF, Eden JA. A systematic review of the reproductive system effects of metformin in patients with polycystic ovary syndrome. Fertil Steril 2003;79:1–13.

[60] Lord JM, Flight IHK, Norman RJ. Metformin in polycystic ovary syndrome: systematic review and meta-analysis. BMJ 2003;327:951–7.

[61] Glucek CJ, Wang P, Kobayashi S, et al. Metformin therapy throughout pregnancy reduces the development of gestational diabetes in women with polycystic ovary syndrome. Fertil Steril 2002;77:520–5.

[62] Glueck CJ, Wang P, Goldenberg N, et al. Pregnancy outcomes among women with polycystic ovarian syndrome treated with metformin. Hum Reprod 2002;17:2858–64.

[63] Glueck CJ, Goldenberg N, Wang P, et al. Metformin during pregnancy reduces insulin, insulin resistance, insulin secretion, weight, testosterone and development of gestational diabetes: prospective longitudinal assessment of women with polycystic ovary syndrome from preconception throughout pregnancy. Hum Reprod 2004;19:510–21.

[64] Vanky E, Salvesen KA, Helmstad R, et al. Metformin reduces pregnancy complications without affecting androgen levels in pregnant polycystic ovary syndrome women: results of a randomized study. Hum Reprod 2004;19:1734–40.

[65] Dorman JS, Steenkiste AR, Foley TP, et al. Menopause in type 1 diabetic women. Is it premature? Diabetes 2001;50:1857–62.

[66] Eisenberg E. Menopause and diabetes. In: Reece EA, Coustan DR, Gabbe SG, editors. Diabetes in women: adolescence, pregnancy and menopause. 3rd edition. Philadelphia: Lippincott Williams & Wilkins; 2004. p. 441–50.

[67] Malacara JM, Huerta R, Rivera B, et al. Menopause in normal and uncomplicated NIDDM women: physical and emotional symptoms and hormone profile. Maturitas 1997;28:35–45.

[68] Lopcz-Lopez R, Huerta R, Malacara JM. Age at menopause in women with type 2 diabetes mellitus. Menopause 1999;6:174–8.

[69] Hulley S, Grady D, Bush T, et al. Randomized trial of estrogen plus progestin for secondary prevention of coronary heart disease in postmenopausal women: Heart and Estrogen/Progestin Replacement Study (HERS) research group. JAMA 1998;280:605–13.

[70] Writing Group for the Women's Health Initiative Investigators. Risks and benefits of estrogen plus progestin in healthy postmenopausal women: principal results from the Women's Health Initiative randomized controlled trial. JAMA 2002;288:321–33.

[71] Crespo CJ, Smit E, Snelling A, et al. Hormone replacement therapy and its relationship to lipid and glucose metabolism in diabetic and non-diabetic postmenopausal women: results from the Third National Health and Nutrition Examination Survey (NHANES III). Diabetes Care 2002;25:1675–80.

[72] Giardina EG. Call to action: cardiovascular disease in women. J Womens Health 1998;7: 37–43.

[73] Lundberg V, Stegmayr B, Asplund K, et al. Diabetes as a risk factor for myocardial infarction: population and gender perspectives. J Intern Med 1997;241:485–92.

[74] Howard BV, Cowan LD, Go O, et al. Adverse effects of diabetes on multiple cardiovascular disease risk factors in women. The Strong Heart Study. Diabetes Care 1998;18:1258–65.

[75] Barrett-Connor E, Ferrara A. Isolated postchallenge hyperglycemia and the risk of fatal cardiovascular disease in older women and men. Diabetes Care 1998;21:1236–9.

[76] Albert C. Sex differences in cardiac arrest survivors. Circulation 1996;93:1170–6.

[77] Berra K. Women, coronary heart disease and dyslipidemia: does gender alter detection, evaluation or therapy? J Cardiovasc Nurs 2000;14:59–78.

[78] Tuominen JT, Impivaara L, Puukka P, et al. Bone mineral density in patients with type 1 and type 2 diabetes. Diabetes Care 1999;22:1196–200.

[79] Olmos JM, Gonzalez-Castrillon JJL, Garcia MT, et al. Bone densitometry and biochemical bone remodeling markers in type 1 diabetes mellitus. Bone Miner 1994;26:1–8.

[80] Schwartz AV. Diabetes mellitus: does it affect bone? Calcif Tissue Int 2003;73:515–9.

ELSEVIER
SAUNDERS

Nurs Clin N Am 41 (2006) 567–588

NURSING
CLINICS
OF NORTH AMERICA

Lifestyle Intervention for Prevention and Treatment of Type 2 Diabetes

Carmen D. Samuel-Hodge, PhD, MS, RD[a],*,
Felicia Hill-Briggs, PhD, ABPP[b], Tiffany L. Gary, PhD[c]

[a]Department of Nutrition, Schools of Medicine and Public Health,
University of North Carolina at Chapel Hill, 1700 Martin Luther King Jr. Boulevard,
Chapel Hill, NC 27599, USA
[b]Department of Medicine, Johns Hopkins University School of Medicine,
2024 East Monument Street, Baltimore, MD 21205, USA
[c]Department of Epidemiology, Bloomberg School of Public Health, Johns Hopkins University,
615 North Wolfe Street, Baltimore, MD 21205, USA

In the United States, and indeed globally, the rapidly increasing number of people who have diabetes and the accompanying burden of premature illness, death, and economic and societal costs constitute a major public health crisis that is expected to worsen in the next several decades [1,2]. As a nation, the only reasonable approach to stem the tide of this diabetes epidemic is to implement effective approaches for prevention of new cases and to intervene to prevent the morbidity and mortality attributable to secondary complications in individuals who already have the disease. Because the epidemic of type 2 diabetes is fueled largely by an obesity epidemic, the attention of public health experts is set on lifestyle factors (ie, diet and physical activity) as the primary modifiable contributing factors.

Lifestyle interventions are one effective approach to prevention and treatment of diabetes. These lifestyle interventions target diet and physical activity behaviors and seek to modify one or more aspects to produce improvements in metabolic outcomes and other health benefits. Because a number of reviews, meta-analyses, and clinical guidelines provide excellent details of the effectiveness of lifestyle interventions, the focus in this article is on summarizing the available evidence and describing what still remains

* Corresponding author. Department of Nutrition, Schools of Medicine and Public Health, University of North Carolina at Chapel Hill, 1700 Martin Luther King Jr. Boulevard, Room 246, CB #7426, University of North Carolina at Chapel Hill, Chapel Hill, NC 27599.

E-mail address: Carmen_samuel@unc.edu (C.D. Samuel-Hodge).

0029-6465/06/$ - see front matter © 2006 Elsevier Inc. All rights reserved.
doi:10.1016/j.cnur.2006.08.001   *nursing.theclinics.com*

unknown about lifestyle interventions for prevention and treatment of type 2 diabetes in adults. The aim is to start with the summary data describing the current evidence concerning the effectiveness of lifestyle intervention and then to explore some possible implications related to translation of the available research into clinical practice, community interventions, and public health policy.

Lifestyle interventions

Lifestyle factors such as diet, physical activity, cigarette smoking, alcohol use, sexual practices, and stress management play a significant role in the health and well-being of the public [3]. Although these factors are all individual behaviors influenced by biologic, psychologic, and other intrapersonal factors, they also are influenced by external contextual factors. Many behavioral theories and health-promotion planning models, therefore, seek to provide a better understanding of lifestyle behaviors through multilevel and socioecologic models that account for multiple influences. These socioecologic frameworks propose that individual behaviors are best understood in the context of influences from friends, family and small groups, systems and culture, community, and policies [3–6]. Accordingly, if individual behaviors and, by extension, group behaviors are influenced by this multitude of factors, any attempts to modify daily lifestyle behaviors through interventions are by nature complex and challenging—particularly if long-term behavior changes are the ultimate goal. Lifestyle interventions to prevent or treat diabetes in adults have used a variety of approaches to modify the behaviors of individuals at risk for or diagnosed as having diabetes. Of the lifestyle behaviors, diet and physical activity have been the behaviors most often targeted by diabetes interventions. The effectiveness demonstrated by interventions focused on these lifestyle behaviors is summarized here.

Lifestyle intervention trials for diabetes prevention

In the United States, the cumulative lifetime risk of developing diabetes for individuals born in 2000 is estimated at 32.8% for men and 38.5% for women, with much higher risk estimates for Hispanics (45.4% and 52.5% for men and women, respectively) and non-Hispanic blacks (40.2% and 49.0% for men and women, respectively) [7]. With a diagnosis of diabetes in midlife, individuals can expect to pay a substantial price in life-years lost (11.6 and 14.3 life-years lost in men and women diagnosed at age 40 years, respectively), and society pays billions in health care costs [7]. Preventing even a small proportion of new cases would lessen the population burden of diabetes, saving thousands of lives and billions of dollars in health care costs.

Lifestyle interventions to prevent diabetes have taken two general approaches: the targeting of high-risk individuals and population-based

approaches. Because obesity is arguably the strongest risk factor for developing diabetes [8,9], many prevention efforts have focused on preventing obesity or promoting weight loss in overweight or obese individuals. Lifestyle risk factors of diet and physical activity relate directly to weight status, so such factors become the primary focus of both approaches to diabetes prevention.

The strength of the evidence for diet and physical activity as risk factors for diabetes has been summarized by the World Health Organization [10] and is presented in Table 1. From this ranking of the evidence, the risk factors for diabetes with the strongest or most convincing evidence include physical inactivity, overweight, and obesity. The evidence available for all dietary factors ranges from "probable" to "insufficient". Evidence for the roles of saturated fats and dietary fiber (nonstarch polysaccharides) is most convincing but is given a "probable" rating because of inconsistencies between results from experimental versus prospective cohort studies. Although there is still much to learn about the best dietary pattern to prevent diabetes, the available evidence suggests that caloric balance (as a function of dietary intake and expenditure through physical activity) is important to weight status and ultimately influences diabetes risk.

Drawing from the available evidence concerning the role of weight, diet, and physical activity, a number of lifestyle interventions for the prevention of diabetes have been conducted. Summaries of these prevention efforts are provided by a number of reviews and meta-analyses [11–15]. The strongest evidence that the onset of diabetes can be prevented comes from four large-scale trials [16–20] conducted during the last 3 decades among high-risk individuals (Table 2). High-risk individuals in these trials had one or more of these characteristics: body mass index (BMI) indicating overweight or obesity, fasting blood glucose levels above normal (impaired fasting glucose); or elevated postprandial blood glucose (impaired glucose tolerance). Of the four trials, the largest and most recent lifestyle intervention took place in the United States and was the only trial to include a racially and ethnically diverse study population (45% minority populations) [19]. All trials involved clinic- or center-based interventions with participants aged, on average, from their mid-forties to fifties and with follow-up durations of about 2 to 6 years. Most interventions had a modest weight-loss goal (5% or more of initial weight) to be achieved through dietary restriction (decreased calories and fat and increased dietary fiber) and increased moderate intensity physical activity. The two more recent trials included more behavioral intervention components (including problem-solving and stress-management skills, stimulus control, cognitive restructuring, motivational interviewing principles, and relapse prevention), with the most intense behavioral intervention in the Diabetes Prevention Program (DPP) trial. Large variability in interventions, however, is seen in intervention duration, number of intervention visits, and intervals between contacts.

These four trials provide sufficient evidence that the onset of diabetes can be prevented or delayed by about 33% to 58% in high-risk individuals using

Table 1
Lifestyle interventions: comparison of four large prevention trials

Study characteristics	Malmö study	Da qing study	Finnish diabetes prevention study	Diabetes prevention program
Study population				
Setting	Sweden (population-based health screening of 6,956 men, with clinic-based intervention)	China (community screening, with intervention in 33 health care clinics)	Finland (5 study centers)	United States (27 study centers)
Number	N = 415	N = 557	N = 522	N = 3234
Age in years, mean (SD)	48.1 (0.7)	45.0 (9.1)	55.0 (7.0)	50.6 (10.7)
Sex (% female)	0	47.0	67.0	67.7%
Inclusion criteria	IGT and early-stage type 2 diabetes patients	Adults with IGT: 2-h postprandial BG ≥ 120 and <200 mg/dL	Overweight adults with IGT: 2-h postprandial PG 140–200 mg/dL and FG < 140 mg/dL	Overweight adults with prediabetes: BMI > 24, FPG 95–125 and 2-h 75 g OGTT PG 140–199 mg/dL
Interventions				
Duration (years)	6	6	3.2 (average)	1.8–4.6
Number of contacts (type)	Not reported (individual and group face-to-face)	30 (group and individual face-to-face)	15 (group and individual face-to-face)	40 (individual face-to-face, with some group contacts)
Frequency	6 months each of dietary treatment and supervised physical training during first 12 months;	Weekly for 1 month, monthly for 3 months, then every 3 months thereafter	7 sessions in 1st year, then every 3 months	16 lessons in first 24-weeks, then monthly contacts

Facilitator	Case manager (lifestyle coach), usually a dietitian	Dietitian	Physician and team	Team of physician, nurse, dietitian, and physiotherapist
Dietary intervention	Goal of 7% weight loss; low-calorie and low-fat diet	Weight-loss goal of $\geq 5\%$ body weight; low fat and high fiber diet: $< 30\%$ fat calories, $< 10\%$ saturated fats, and increased fiber (15 g/1000 kcal)	BMI < 25: limit of 25–30 kcal/kg (25%–30% fat; 50%–65% carbohydrates, 10%–15% protein) BMI > 25: 0.5–1 kg/mo weight loss to reach BMI of 23	Limit intake of simple carbohydrates with increase in dietary fiber
Physical activity intervention	150 min/wk moderate-intensity exercise (700 kcal/wk expenditure); supervised sessions twice weekly; supplemental group sessions	30 min/d (210 min/wk) moderate-intensity physical activity; supervised strength-training sessions	Daily activity of 1–2 units based on intensity. 1 units = 30 minutes mild activity, 20 minutes moderate activity or 10 minutes strenuous activity	Supervised physical training
Behavioral intervention	Goal setting, individual case managers, self-monitoring of weight, dietary intake, and physical activity, individualization, culturally sensitive materials and strategies, motivational interviewing techniques *(continued on next page)*	Food records and goal setting	None	None reported

Table 1 (*continued*)

Study characteristics	Malmo study	Da qing study	Finnish diabetes prevention study	Diabetes prevention program
Significant outcomes				
Weight, cholesterol, blood pressure, other	Reduction in body weight of 2.3%–3.7% at 5-year follow-up (at 1-year follow-up, mean weight loss was >6 kg); 50% of IGT patients had normalized glucose tolerance, and 50% of patients who had diabetes were in remission at 6-year follow-up	Incidence of diabetes reduced 31% (diet-only), 46% (physical activity-only), and 42% in diet + physical activity groups compared with controls; −0.9 to −1.6 change in BMI among overweight participants at 6-year follow-up	Mean weight loss of 4.2 kg in lifestyle group; 58% reduction in the incidence of diabetes; significant changes in waist circumference, plasma glucose, 2-h serum insulin and PG after oral glucose challenge, blood pressure, and serum triglycerides	Mean weight loss of 6.0 kg at 1-year follow-up; 58% reduction in the incidence of diabetes in lifestyle group

Abbreviations: BG, blood glucose; BMI, body mass index; FG, fasting glucose; FPG, fasting plasma glucose; IGT, impaired glucose tolerance; OGTT, oral glucose tolerance test; PG, plasma glucose.

Table 2
Diet, physical activity, weight, and type 2 diabetes prevention: strength of evidence and recommendations

	Risk	Strength[a] or Level[b] of Evidence
Dietary		
Saturated fatty acids	Increased	Probable
High intake of dietary fiber (nonstarch polysaccharides)	Decreased	Probable
Fruits (including berries) and vegetables	Decreased (based on nonstarch polysaccharides contributions)	Probable
Trans fatty acids	Increased	Possible
Total fat	Increased	Possible
Low glycemic index foods	Decreased	Possible
Exclusive breastfeeding	Decreased	Possible
Moderate alcohol consumption	Decreased	Insufficient
Vitamin E, chromium, and magnesium	Decreased	Insufficient
Physical activity		
Regular physical activity	Decreased	Convincing
Physical inactivity/sedentary lifestyle	Increased	Convincing
Weight		
Abdominal obesity	Increased	Convincing
Overweight and obesity	Increased	Convincing
Intentional weight loss in overweight or obese people	Decreased	Convincing
Recommendations for prevention or delay[b]		
Modest weight loss and participation in regular physical activity for individuals at high risk for developing diabetes		Best evidence (A)
Modest weight loss and increase in physical activity for individuals who have impaired glucose tolerance		Best evidence (A)
Modest weight loss and increase in physical activity for individuals who have impaired fasting glucose		Limited evidence (E)
Follow-up counseling seems to be important to success of lifestyle interventions (sustaining behavior changes)		Good evidence (B)

[a] World Health Organization strength of evidence: convincing = strong evidence based on epidemiologic studies showing consistent association between exposure and disease, with little or no evidence to the contrary; probable = evidence based on epidemiologic studies showing fairly consistent associations between exposure and disease; possible = evidence based mainly on findings from cross-sectional studies and supportive experimental data; insufficient = evidence based on findings of a few studies that are suggestive but insufficient to establish an association between exposure and disease.

[b] Amreican Diabetes Association levels of evidence: A = clear evidence from well-conducted, generalizable, randomized, controlled trials that are adequately powered; B = supportive evidence from well-conducted cohort studies; C = supportive evidence from poorly controlled or uncontrolled studies; E = expert consensus or clinical experience.

lifestyle interventions of varying intensities, durations, facilitators, and intervention components. Modest weight loss, modifications in diet (caloric and macronutrient composition), and increasing moderate-intensity physical activity all contribute to this reduction in diabetes onset and improved disease risk-factor profiles observed over a period of 2 to 6 years.

In addition to these large-scale trials, a number of smaller randomized, controlled trials (RCTs) of lifestyle interventions (for weight loss) in adults who had prediabetes provide further evidence of the effectiveness of modest weight loss in delaying diabetes onset. In the recent Cochrane review [11] of nine RCTs (including three of the large trials mentioned previously) with weight-loss interventions among adults who had prediabetes, intervention durations varied from 4 weeks to 10 years, with 4 to 78 contacts provided mainly by dietitians. The dietary interventions focused on caloric and fat restrictions, and physical activity interventions varied from supervised weekly physical activity sessions to advice or counseling. Behavioral components were included in more than half of the interventions; common strategies included goal setting, stress management, coping skills, and self-feedback (diet and physical activity diaries). The findings from this review are consistent with other reviews that show average weight loss of 2.8 kg (3.3% of body weight) at 1-year follow-up, with more intense programs (eg, the DPP) producing greater weight loss and weight-loss maintenance. Moreover, these studies suggest that prolonged and frequent contacts are needed for long-term successful weight loss. Besides the weight loss, a small number of interventions demonstrated modest improvements in blood pressure, blood lipids, and glucose, although the magnitude of change generally was not statistically significant in between-group comparisons.

In addition to the clinic- and center-based approaches among high-risk individuals, a number of studies have sought to approach diabetes prevention through population-based or public health approaches. Such population-based approaches attempt to reduce risk factors or causes of the disease. This population approach may take the form of local or community-based interventions that involve participation and collaboration among multiple local entities responsible for or affected by the issue of interest. Population approaches to diabetes prevention also may be initiated on a larger scale through governmental agencies seeking to address diabetes primary prevention on a state or national level. Whether on a local, state, or national level, efforts to prevent diabetes can be focused broadly to address contributing factors at different stages along the life-stage continuum, even starting with prenatal influences [21]. Because this article focuses on lifestyle interventions for diabetes prevention, diabetes prevention efforts initiated by national, governmental, and nonprofit organizations are not discussed, even though their impact on raising diabetes awareness and providing resources for community-based interventions should be recognized as potentially enhancing.

The Centers for Disease Control and Prevention, Division of Diabetes Translation recently conducted a review of community-based interventions to prevent type 2 diabetes [15]. Their search of the literature yielded 16 reports published in peer-reviewed journals between 1990 and 2001 and representing many populations and countries. Study designs were primarily quasi-experimental (only one was a RCT). Most of the interventions targeted adults (six focused on youth), and half were conducted in the United States. All but one of the interventions focused on both diet and physical activity, and many were designed to enhance the participation of the community in planning and implementation of the interventions, with attention given to including culturally meaningful program components and formats. Intervention components mainly targeted individual-level factors such as awareness (knowledge), attitudes, and individual behavioral changes; only one mentioned policy or organizational-level intervention components. Many included media campaigns as part of their activities to increase awareness. Components related to dietary behaviors of adults included opportunities for nutrition education such as food demonstrations, grocery tours, and recipe exchanges. Physical activity approaches included residential walking programs, exercise clubs and programs, and creating exercise facilities.

Few results were reported from the 10 studies among adults (with study durations ranging from 1–10 years). Only one study measured or reported the effect of the intervention on diabetes prevalence (reported as no change); three reported improvements in knowledge; five indicated positive behavioral changes (only two of these outcomes, however, were significantly different when comparisons were made between rather than within groups); and half did not report results in clinical markers such as BMI, weight, and blood pressure. Results for clinical markers were inconsistent for changes in blood pressure, weight, and BMI, with no change, increased, and decreased outcome values among intervention group participants. The authors of this review concluded that community-based diabetes prevention intervention research is in its beginning phases as reflected by the small number of studies, and several barriers to conducting well-designed research exist [15].

Considering the research findings from both high-risk and population approaches to diabetes prevention, a number of implications can be drawn relative to public health policy and future research. Implications for public health policy relate to issues of screening to identify the persons who have undiagnosed diabetes and individuals who have prediabetes, treatment decisions given the current health care system, and environmental policy changes to increase opportunities for health-promoting food and physical activity choices. Additional research is needed to:

1. Define targets for screening and diabetes prevention interventions. The US Preventive Services Task Force [22] considers the current evidence

insufficient to recommend for or against routinely screening for type 2 diabetes in asymptomatic adults who have type 2 diabetes, impaired fasting glucose, or impaired glucose tolerance. They do, however, recommend screening for adults who have hypertension or hyperlipidemia. Because the cost effectiveness of intervention strategies is still unclear [23], decisions about which individuals to treat and when to initiate treatment are difficult, and further study is warranted. Moreover, because 18.6 million Americans are estimated to have prediabetes or undiagnosed diabetes, providing treatment would be challenging in an already stretched health care system [13].
2. Evaluate the effects and costs of varying options for the health care system to deliver, coordinate access to, or otherwise link high-risk patients to lifestyle-intervention programs or resources [13]. Issues of who should deliver the interventions (physician or other ancillary staff), who should have oversight, where interventions should be conducted, and who should pay for these programs (patients, health insurer, or other payer) need to be addressed. Already, there are some research data on the potential for outcome-driven insurance reimbursement for short-term weight loss [24] and the willingness of some insurance providers to offer weight-management programs to their members [25].

The environmental and policy implications of the diabetes prevention research data target strategies related to obesity prevention in both adult and childhood.

1. Implement policies that increase the chances of being active and eating more healthful foods through improved access to safe places for physical activity, walkable neighborhoods, and local markets that offer healthful food choices. There is sufficient evidence to recommend environmental and policy approaches to increasing physical activity through the creation of and enhanced access to places for physical activity combined with informational outreach activities; point-of-decision prompts; and street- and community-scale urban design and land use policies and practices [26]. There is insufficient evidence concerning the effectiveness of policies and practices related to transportation and travel; additional research is also suggested in these areas: (1) understanding community characteristics needed for optimal implementation of policy and environmental interventions; (2) identifying variations, if any, in the effectiveness of policy and environmental interventions in different socioeconomic groups and access settings (eg, work site versus community facility) [27]. Recommendations for policy and environmental approaches targeting the food environment from the Task Force on Community Preventive Services are not yet available, but the Institute of Medicine has recommended a number of immediate steps for obesity prevention that target actions of federal, state, and local governments as well as industry and media [28]. These immediate steps include

developing standards for foods and beverages sold in schools and guide-lines for advertising and marketing to children; expanding consumer nutrition information and providing clear and consistent media messages; and working with communities to support partnerships that expand the availability of and access to healthful foods [28].

2. Target diabetes prevention through prevention of childhood obesity. Although there currently is little conclusive evidence that making changes in the nutrition environment will reduce rates of obesity, and research into the link between the built environment and childhood obesity is still in its infancy [29], there is sufficient evidence to support the relationship between the built environment and healthy lifestyle behaviors [29,30]. Moreover, policy-level interventions that target the critical periods during the life cycle, (eg, fetal, infant, childhood, pregnancy, and lactation) are now seen as important to modifying lifetime risk of obesity [21]. Such policy-level interventions would include hospital policies that increase the initiation and duration of breastfeeding; worksite policies that support breastfeeding; and child-care and school environments that encourage and support physical activity throughout the day [21].

In terms of future research implications, additional studies are needed [11,13–15] to:

1. Determine the most effective intensity, frequency, and duration of physical activity to prevent diabetes
2. Improve the level of evidence for dietary factors associated with diabetes and determine an optimal dietary composition related to macronutrients (eg, optimal levels of carbohydrates, protein, total fat, and fatty acid composition)
3. Determine the effectiveness of lifestyle interventions in obese adults who have normoglycemia, impaired fasting glucose, but no glucose intolerance. Efficacy studies have not yet been conducted in these groups [13].
4. Determine the effectiveness of lifestyle interventions when nonselective community recruitment is used and interventions are conducted in diverse community settings
5. Identify the role of physical activity independent of weight loss on diabetes prevention in individuals who have prediabetes
6. Determine the level of effectiveness of lifestyle interventions for weight loss in combination with pharmacologic or surgical treatment or public health (physical and social environmental change) interventions
7. Determine how best to maintain lifestyle behavior changes over the long term: intervention format, frequency, and duration of follow-up contacts
8. Determine the long-term outcomes (cardiovascular events and mortality) of sustained lifestyle changes. Later findings from the Malmo study population indicate that the 12-year mortality was reduced by about half (6.5 versus 14.0 per 1000 person-years at risk) in men who had

impaired glucose tolerance who participated in the lifestyle intervention compared with those who did not [31]. Additional data from studies such as the DPP [32] and Action for Health in Diabetes (Look AHEAD) study [33] will help answer this question.

9. Improve the quality of study designs, lifestyle interventions, and study measurements (of both processes and outcomes) used in population-based lifestyle interventions. Measurements in population-based interventions should assess community or environmental indicators of change, such as patterns of food purchase, use of physical activity resources, and organizational food and physical activity policies.

Lifestyle interventions for diabetes treatment

For individuals who already have diabetes, managing lifestyle behaviors is considered the cornerstone of treatment. Effective treatment approaches for type 2 diabetes lifestyle interventions would have to produce clinically meaningful improvements in glycemic control, weight, blood pressure, or blood lipid profiles and have an impact on the onset or progression of secondary complications of diabetes such as retinopathy, neuropathy, nephropathy, and cardiovascular disease. Results from the 20-year United Kingdom Prospective Diabetes Study (UKPDS) [34] published in 1998 provided the first strong evidence that intensive blood glucose or blood pressure control achieved through pharmacologic approaches significantly reduces the risk of microvascular complications (an overall 25% reduction in complication rates) but has little effect on macrovascular events [35]. Since then a number of studies have evaluated the effects of nonpharmacologic approaches such as lifestyle interventions on glycemic control and other clinical outcomes. This section primarily presents the findings from systematic reviews and meta-analyses of lifestyle interventions in patients who had type 2 diabetes. Some of the more recent research in lifestyle interventions for the treatment of diabetes is included to supplement the review data but does not represent an exhaustive listing of relevant research.

Lifestyle interventions to treat patients who have diabetes are similar to those for prevention in that they also focus primarily on diet and physical activity behaviors and often target weight loss, glycemic control as measured by hemoglobin A1c, or reduction in cardiovascular risk factors as primary outcomes. A number of meta-analyses and reviews offer summaries of the research data on lifestyle interventions in diabetes treatment [36–39]. From a total of 63 included articles, Gary and colleagues [39] analyzed data from 18 RCTs published between 1984 and 1999 and generated pooled effect size estimates for glycohemoglobin; no standardized effect sizes for weight loss or fasting blood glucose were possible with data reported. These 18 RCTs included 2720 participants in interventions lasting 1 to 26 months (median, 5 months). Total intervention visits ranged from 8 to 52 (median, 8.5 visits); the largest proportion of interventions

were facilitated by nurses (39%), included group (52%) or individual (65%) counseling, and focused the educational component on dietary behaviors (reduction in calories and total fat intake) (70%) and physical activity (57%). Gary and colleagues [39] concluded from their review that educational and behavioral interventions produced modest improvements in glycemic control as measured by glycohemoglobin (total glycohemoglobin, hemoglobin A1, hemoglobin A1c), with a pooled effect size of −0.43%. Stratified analysis showed that effect sizes varied significantly, with the largest reductions observed in studies in which the focus was on diabetes medications (−0.72%), followed by physical activity (−0.69%), diet (−0.51%), and blood glucose self-monitoring (−0.21%) [39]. Their analysis also showed physician-led interventions had the greatest effect size for glycohemoglobin reduction (−1.80) and that group and individual counseling produced similar effects.

The meta-analysis of Norris and colleagues [36,37] summarizes the findings from studies that have looked at the long-term effectiveness of lifestyle and behavioral (ie, nonpharmacologic) weight-loss interventions in adults who had type 2 diabetes. The Cochrane review [36] included 22 weight-loss interventions (with 4659 participants and 1–5 years of follow-up) evaluated in RCTs published before May 2004. This review demonstrated the following main results:

1. Weight-loss interventions using dietary, physical activity, and behavioral strategies produced small improvements in weight (1.7-kg pooled weight loss, representing 3.1% of body weight, at 1 year or longer) when compared with usual care. The magnitude of weight loss was attenuated by weight loss in the usual-care or comparison group.
2. Similar to the weight-loss experiences in adults who had prediabetes, comprehensive, intensive group-based diet and behavioral programs produced a mean weight loss of 8 to 10 kg in 6 months, with a regain of 30% to 35% at 1 year.
3. Interventions using very-low-calorie diets produced greater weight loss (3.0 kg more) than those with low-calorie diets. Likewise, interventions with higher-intensity physical activity led to greater weight loss (3.9 kg more) than interventions with lower-intensity or no physical activity component.
4. Changes in hemoglobin A1c as a measure of glycemic control (pooled effect of a 0.3% reduction) corresponded directly to changes in weight but were not significantly different when compared between groups.

Norris and colleagues [36,37] concluded that although lifestyle interventions can produce modest weight loss in adults who have type 2 diabetes and this level of weight loss is accompanied by health benefits, it is difficult to achieve long-term weight-loss maintenance. Because of the limited quality

and quantity of research data available for this review, the authors noted two implications for practice:

1. Because of the observed difficulty in sustaining weight loss among patients who have diabetes, other strategies, such as pharmacotherapy or surgery, may be needed in conjunction with lifestyle interventions to achieve sustained weight loss or control.
2. There is much to be learned about implementing dietary, physical activity, and behavioral interventions for weight loss and control in the long term and about whether intensive and long-term interventions such as the DPP will have similar effectiveness among adults who have diabetes.

The second implication for practice also is reflected in the joint position statement of organizations such as the American Diabetes Association (ADA), the North American Association for the Study of Obesity, and the American Society for Clinical Nutrition [40]. Their position is that the available evidence indicates that moderate weight loss (5% of body weight) can improve insulin action, decrease fasting blood glucose concentrations, and reduce the need for diabetes medications. Beyond the benefits in glycemic control, weight loss also improves cardiovascular risk factors through reductions in blood pressure, improved serum lipids (reductions in triglycerides and in total and low-density lipoprotein cholesterol and increased serum high-density lipoprotein cholesterol), and reductions in markers of inflammation. For obese patients who have longstanding diabetes or severe pancreatic B-cell dysfunction, weight loss may not produce the same level of benefit in glycemic control [40].

In addition to the implications for practice, the data presented have a number of implications for future research [36,37]:

1. A focus on conducting longer-term (sustained) interventions for weight loss and control
2. Conduct of intervention research to manage or maintain the weight of persons who have diabetes but who are not overweight
3. Evaluation of long-term health and quality-of-life outcomes
4. Determination of the economic efficiency of effective long-term weight-loss interventions
5. Improvement in the conduct of studies to minimize dropouts or attrition, improve the follow-up of dropouts, compare baseline characteristics of dropouts to completers, and report intention-to-treat analyses

On the basis of the available evidence, the shorter-term effectiveness of lifestyle interventions as part of diabetes treatment has been demonstrated, but there remain a number of unanswered questions that deal with the chronic nature of diabetes treatment and the need for interventions (particularly weight-loss interventions) whose effectiveness can be sustained over the long term. Similarly, there is much to learn about the longer-term outcomes of interventions, such as their impact on reducing the incidence and

mortality from cardiovascular disease, which remains the most common cause of death among persons who have diabetes. One trial currently underway aims to answer many of these important questions. The ongoing Look AHEAD study [33] will evaluate the long-term consequences of intentional weight loss in overweight or obese patients who have type 2 diabetes. The primary study outcome is time to incidence of a major cardiovascular disease–related event (ie, cardiovascular morbidity and mortality), with study follow-up planned to last until 2012. Look AHEAD includes an intensive weight-loss intervention designed to achieve and maintain weight loss through reduced caloric intake and increased physical activity over 4 years at 16 clinical centers. The intensive lifestyle intervention represents an adaptation of the DPP intervention components and strategies and group behavioral programs. The intervention includes 42 contact visits (three or four visits per month) during the first year, two contacts per month in the second year, and two contacts per year thereafter. In the first year, the lifestyle intervention is designed to achieve a weight loss of 7% of initial weight, with calorie goals of 1200 to 1800 kcal/day depending on initial body weight and a goal of 175 minutes/week of moderate physical activity.

Lifestyle interventions for the treatment of diabetes generally are multicomponent programs focused on diet, physical activity, and behavioral factors. Considering the highest quality evidence available, lifestyle recommendations for treatment of type 2 diabetes are summarized in Table 3 [23,41]. Despite the focus on dietary behavior changes in lifestyle interventions for patients who have diabetes, there still is not sufficient high-quality evidence to recommend an optimal dietary pattern for weight loss, metabolic control, and improvement in cardiovascular risk factors in people who have type 2 diabetes. In a recent Cochrane systematic review, the authors concluded that "There is no high quality data on the efficacy of the dietary treatment of type 2 diabetes, however, the data available indicate that the adoption of exercise appears to improve glycated hemoglobin at 6 and 12 months in people with type 2 diabetes" [38]. Consistent with this lack of a strong evidence base to guide dietary recommendations, only 5 of 15 specific dietary recommendations in the 2006 ADA position statement on medical nutrition therapy are level A recommendations (ie, based on clear evidence from well-conducted randomized trials). The majority (seven recommendations) are designated level E (ie, based on expert consensus or clinical experience) [23]. The ADA statement further notes that "although numerous studies have attempted to identify the optimal combination of macronutrients for those with diabetes, it is unlikely that any one such combination of macronutrients exists" [23]. Consequently, further research is needed on the dietary composition that should be promoted in lifestyle interventions to achieve optimal effects on metabolic control and improvement in cardiovascular risk factors in persons who have type 2 diabetes, especially given that most people who have diabetes die of heart disease and stroke.

Table 3
Highest evidence lifestyle recommendations in the treatment of type 2 diabetes*

Lifestyle component	Recommendation for persons who have diabetes	Evidence-based benefit
Physical activity	At least 150 min/wk of moderate-intensity aerobic activity and/or 90 min/wk of vigorous activity. Activity should occur 3 d/wk, with no more than 2 consecutive days without activity. Unless contraindicated, all persons should perform resistance exercises at least 3 times/wk: all muscle groups, three sets of 8–10 repetitions at a weight that cannot be lifted more than 8–10 times.	Improvement in glycemic control, reduction of cardiovascular risk factors, contribution to weight loss, and improvement in well-being
Nutrition	Total grams of carbohydrate should be monitored, using carbohydrate counting or exchanges, for glycemic control. Saturated fat should be limited to <7% of total calories. Non-nutritive sweeteners (acesulfame, aspartame, neotame, saccharine, sucrolose) are safe within -determined daily intake levels. Routine antioxidant supplements, such as vitamin E, vitamin C, and beta-caroten, are not recommended because of insufficient evidence of efficacy and long-term safety concerns. If possible, avoid or limit alcohol intake because the effect of alcohol on blood glucose is complex and difficult to predict or anticipate. If drinking, limit alcohol intake to a moderate amount: ≤1 drink/d for adult women and ≤2 drinks/d for adult men; 1 drink = 12 oz beer, 5 oz wine, 1.5 oz distilled spirits	Prevention and treatment of chronic diabetes complications by helping patients attain and maintain optimal control of blood sugar and hemoglobin A1c levels, low-density lipoprotein and high-density lipoprotein cholesterol, triglyceride levels, blood pressure, and weight
Smoking cessation	All patients are advised not to smoke.	Reduction in risk of premature death from macrovascular disease and premature development of microvascular complications

* American Diabetes Association level of evidence A (clear evidence from well-conducted, generalizable, randomized, controlled trials that are adequately powered). *Adapted from* the American Diabetes Association. Clinical Practice Recommendations. Diabetes Care 2006;29:S1–85; and the American Association of Clinical Endocrinologists. Medical Guidelines for the Management of Diabetes Mellitus. Endocr Pract 2002;8:S41–82.

Although not specific to diabetes, recent findings from the Women's Health Initiative [42] that a low-fat diet had no effect on heart disease rates offer some indication that total fat content should not be the sole focus. In fact, reviews of dietary intervention trials [43] and recommendations from the Institute of Medicine [44], the American Heart Association [45], and Adult Treatment Panel III [46] show a shift from a focus on total fat intake to guidelines targeting the type or quality of fat and carbohydrate intake. The Omniheart randomized trial [47] recently has provided evidence of benefits to blood pressure and lipid profiles from partially replacing some dietary carbohydrate with either unsaturated fat or plant protein. In summary, additional evidence is needed to support specific dietary recommendations for the treatment of diabetes, but dietary factors remain central to lifestyle interventions.

Translation of lifestyle intervention research

This article has presented evidence for the effectiveness of lifestyle interventions in the treatment of type 2 diabetes along with a number of questions that remain regarding implications for practice and future research. These implications are central to the issue of translating and disseminating what is known from efficacy trials into real-world settings and circumstances so that benefits are realized at the population level and particularly among populations at highest risk. Diabetes translational research involves comprehensive applied research that takes available knowledge and makes it useful in everyday clinical and public health practice; translation research focuses on finding solutions to real-world problems in different settings and situations [48]. The road from research to practice generally starts with efficacy trials (eg, DPP and UKPDS), which are followed by effectiveness trials that seek to show how programs perform in real-world settings, and ultimately ends with dissemination of effective programs and interventions. Translational research extends from effectiveness to dissemination research.

Unfortunately, the road from clinical trials to practice can be very long. Some estimate that it takes almost 2 decades to translate original clinical research in benefits of patient care [49]. One example of this translation gap is the current estimates of adults in the United States who meet the ADA clinical practice recommendations [50]. Although it has been known since the 1998 UKPDS trial results that control of blood glucose, obesity, and hypertension are beneficial to individuals who have type 2 diabetes and those at high risk of developing the disease, the proportion of persons who have diabetes and who meet recommended clinical goal levels is woefully inadequate. Using data from the 1999 to 2002 National Health and Nutrition Examination Survey, Resnick and associates [50] found that among the clinical measures, 49.8% had hemoglobin A1c levels below 7%; 27.4% were considered at low risk for high-density lipoprotein cholesterol, 36% for low-density lipoprotein cholesterol, and 65% for triglycerides; and only 39.6% met the recommendation for blood pressure control. A mere

28.2% reported engaging in the recommended level of physical activity, and recommended dietary intakes of saturated fats, unsaturated fats, and fibers were met by 48.3%, 28.3%, and 18.3%, respectively. Thus, although the knowledge gained from clinical trials has been used to develop guidelines and clinical recommendations, there are a number of challenges to implementing these recommendations in practice settings so that patients who have diabetes realize full benefits.

The challenges to diabetes translation research include numerous barriers to instituting public policies that affect the food and physical activity environments, access to and cost of preventive care, and barriers to diabetes care on the level of health care providers, patients, and the health care system [48,51]. Some priority areas for diabetes translation include [48,51]

1. Public health and policy efforts: Needed are efforts to increase the public's awareness and understanding of diabetes (eg, those of the National Diabetes Education Program [52]), public health policies that address diabetes prevention and support through increased availability of healthful food choices, promotion of incentives and opportunities to be physically active, and improved insurance coverage for interventions leading to changes in lifestyle behavior.
2. Community-based participatory translational efforts: Partnerships are needed among researchers, community members, and governmental/private agencies to increase the likelihood of implementing successful and sustainable interventions that build on the knowledge and participation of all partners.
3. Chronic-care model for system changes: Translation research is needed specific to each of the elements required for effective treatment of diabetes (systems of care and disease management that recognize diabetes as a chronic condition and organize diabetes care around elements of the community, the health care system, support for patient self-management, design of care delivery, decision support, and clinical information systems [53].
4. Diabetes translation interventions: Research in diverse populations and real-world settings is needed. These diverse groups should include vulnerable populations such as older patients who have diabetes, minority populations, and socially and economically disadvantaged groups. Recent examples of such translation research include a lifestyle intervention for weight loss among patients who have diabetes living in medically underserved rural communities [54] and a moderately intense and lower-cost behavioral weight-loss intervention in a primary care setting [55].
5. Attention to external validity and practical clinical trials: Priority should be given to the conduct of trials that are relevant to practicing clinicians, administrative decision makers, and policymakers (ie, externally valid interventions). Practical clinical trials [56] would provide

information relative to issues such as enrolling a broad and representative sample, testing interventions in different organizational settings, comparing clinically relevant treatment options (not just comparing treatment versus no treatment), and measuring a broad set of health outcomes such as contextual factors, population reach, protocol implementation, quality-of-life and economic outcomes, behavior changes in staff and patients, adoption, and maintenance. The Reach, Effectiveness, Adoption, Implementation, & Maintenance (RE-AIM) framework [57–59] provides guidance in reporting on intervention generalizations across diverse populations, settings, and duration.

Lifestyle interventions have demonstrated effectiveness in the primary prevention of diabetes and the secondary prevention of its complications. To realize the potential benefits of interventions such as the DPP, much needs to be done in translating this evidence into practice. Generating real-world data from diverse populations and settings remains a high priority that comes with many challenges. In the context of a diabetes epidemic concurrent with an obesity epidemic, national efforts to address the prevention, control, and management of diabetes have begun. In identifying obesity as the target, government agencies such as the Centers for Disease Control and Prevention have begun to employ system dynamics modeling [60,61] as a tool to project future trends (through 2050) in diabetes prevalence and to enhance the design and evaluation of intervention strategies on national, state, and local levels. Such modeling provides opportunities for policy testing using sample simulations (eg, addressing questions such as the likely impact of a purely downstream approach with clinical management of diagnosed prediabetes and diabetes increased to a level of 90% of cases, of a purely upstream approach, with caloric intake of the population reduced by 3% (or about 74 calories/person/day), or of policies directed at both clinical management and the food environment, that is, a balanced approach). Using such simulations, the value of upstream or prevention approaches become evident, but these benefits may take 10 to 15 years before they are manifested in symptoms or disease prevalence. Using a balanced or mixed approach seems to be the best policy option in the longer term [60].

References

[1] World Health Organization. Diabetes. Available at: http://www.who.int/dietphysicalactivity/publications/facts/diabetes/en/print.html. Accessed July 27, 2006.

[2] Cowie CC, Rust KF, Byrd-Holt DD, et al. Prevalence of diabetes and impaired fasting glucose in adults in the US population. Diabetes Care 2006;29(6):1263–8.

[3] Gielen AC, McDonald EM. Using the PRECEDE-PROCEED planning model to apply health behavior theories. In: Glanz K, Rimer BK, Lewis FM, editors. Health behavior and health education: theory, research, and practice. 3rd edition. San Francisco (CA): Jossey-Bass; 2002. p. 409–36.

[4] Fisher EB, Brownson CA, O'Toole ML, et al. Ecological approaches to self-management: the case of diabetes. Am J Public Health 2005;95(9):1523–35.

[5] Baranowski T, Perry CL, Parcel GS. How individuals, environments, and health behavior interact: social cognitive theory. In: Glanz K, Rimer BK, Lewis FM, editors. Health behavior and health education: theory, research, and practice. 3rd edition. San Francisco (CA): Jossey-Bass; 2002. p. 165–84.

[6] Sallis JF, Owen N. Ecological models of health behavior. In: Glanz K, Rimer BK, Lewis FM, editors. Health behavior and health education: theory, research, and practice. 3rd edition. San Francisco (CA): Jossey-Bass; 2002. p. 462–84.

[7] Narayan KM, Boyle JP, Thompson TJ, et al. Lifetime risk of diabetes mellitus in the United States. JAMA 2003;290(14):1884–90.

[8] Colditz GA, Willet WC, Rotnitzky A, et al. Weight gain as a risk factor for clinical diabetes mellitus in women. Ann Intern Med 1995;122:481–6.

[9] Chan JM, Stampfer MJ, Rimm EB, et al. Obesity, fat distribution, and weight gain as risk factors for clinical diabetes in men. Diabetes Care 1994;17:961–9.

[10] WHO/FAO. Diet, nutrition and the prevention of chronic diseases: report of a joint WHO/ FAO expert consultation. World Health Organ Tech Rep Ser 2003;916:72–9;147–9.

[11] Norris SL, Zhang X, Avenell A, et al. Long-term non-pharmacological weight loss interventions for adults with prediabetes. Cochrane Database Syst Rev 2005;18(2):CD005270.

[12] Norris SL, Zhang X, Avenell A, et al. Long-term effectiveness of weight-loss interventions in adults with pre-diabetes: a review. Am J Prev Med 2005;28(1):126–39.

[13] Centers for Disease Control and Prevention Primary Prevention Working Group. Primary prevention of type 2 diabetes mellitus by lifestyle intervention: implications for public policy. Ann Intern Med 2004;140(11):951–7.

[14] Bazzano LA, Sedula M, Liu S. Prevention of type 2 diabetes by diet and lifestyle modification. J Am Coll Nutr 2005;24(5):310 9.

[15] Satterfield DW, Volansky M, Caspersen CJ, et al. Community-based lifestyle interventions to prevent type 2 diabetes. Diabetes Care 2003;26(9):2643–52.

[16] Eriksson KF, Lindgarde F. Prevention of type 2 (non-insulin-dependent) diabetes mellitus by diet and physical exercise. The 6-year Malmo feasibility study. Diabetologia 1991; 34(12):891–8.

[17] Pan XR, Li GW, Hu YH, et al. Effects of diet and exercise in preventing NIDDM in people with impaired glucose tolerance: The Da Qing IGT and diabetes study. Diabetes Care 1997; 20(4):537 44.

[18] Toumilehto J, Lindstrom J, Eriksson JG, et al. Prevention of type 2 diabetes mellitus by changes in lifestyle among subjects with impaired glucose tolerance. N Engl J Med 2001; 344(18):1343–50.

[19] The Diabetes Prevention Program (DPP) Research Group. The Diabetes Prevention Program (DPP): description of lifestyle intervention. Diabetes Care 2002;25(12):2165–71.

[20] Knowler WC, Barrett-Connor E, Fowler SE, et al. Reduction in the incidence of type 2 diabetes with lifestyle intervention or metformin. N Engl J Med 2002;346:393–403.

[21] Johnson DB, Gerstein DE, Evans AE, et al. Preventing obesity: a life cycle perspective. J Am Diet Assoc 2006;106(1):97–102.

[22] Screening for type 2 diabetes mellitus in adults. What's new from the USPSTF? AHRQ Publication # APPIP03–0005, February 2003. Rockville (MD): Agency for Healthcare Research and Quality; 2003.

[23] American Diabetes Association. Standards of medical care in diabetes 2006. Diabetes Care 2006;26(Suppl 1):S4–42.

[24] Hubbert KA, Busey BF, Allison DB, et al. Effects of outcome-driven insurance reimbursement on short-term weight control. Int J Obes 2003;27:1423–9.

[25] Blue Cross Blue Shield of North Carolina. Get fit blue. Available at: http://www.bcbsnc.com/ members/health-wellness/blue-extras/getfitblue/. Accessed June 6, 2006.

[26] US Preventive Services Task Force Guide to community preventive services—promoting physical activity. Available at: http://www.thecommunityguide.org/pa/pa. Accessed July 27, 2006.

[27] US Preventive Services Task Force. Guide to community preventive services—physical activity research issues. Avaliable at: http://www.thecommunityguide.org/pa/pa-res-qs.html. Accessed July 27, 2006.

[28] Koplan JP, Liverman CT, Kraak VI, editors. Preventing childhood obesity: health in the balance. Washington (DC): National Academies Press; 2005. p. 1–22.

[29] Sallis JF, Glanz K. The role of built environments in physical activity, eating, and obesity in childhood. Future Child 2006;16(1):89–108.

[30] Rose D, Richards R. Food store access and household fruit and vegetable use among participants in the US Food Stamp Program. Public Health Nutr 2004;7(8):1081–8.

[31] Eriksson KF, Lindgarde F. No excess 12-year mortality in men with impaired glucose tolerance who participated in the Malmo Preventive Trial with diet and exercise. Diabetologia 1998;41:1010–6.

[32] Ratner RE. The Diabetes Prevention Program research. An update on the Diabetes Prevention Program. Endocr Pract 2006;12(Suppl 1):20–4.

[33] The Look AHEAD Research Group. Look AHEAD (Action for Health in Diabetes): design and methods for a clinical trial of weight loss for the prevention of cardiovascular disease in type 2 diabetes. Control Clin Trials 2003;24:610–28.

[34] United Kingdom Prospective Diabetes Study Group. Intensive blood glucose control with sulfonylureas or insulin compared with conventional treatment and risk of complications in patients with type 2 diabetes. Lancet 1998;352:837–53.

[35] Leslie RD. United Kingdom prospective diabetes study (UKPDS): what now or so what? Diabetes Metab Res Rev 1999;15(1):65–71.

[36] Norris SL, Zhang X, Avenell A, et al. Long-term non-pharmacological weight loss interventions for adults with type 2 diabetes mellitus. Cochrane Database Syst Rev 2005;2: CD004095.

[37] Norris SL, Zhang X, Avenell A, et al. Long-term effectiveness of lifestyle and behavioral weight loss interventions in adults with type 2 diabetes: a meta-analysis. Am J Med 2004; 117:762–74.

[38] Moore H, Summerbell C, Hooper L, et al. Dietary advice for treatment of type 2 diabetes mellitus in adults. Cochrane Database Syst Rev 2004;(2):CD004097.

[39] Gary TL, Genkinger JM, Guallar E, et al. Meta-analysis of randomized educational and behavioral interventions in type 2 diabetes. Diabetes Educ 2003;29(3):488–501.

[40] Klein S, Sheard NF, Pi-Sunyer X, et al. Weight management through lifestyle modification for the prevention and management of type 2 diabetes: rationale and strategies: a statement of the American Diabetes Association, the North American Association for the Study of Obesity, and the American Society for Clinical Nutrition. Diabetes Care 2004;27(8): 2067–73.

[41] American Association of Clinical Endocrinologists. The American Association of Clinical Endocrinologists medical guidelines for the management of diabetes mellitus: the AACE system of diabetes self-management—2002 update. Endocr Pract 2002;8(Suppl 1): 41–82.

[42] Howard BV, Manson JE, Stefanick ML, et al. Low-fat dietary pattern and weight change over 7 years: the Women's Health Initiative Dietary Modification Trial. JAMA 2006;295: 39–49.

[43] Hu FB, Willett WC. Optimal diets for prevention of coronary heart disease. JAMA 2002; 288:2569–78.

[44] Institute of Medicine. Dietary reference intakes for energy, carbohydrate, fiber, fat, fatty acids, cholesterol, protein, and amino acids. Available at: http://www.ionedu/report.asp?id=4340. Accessed July 27, 2006.

[45] Poirier P, Giles TD, Bray GA, et al. Obesity and cardiovascular disease: pathophysiology, evaluation, and effect of weight loss—an update of the 1997 American Heart Association scientific statement on obesity and heart disease from the obesity committee of the Council on Nutrition, Physical Activity, and Metabolism. Circulation 2006;113:898–918.

[46] National Cholesterol Education Program Adult Treatment Panel III. Executive summary of the third report of the National Cholesterol Education Program (NCEP) expert panel on detection, evaluation, and treatment of high blood cholesterol in adults (adult treatment panel III). JAMA 2001;285:2486–97.

[47] Appel LJ, Moore TJ, Obarzanek E, et al. Effects of protein, monounsaturated fat, and carbohydrate intake on blood pressure and serum lipids: results of the OmniHeart randomized trial. JAMA 2005;294:2455–64.

[48] Narayan KMV, Benjamin E, Gregg EW, et al. Diabetes translation research: where are we now and where do we want to be? Ann Intern Med 2004;140(11):958–63.

[49] National Institutes of Health. Proceedings from the Conference From Clinical Trials to Community: the Science of Translating Diabetes and Obesity Research. Bethesda (MD): National Institutes of Health; 2004.

[50] Resnick HE, Foster GL, Bardsley J, et al. Achievement of American Diabetes Association clinical practice recommendations among US adults with diabetes, 1999–2002. Diabetes Care 2006;29(3):531–7.

[51] Garfield SA, Malozowski S, Chin MH, et al. Considerations for diabetes translational research in real-world settings. Diabetes Care 2003;26(9):2670–4.

[52] National Diabetes Education Program. Available at: http://www.ndep.nih.gov. Accessed July 27, 2006.

[53] Wagner EH, Austin BT, Von Korff M. Organizing care for patients with chronic illness. Milbank Q 1996;74:511–44.

[54] Mayer-Davis EJ, D'Antonio AM, Smith SM, et al. Pounds off with empowerment (POWER): a clinical trial of weight management strategies for black and white adults with diabetes who live in medically underserved rural communities. Am J Public Health 2004;94(10):1736–42.

[55] Wolf AM, Conaway MR, Crowther JQ, et al. Translating lifestyle intervention to practice in obese patients with type 2 diabetes. Diabetes Care 2004;27:1570–6.

[56] Glasgow RE, Magid DJ, Beck A, et al. Practical clinical trials for translating research to practice: Design and measurement recommendations. Med Care 2005;43(6):551–7.

[57] Glasgow RE, Nelson CG, Strycher LA, et al. Using RE-AIM metrics to evaluate diabetes self-management support interventions. Am J Prev Med 2006;30(1):67–73.

[58] Klesges LM, Estabrooks PA, Dzewaltowski DA, et al. Beginning with the application in mind: designing and planning health behavior change interventions to enhance dissemination. Ann Behav Med 2005;29(2 Suppl):66–75.

[59] Dzewaltowski DA, Estabrooks PA, Klesges LA, et al. Behavior change intervention research in community settings: how generalizable are the results? Health Promot Int 2004;19(2):235–45.

[60] Homer JB, Hirsch GB. System dynamics modeling for public health: background and opportunities. Am J Public Health 2006;96(3):19–25.

[61] Jones AP, Homer JB, Murphy DL, et al. Understanding diabetes population dynamics through simulation modeling and experimentation. Am J Public Health 2006;96(3):488–94.

NURSING
CLINICS
OF NORTH AMERICA

Nurs Clin N Am 41 (2006) 589–604

Pharmacologic Interventions for Type 1 and Type 2 Diabetes

James A. Fain, PhD, RN, BC-ADM, FAAN[a],*,
David K. Miller, RN, MSEd, BSN, BC, CDE[b]

[a]College of Nursing, University of Massachusetts Dartmouth, 285 Old Westport Road,
North Dartmouth, MA 02747–2300, USA
[b]Health Education and Life Promotion, 16122 NE Lakeshore Drive South, Suite 200,
Hope, IN 47246, USA

A variety of pharmacologic interventions are available to treat people with type 1 and type 2 diabetes. For people with type 1 diabetes, the problem is that the pancreas no longer produces insulin, making it necessary for them to inject insulin on a daily basis to compensate for the loss of an endogenous source. For people with type 2 diabetes, there is a dual defect of insulin resistance or decreased sensitivity to insulin in the liver, muscle, and tissue, and impaired insulin secretion. Several oral diabetes medications have been developed that function at specific sites in the body, targeting not only the production and release of insulin but also muscle sensitivity and hepatic glucose production. A list of currently prescribed oral diabetes medications is shown in Table 1.

This article provides an update of pharmacologic interventions for diabetes, including a discussion of the drug classifications (eg, sulfonylureas, biguanides, meglitinide analogues, α-glucosidase inhibitors, thiazolidinediones [TZD], and insulin) with specific examples of each, and their background, dosing, and side effects. Combination therapy is reviewed, and information is provided on two new therapeutic classes of diabetes medications referred to as "incretin mimetics" and "antihyperglycemics."

* Corresponding author.
E-mail address: jfain@umassd.edu (J.A. Fain).

Table 1
Oral diabetes medications in the management of type 2 diabetes

Drug classification	Generic (brand name)	Mode of action
Sulfonylureas		
First generation	Chlorpropamide (Diabinese)	Stimulates beta cells to produce and release insulin
	Tolazamide (Tolinase)	
	Tolbutamide (Orinase)	
Second generation	Glyburide (Micronase, DiaBeta)	
	Glipizide (Glucotrol)	
	Glipizide, long-acting (Glucotrol XL)	
	Glimepiride (Amaryl)	
Biguanides	Metformin (Glucophage)	Slows the rate at which the liver releases stored glucose
	Metformin, long-acting (Glucophage XR)	
Meglitinide analogues	Repaglinide (Prandin)	Stimulates pancreas to release more insulin in a quick burst in response to food
	Nateglinide (Starlix)	
Alpha-glucosidase inhibitors	Acarbose (Precose)	Blocks an enzyme that slows or delays the digestion of carbohydrates
	Miglitol (Glyset)	
Thiazolidinediones	Rosiglitazone (Avandia)	Decreases insulin resistance in muscle cells
	Pioglitazone (Actos)	
Combination therapy	Glyburide/metformin (Glucovance)	
	Glipizide/metformin (Metaglip)	
	Rosiglitazone/metformin (Avandamet)	

Sulfonylureas

Background

Sulfonylureas are among the most widely used type of medications to treat type 2 diabetes. This class of oral diabetes medications was introduced in the mid 1950s, has been on the market the longest, and is the least expensive. Sulfonylureas lower blood glucose levels by stimulating the pancreas to produce and release insulin; the beta cells must be functioning for these medications to work. Over time, however, beta cell function starts to decline. Results of the United Kingdom Prospective Diabetes Study indicated that beta cell function declines progressively in patients with type 2 diabetes [1]. The inability of sulfonylureas to maintain control of blood glucose levels after initial success is referred to as "secondary failure" [2].

Sulfonylureas are members of a larger class of medications known as "insulin secretagogues." Insulin secretagogues exert their effects by increasing

the secretion of insulin by the islet cells of the pancreas. Sulfonylureas are classified as first-generation or second-generation medications. First-generation sulfonylureas include tolbutamide (Orinase); chlorpropamide (Diabinese); tolazamide (Tolinase); and acetohexamide (Dymelor). This group of sulfonylureas are less potent than second-generation sulfonylureas, must be given in higher doses, and often interact with other drugs.

Second-generation sulfonylureas include glyburide (Diabeta, Micronase); glipizide (Glucotrol/Glucotrol XL); and glimepiride (Amaryl). They are associated with fewer side effects and drug interactions than the first-generation sulfonylureas. Among all of the second-generation sulfonylureas, glipizide has the shortest duration of action and poses the least risk of hypoglycemia. Glipizide is usually administered twice a day; the delayed-release formulation (Glucotrol XL) is administered once daily. Glyburide and glimepiride are longer-acting oral medications. If two sulfonylureas are being administered simultaneously, and one is a second-generation medication, there is little evidence to suggest any benefits from switching to another second-generation sulfonylurea. Sulfonylureas generally lower hemoglobin A_{1C} values by 1% to 2% [3].

Dosing

First-generation sulfonylureas are seldom used as initial treatment for people with diabetes because high doses are required to achieve the same effect as produced by lower doses of second-generation sulfonylureas. Treatment with sulfonylureas should be initiated at low doses and titrated upward every 1 to 4 weeks as needed for an optimal glycemic response. Maximum effect has been shown with 50% of the maximum recommended doses.

Side effects

Few side effects generally occur with sulfonylureas; the most commonly reported ones are hypoglycemia and weight gain. Caution should be used when administering sulfonylureas to older people with decreased renal function. Glimepiride has been associated with a lower incidence of hypoglycemia than glyburide, which currently is the most commonly prescribed sulfonylurea in the United States [4]. Because there is a sulfonyl compound in sulfonylureas, hypersensitivity can occur in people with sulfur allergies, so sulfonylureas should be prescribed with caution in this patient population.

Biguanides

Background

Until 1994, sulfonylureas were the only oral medications available to treat people with type 2 diabetes. In December 1994, the US Food and

Drug Administration (FDA) approved the use of metformin (Glucophage) for type 2 diabetes. This first-line diabetes medication is indicated in people who are obese and have known insulin resistance. Metformin belongs to the class of drugs called biguanides, which lower blood glucose levels by inhibiting the release of stored glucose from the liver. Biguanides also reduce the absorption of glucose from food being digested in the small intestines, causing an anorexiant effect that can result in a small weight loss, a potential advantage for people who are obese.

Because metformin acts to decrease glucose release rather than increase insulin activity, there is little risk of hypoglycemia when taken alone. Biguanides generally reduce hemoglobin A_{1C} values by 1.5% to 1.8%, and may also beneficially affect lipid profiles and body weight [3]. Metformin is particularly useful for people who are allergic to sulfa drugs and cannot take sulfonylureas.

Dosing and side effects

People starting on metformin may experience side effects that mostly involve the gastrointestinal (GI) tract, including nausea, diarrhea, bloating, and abdominal cramps. GI side effects can be diminished to some extent by initiating therapy at a low dose and gradually increasing the dose over time. Metformin should be started at 500 mg twice a day (with meals) and gradually increased after a week or two to 1000 mg twice a day. Some people experience fewer GI effects on the long-acting metformin formulation. A small percentage of people may experience a metallic taste in the mouth.

A rare side effect associated with metformin is an increased risk of lactic acidosis. Because metformin is excreted 100% by the kidneys, renal insufficiency can easily lead to accumulation of metformin and subsequent development of lactic acidosis. It is important for kidney and liver function tests to remain normal for people who take metformin. Patients should be monitored when therapy is initiated and annually thereafter. For individuals undergoing a contrast study or acute hospitalization for any condition that could compromise renal function, metformin should be discontinued 48 hours before the procedure and restarted after renal function as been re-evaluated.

Thiazolidinediones

Background

TZDs are a relatively new class of diabetes medications that were first introduced in the United States in 1997. TZDs act primarily by decreasing peripheral insulin resistance, affecting muscle and adipose tissue. TZDs are sometimes referred to as insulin sensitizers because of their ability to

enhance insulin action at the muscle and adipose tissue level. To a lesser extent, TZDs also decrease hepatic glucose output.

The first medication in this class of drugs was troglitazone (Rezulin). After a couple of years, troglitazone was removed from the market because of the occurrence of severe liver toxicity and liver failure associated with its use [5]. Two TZDs that are currently on the market are rosiglitazone (Avandia) and pioglitazone (Actos). These medications have a lower incidence of hepatotoxicity than the first-generation medication, troglitazone.

In addition to decreasing peripheral insulin resistance, TZDs impact the lipid profile by decreasing triglycerides and increasing high-density lipoprotein cholesterol levels. Pioglitazone has a more overall positive effect on lipids than rosiglitazone and tends to lower triglycerides. Both drugs have a positive effect on lipids by increasing high-density lipoprotein cholesterol concentrations [6]. TZDs generally lower hemoglobin A_{1C} values by 0.7% to 1.75% [3].

Dosing

Pioglitazone and rosiglitazone are approved as first-line therapy in diabetes, alone or in combination with other oral diabetes medication. Both drugs are effective at their maximum dose and work within 1 to 2 hours after administration. Doses of pioglitazone range from 15 to 45 mg per day, and doses of rosiglitazone range from 4 to 8 mg per day. Because of a slow onset of action, TZDs may take up to 4 weeks to decrease blood glucose levels and up to 12 weeks to achieve a maximum glycemic benefit.

Side effects

The most common side effects of pioglitazone and rosiglitazone are weight gain and fluid retention. Weight gain seems to be associated with higher doses. People with mild to moderate edema, such as ankle swelling and puffiness, may benefit from a low dose of a mild diuretic, such as thiazide (eg, 12.5–25 mg), or a decreased dose of pioglitazone or rosiglitazone. Because of the potential for fluid retention, TZDs should be avoided in people with class III or IV heart disease (per New York Heart Association classification) [6].

Pioglitazone and rosiglitazone have a much lower incidence of liver toxicity than the first-generation TZD, troglitazone. Liver function tests should be performed before initiating treatment, however, every 2 months for the first year, and then every 3 to 6 months thereafter [5]. Pioglitazone and rosiglitazone should not be used in a person whose baseline serum transaminase levels are more than 2.5 times over the upper limit of normal.

α-Glucosidase inhibitors

Background

α-Glucosidase inhibitors were first introduced in the United States in the mid-1990s. This class of oral diabetes medications lowers postprandial blood

glucose levels primarily by slowing the absorption of carbohydrates. α-Glucosidase inhibitors act locally in the small intestines by inhibiting the enzyme α-glucosidase. Two α-glucosidase inhibitors currently on the market are acarbose (Precose) and miglitol (Glycet). Because α-glucosidase inhibitors do not affect insulin levels, they do not cause hypoglycemia when taken alone.

Dosing

α-Glucosidase inhibitors can be used as first-line therapy or in combination with other oral diabetes medications. As monotherapy, acarbose decreases fasting blood glucose levels by 25 to 30 mg/dL and hemoglobin A_{1C} values by 0.5% to 1% [3]. The greatest benefit of acarbose is a 40 to 50 mg/dL decrease in postprandial glucose levels. Therapy with α-glucosidase inhibitors should be initiated at the lowest possible dose and given once daily. Dosing should be increased gradually to two or three times a day if the patient tolerates the medication. The maximum dose of acarbose is based on the patient's weight. For patients who weigh 60 kg or less, the maximum dose is 50 mg three times a day. For patients who weigh over 60 kg, the maximum dose is 100 mg three times a day.

Side effects

α-Glucosidase inhibitors have a high rate of being discontinued because of flatulence and other GI symptoms (eg, bloating, abdominal discomfort, and diarrhea). Most GI symptoms occur because of the incomplete breakdown of carbohydrates in the small intestine and the subsequent action of bacteria on undigested carbohydrates in the colon. Starting at a lower dose and gradually increasing the dose until the patient builds tolerance may help diminish the GI side effects. Hypoglycemia does not usually occur with these medications unless they are taken in combination with sulfonylureas, meglitinides, or insulin. If hypoglycemia occurs, only pure glucose (which can be absorbed without enzymatic degradation) or milk is absorbed quickly enough to treat the hypoglycemia. Glucose tablets or gels are the preferred treatment [7]; juices and soft drinks are not effective because their absorption is greatly reduced.

Meglitinide analogues

Background

Meglitinides were introduced as new class of nonsulfonylurea insulin secretagogues in the early 1990s. Meglitinides act primarily by increasing insulin secretion by the pancreas. A functioning pancreas is necessary because this medication causes a quick burst of insulin to be released, raising plasma insulin levels for 1 to 2 hours. This rapid onset of action stimulates the beta

cell at the first-phase insulin response, which often is lacking in people with type 2 diabetes, and causes a decrease in the postprandial glucose spike. Meglitinides improve insulin secretion by binding to a different site than sulfonylureas. The two meglitinides currently on the market in the United States are repaglinide (Prandin) and nateglinide (Starlix).

Dosing

Repaglinide is indicated for use as monotherapy or in combination with other oral diabetes medications, such as metformin. Repaglinide is taken 15 minutes before meals, with a starting dose of 0.5 mg with each meal, and is titrated upward to a total dose of 16 mg per day based on glycemic response. The number of meals eaten determines the number of daily doses. Such dosing is advantageous for people who eat small frequent meals or those who choose to eat only two meals a day. People should be instructed to dose and then eat; if they do not eat, they should not take the medication. Also, if they forget to take their dose of meglitinide before a meal, they should be instructed to not take the medication afterward. Nateglinide has a more rapid onset of action and is dosed at 120 mg per meal. Occasionally, people may be started with 60 mg per meal with each meal if their hemoglobin A_{1C} values are close to normal.

Side effects

As with sulfonylureas, the most common side effect of meglitinides is hypoglycemia. People taking nateglinide were found to have a slight increase in uric acid, which was of no clinical consequence [3].

Combination therapy

Background

Combined treatment with two or more oral diabetes medications may be appropriate for people who are unable to achieve glycemic control with monotherapy. Instead of stopping one medication and replacing it with another medication, an additive benefit has been demonstrated from taking two medications at the same time and has led to the growing popularity of combination therapy.

The most commonly used combination of oral diabetes medications is metformin plus a sulfonylurea [8]. Metformin-glyburide (Glucovance) was one of the first fixed-dose combination medications approved by the FDA. This distinct new drug, however, may not be clinically beneficial to all individuals. The weight-sparing relative effect of metformin is sometimes lost because the weight gain associated with this combination therapy is equal to that with glyburide alone and more than with metformin alone.

In addition, the plasma levels of glyburide peak earlier, causing a more pronounced hypoglycemic effect and glyburide causes more weight gain than some of the other sulfonylureas [3].

Incretin-based therapies

Although the five major classes of oral medications previously discussed are available for the treatment of type 2 diabetes, each class has distinct benefits and concerns associated with its use. Likewise, many of the oral medications are aimed at only one aspect of the underlying pathogenesis of type 2 diabetes. Multiple medications are often needed to achieve optimal glycemic control. Given that type 2 diabetes is a progressive disease complicated by side effects associated with various pharmacologic interventions (eg, hypoglycemia and weight gain), newer medications are needed that target multiple aspects of the underlying pathogenesis of type 2 diabetes.

A new therapeutic class of medications based on incretin hormones has been developed. Incretin hormones are GI hormones that are released following food ingestion. The incretin effect that has been observed led to the hypothesis that GI factors play an important role in stimulating insulin secretion.

Background

Two major incretin hormones have been identified: glucagon-like peptide-1 and glucose-dependent insulinotropic polypeptide. Both hormones play a major role in stimulating insulin secretion and facilitating homeostasis following food ingestion. Synthesis of glucagon-like peptide-1 occurs in the L cells, which are located in the ileum and colon, whereas glucose-dependent insulinotropic polypeptide is released by K cells in the duodenum and proximal jejunum. Secretion of both incretins is impaired in people with type 2 diabetes. Both hormones are also rapidly inactivated by dipeptidyl-peptidase–IV [9,10].

The first incretin-based medication to be approved by the FDA was exenatide (Byetta). Exenatide, an incretin mimetic, is a glucagon-like peptide-1 receptor agonist that is resistant to the effects of dipeptidyl-peptidase–IV. This medication is indicated for use in people with type 2 diabetes who are not adequately controlled with a sulfonylurea, metformin, or combination of both. Exenatide is an analogue of glucagon-like peptide-1 and is derived from a compound found in the saliva of the Gila monster, a lizard located in the southwestern part of the United States. This analogue enhances insulin secretion in response to elevated blood glucose levels.

Dosing

The recommended starting dose of exenatide is 5 µg twice a day, titrating up to 10 µg twice a day after 1 month if well tolerated. Individuals may take

exenatide within 60 minutes before the morning and evening meals, and continue taking their other oral medications. If, however, an individual is taking a sulfonylurea, the dose may need to be decreased by 50% because of the potential for hypoglycemia. Exenatide is delivered in a fixed dose, and no other adjustments are needed based on the meal plan or physical activity [11].

Side effects

There is a risk of hypoglycemia when exenatide is used with a sulfonylurea, or with a combination of a sulfonylurea and metformin. Exenatide also is associated with mild to moderate GI symptoms, such as nausea, vomiting, and diarrhea.

Further development of incretin-based therapies

Several new incretin-based medications are currently in development and undergoing clinical testing. Medications in this therapeutic class inhibit the action of dipeptidyl-peptidase–IV, increasing the activity of glucagon-like peptide–1. Vildagliptin, a dipeptidyl-peptidase–IV inhibitor, has shown favorable effects in clinical research by demonstrating a 0.7% reduction in hemoglobin A_{1C} values. It has been tolerated well by individuals and has a low incidence of hypoglycemia, nausea, and vomiting [12]. Vildagliptin will probably be the first dipeptidyl-peptidase–IV inhibitor available for clinical use; similar dipeptidyl-peptidase–IV inhibitors, such as sitaglitin and saxagliptin, are currently in development.

Pramlintide

Background

Pramlintide (Symlin) is a new class of diabetes medication referred to as an "antihyperglycemic" approved by the FDA in March 2005. Pramlintide is an injectable diabetes medication for use in people with type 1 and type 2 diabetes. Symlin acts primarily by regulating glucose concentrations in the postprandial state; enhances satiety, leading to weight loss; decreases mealtime insulin requirements; and improves glycosylated hemoglobin [13]. For people with type 1 diabetes, Symlin is an additional treatment for use with mealtime insulin for those who have failed to achieve desired glucose control despite optimal insulin therapy. For people with type 2 diabetes, Symlin is an additional treatment for use with mealtime insulin for those who have failed to achieve desired glucose control despite optimal insulin therapy, with or without a sulfonylurea agent or metformin. In addition to regulating postmeal increase in glucose concentrations, symlin slows gastric emptying and suppresses glucagon secretion [13].

Symlin is a synthetic analogue of the hormone amylin. Amylin is a naturally occurring hormone located in the beta cells of the pancreas and secreted with insulin in response to meals. Like insulin, amylin is absent or deficient in people with diabetes. Amylin and insulin work together with glucagon to maintain normal glucose concentrations. Insulin and amylin concentrations normally increase, whereas glucagon levels decrease after meals. Amylin slows gastric emptying and suppresses glucagon secretion.

Dosing

Pramlintide is administered subcutaneously like insulin and given immediately before meals. People with type 1 diabetes start at 15 μg (2.5 units) before each meal. Increase the dose another 15 μg (2.5 units) after 3 days if there are no signs of nausea. Continue to increase the dose another 15 μg (2.5 units) up to a maximum of 60 μg (10 units). People with type 2 diabetes start at 60 μg (10 units) before meals, increasing to a maximum of 120 μg (20 units). Symlin cannot be mixed in the same syringe as insulin [14].

Side effects

The most common side effect associated with taking Symlin is nausea. Begin taking Symlin at a lower dose to minimize nausea. Do not increase the dose of Symlin until the nausea has subsided. Take Symlin with at least 30 g of carbohydrates or 250 calories [14]. When Symlin is used with insulin there is an increased risk of hypoglycemia, particularly in people with type 1 diabetes. If hypoglycemia does occur the insulin dose, and not Symlin, is the cause. Lowering the bolus insulin (mealtime insulin) by 30% to 50% is recommended to help resolve hypoglycemia.

Symlin is not recommended for people who do not follow their current insulin regimen or check their blood glucose levels three or more times a day, have a history of hypoglycemia requiring assistance, are diagnosed with gastroparesis, and use medications that stimulate GI motility, and pediatric patients or pregnant women [14].

Insulin

Background

Insulin is a hormone produced and released by the pancreas in different amounts throughout the day. Insulin allows the cells of the body to absorb glucose from the bloodstream to use for energy or to store in the cells for later use. A variety of insulin preparations are available for use in people with type 1 and type 2 diabetes. Preparations are either human insulin, produced by recombinant DNA technology (often called genetic engineering), or insulin analogues, produced by altering the insulin molecule to provide

an immediate onset of action or long-acting and virtually peakless action. Insulins are classified according to their actions (eg, rapid-acting, short-acting, intermediate-acting, and long-acting insulins). A comparison of the onset, peak, and duration of action of the various types of human insulins and analogues is shown in Table 2.

The goal of insulin therapy is to provide insulin in a fashion that closely mimics the body's natural secretion of insulin from the pancreas in the fasting and fed states in a healthy person without diabetes. There should be a relatively constant 24-hour secretion of a small amount of insulin, or basal insulin, supplemented by a quick burst of bolus insulin to cover mealtimes [15].

Basal insulin

Approximately 50% to 60% of total insulin requirements should be basal insulin, with approximately 40% to 50% given before meals. Neutral protamine hagedorn (NPH) insulin is an intermediate-acting insulin that has an extended activity because of the presence of protamine. Because of the extended action, NPH is used as a basal insulin that generally is given once or twice a day, depending on the individual situation. NPH is usually given before breakfast and before dinner or bedtime. Bedtime may be a better time for the second dose of NPH because it would peak later in the morning rather than during the night. NPH has a duration of action that can last up to 12 hours; skipping meals could cause hypoglycemia [16].

A second strategy for providing basal insulin coverage is to administer Ultralente (long-acting insulin) in equal doses before breakfast and dinner. Ultralente insulin is made by combining zinc with human insulin, which slows the rate of absorption after subcutaneous injection. Ultralente is usually given twice a day to provide a more level peak action.

Table 2
Insulin preparations: onset, peak, and duration of action

Types of insulin	Band name	Onset of action	Peak action	Duration of action (h)
Rapid-acting (bolus or mealtime insulin)				
Insulin lispro	Humalog	5–15 min	30–90 min	4–5
Insulin aspart	Novolog	5–15 min	30–90 min	4–5
Insulin glulisine	Apidra	15 min	30–90 min	4–5
Short-acting (bolus or mealtime insulin)				
Regular insulin	Humulin R	30–90 min	2–4 h	5–7
Regular insulin	Novolin R	30–90 min	2–4 h	5–7
Intermediate-acting (basal insulin)				
NPH	Humulin N	1–2 h	6–14 h	16–20
Long-acting (basal insulin)				
Insulin glargine	Lantus	90 min	Peakless	24
Insulin detemir	Levemir	90 min	Peakless	24

Abbreviation: NPH, neutral protamine hagedorn.

Glargine (Lantus) is a long-acting insulin analogue without a peak that provides insulin in a basal pattern for 24 hours. Glargine may be given at breakfast, the evening meal, or bedtime. Whatever time is chosen, it is important that glargine be given at the same time each day. Glargine should not be mixed with other insulins in the same syringe. To assess the effect of glargine, the morning fasting blood glucose level should be measured and the dose of glargine should be titrated upward for 3 to 5 days until a target range is reached. Glargine provides only basal insulin coverage and, in many cases, is used in combination with other insulin preparations or oral medications [16].

Insulin detemir (Levemire) is a new long-acting basal insulin that was approved by the FDA in June 2005. Insulin detemir can be given once a day and in combination with a mealtime insulin dose (bolus insulin). This new insulin looks different from most long-acting insulins because its appearance is clear rather than cloudy like glargine. People who take rapid-acting or short-acting insulin along with insulin detemir need to be aware of the possible confusion that could occur when taking both insulins. Treatment with insulin detemir has resulted in more predictable glycemic control, fewer hypoglycemic episodes, and less weight gain [17].

Bolus insulins

Rapid-acting insulins

Rapid-acting insulin analogues currently available in the United States include insulin lispro (Humalog), insulin aspart (Novolog), and insulin glulisine (Apira). Rapid-acting insulins are used to control postmeal glucose excursions and to cover the meal-related glucose peak, resulting in fewer between-meal hypoglycemic episodes and better postprandial blood glucose levels [15].

Lispro was the first rapid-acting insulin analogue on the market. It starts working in 5 to 15 minutes and peaks within 45 to 90 minutes. Because it has such a quick onset of action, lispro provides better control of postmeal glucose excursions, minimal antibody production, and rapid disposal. Both lispro and aspart are appropriate for general diabetes care and gestational diabetes care. Rapid-acting insulin analogues are the closest to mimicking the body's natural first-phase insulin secretion in response to food. Aspart is another rapid-acting insulin analogue that has an onset of action in less than 15 minutes with a duration of action between 3 and 5 hours.

Premixed insulins

Premixed preparations of insulin have gained popularity in the treatment of type 2 diabetes because of their convenience and simplicity. A list of currently used premixed preparations is shown in Table 3. Mixed insulin preparations contain intermediate-acting insulin (NPH) with either a rapid-acting or short-acting insulin in varying percentages. These

Table 3
Premixed insulins

Combination of insulin	Brand name	Onset of action	Peak action	Duration of action
Insulin lispro protamine				
Lispro (75% is NPL [NPH-like insulin]/25% insulin lispro)	Humalog mix 75/25	15–30 min	30–120 min	14–24
Insulin aspart protamine				
Aspart (70% is NPL [NPH like insulin]/30% is insulin aspart)	Novolog mix 70/30	10–20 min	60–180 min	24
NPH/regular (70% NPH insulin/30% regular insulin)	Humulin 70/30	30–60 min	2–6 h	14–24
NPH/regular (70% NPH insulin/30% regular insulin)	Novolin 70/30	30–60 min	2–6 h	14–24
NPH/regular (50% NPH insulin/50% regular insulin)	Humulin 50/50	30–60 mins	2–6 h	14–24

Abbreviations: NPH, neutral protamine hagedorn; NPL, a novel intermediate acting insulin.

preparations offer the advantage of 24-hour coverage from two injections per day. The short-acting or rapid-acting insulin in the morning dose covers breakfast, and the intermediate-acting insulin covers postlunch and afternoon needs. The second dose in the afternoon covers the evening meal, overnight, and early morning needs. Another advantage of using a premixed preparation is not having to mix the insulins when drawing an injection, and not having to take two injections each time rather than one. Although using premixed insulin preparations may be easier for some people, there may be certain constraints on adjusting glycemic control because of the fixed amounts of both types of insulin in each injection.

Inhaled insulin

Background

Inhaled insulin is an alternative to insulin injections that has been tested for safety and efficacy and approved by the FDA in January 2006 for use with people who have type 1 or type 2 diabetes over the age of 18. Exubera is the first inhaled insulin product to be approved for use in the United States.

Recent technologic advances have made it possible to deliver insulin to the alveolar space through use of an inhaler-type device. Insulin is then rapidly absorbed into the alveolar capillaries and dispersed throughout the systematic circulation. The Exubera inhaler was developed by Nektar Therapeutics (San Carlos, CA) and is about the size of an eyeglass case, weighing about 4 oz.

Inhaled insulin is a short-acting powder form of insulin that is similar to insulin lispro. The onset of action is faster than both insulin lispro and regular insulin, however, with a duration of action that is also longer [18]. Exubera is used as a meal time insulin and given 10 minutes before a meal. People who use Exubera should understand that Exubera is not taken as a substitute for all insulin injections taken every day. People with type 1 diabetes use Exubera in combination with longer-acting injected insulin, whereas people with type 2 diabetes may use Exubera alone as a rapid-acting (mealtime) insulin or in combination with other oral diabetes medications or longer-acting insulins. Data from a small pilot study suggested that when oral diabetes medications failed in people with type 2 diabetes, adding premeal inhaled insulin improved glycemic control [19]. Results of several studies have demonstrated that people with type 1 diabetes have had a decrease in hemoglobin A_{1C} levels compared with those individuals taking insulin injections [20]. Likewise, individuals with type 2 diabetes have experienced similar improvements in glycemic control [21].

Dosing

Exubera comes in 1- or 3-mg dose blister packs. The term "blister pack" refers to the shape and type of dose packet that holds the insulin powder. A 1-mg blister pack is equivalent to approximately 2.5 to 3 units of injected insulin [22]. People who normally inject one or two units of rapid-acting insulin before meals may not be able to use Exubera. One of the most important aspects in using Exubera is to instruct people to monitor glucose levels throughout the day and contact their health care provider if hypoglycemia develops.

Side effects

As with all forms of insulin, a possible side effect of Exubera is hypoglycemia. Use of Exubera may likewise cause a cough, dry mouth, sore throat, chest discomfort, or shortness of breath. Exubera is not recommended in people who smoke or have stopped smoking in the past 6 months, have an unstable or uncontrolled lung disease, or are allergic to insulin.

Summary

Use of oral diabetes medications continues to be an effective component in the treatment of type 2 diabetes. By addressing the defects of insulin deficiency and resistance, people have benefited from taking sulfonylureas, biguanides, meglitinide analogues, α-glucosidase inhibitors, and TZD with desired glucose control that has significantly reduced the risk of diabetes-related complications and improved health. In recent years, newer medications, such as Byetta and Symlin, are available, targeting specific pathophysiologic abnormalities associated with type 2 diabetes. In addition,

use of new insulin therapies (rapid-acting and long-acting insulin analogues) and noninvasive insulin delivery methods (inhaled insulin) have made it possible to improve glycemic control without an increase in hypoglycemic events along with the ability to individualize treatment.

References

[1] UKPDS 16. Overview of 6 years' therapy of type 2 diabetes: a progressive disease. Diabetes 1995;44:1249–58.
[2] Karl DM. Sulfonylureas: new thoughts about old friends. Practical Diabetology 2004;23: 26–9.
[3] Beaser RS. Pharmacotherapy of type 2 diabetes: medications to match the pathology. In: Beaser RS, staff of the Joslin Diabetes Center, editors. Joslin's diabetes deskbook: a guide for primary care providers. 2nd edition. Boston: Joslin Diabetes Center; 2003. p. 143–76.
[4] Holstein A, Plaschke A, Egberts EH. Lower incidence of severe hypoglycemia in patients with type 2 diabetes treated with glimepiride vs. glibenclamide. Diabetes Metab Rev Res 2001;17:467–73.
[5] Harmel AP, Mathur R. Oral antidiabetes agents. In: Harmel AP, Mathur R, editors. Davidson's diabetes mellitus: diagnosis and treatment. 5th edition. Philadelphia: WB Saunders; 2004. p. 71–108.
[6] King AB. A comparison in a clinical setting of the efficacy and side effects of three thiazolidinediones. Diabetes Care 2000;23:557.
[7] White JR, Campbell RK, Yarborough PC. Pharmacologic therapies. In: Franz MJ, editor. A core curriculum for diabetes educators. 5th edition. Chicago: American Association of Diabetes Educators; 2003.
[8] DeFronzo RA. Pharmacologic therapy for type 2 diabetes. Ann Intern Med 1999;131: 281–303.
[9] Drucker DJ. Enhancing incretin action for the treatment of type 2 diabetes. Diabetes Care 2004;26:2929–40.
[10] Drucker DJ. Incretin-based therapies: a clinical need filled by unique metabolic effects. Diabetes Educ 2006;32(Suppl 2):65S–71S.
[11] Siminerio L. Challenges and strategies for moving patients to injectable medications. Diabetes Educ 2006;32(Suppl 2):82S–90S.
[12] Pratley R, Galbreath E. Twelve-week monotherapy with the DDP-4 inhibitor, LAF237 improves glycemic control in patients with type 2 diabetes (T2DM). Diabetes 2004;53(Suppl 2): A83.
[13] Karl DM. Learning to use pramlintide. Practical Diabetology 2006;25:42–6.
[14] Kruger D. Symlin and Byetta: two new antihyperglycemic medications. Practical Diabetology 2006;25:49–52.
[15] Beaser RS. Using insulin to treat diabetes: general principles. In: Beaser RS, staff of the Joslin Diabetes Center, editors. Joslin's diabetes deskbook: a guide for primary care providers. 2nd edition. Boston: Joslin Diabetes Center; 2003. p. 203–32.
[16] Harmel AP, Mathur R. Insulin therapy. In: Harmel AP, Mathur R, editors. Davidson's diabetes mellitus: diagnosis and treatment. 5th edition. Philadelphia: WB Saunders; 2004. p. 109–45.
[17] Vague P, Selam JL, Skeie S, et al. Insulin detemir is associated with more predictable glycemic control and reduced risk of hypoglycemia than NPH insulin in patients with type 1 diabetes on a basal-bolus regimen with premeal insulin aspart. Diabetes Care 2003;26:590–6.
[18] Rave K, Bott S, Heinemann L, et al. Time- action profile of inhaled insulin in comparisons with subcutaneously injected insulin lispro and regular human insulin. Diabetes Care 2005; 28:1077–82.

[19] Weiss SR, Cheng SL, Kourides IA, et al. Inhaled insulin provides improved glycemic control in patients with type 2 diabetes mellitus inadequately controlled with oral agents: a randomized controlled trial. Arch Intern Med 2003;163:2277–82.
[20] Quattrin T, Belanger A, Bohannon NJ, et al. Efficacy and safety of inhaled insulin (Exubera) compared with subcutaneous insulin therapy in patients with type 1 diabetes: results of a 6-month randomized comparative trial. Diabetes Care 2004;27:2622–7.
[21] Hollander PA, Blonde L, Rowe R, et al. Efficacy and safety of inhaled insulin (Exubera) compared with subcutaneous insulin therapy in patients with type 2 diabetes: results of a 6-month, randomized, comparative trial. Diabetes Care 2004;27:2356–62.
[22] Rosenstock J, Zinman B, Murphy LJ, et al. Inhaled insulin improves glycemic control when substituted for or added to oral combination therapy in type 2 diabetes. Ann Intern Med 2005;143:549–58.

ELSEVIER
SAUNDERS

Nurs Clin N Am 41 (2006) 605–623

NURSING
CLINICS
OF NORTH AMERICA

Vulnerable Populations
with Diabetes Mellitus

Alexandra A. García, PhD, RN*,
Sandra Benavides-Vaello, RN, MPAff

School of Nursing, The University of Texas at Austin,
1700 Red River, Austin, TX 78701–1499, USA

Populations who have elevated risk or susceptibility to disease and its resulting complications are called "vulnerable." By definition they experience higher comparative mortality rates, prevalence of disease, and diminished quality of life. Vulnerable populations include members of racial and ethnic minority groups, those who are of low-income, or those who are rural-dwelling. Having few resources contributes to their lower social status and relative lack of personal, social, or political power. They may be discriminated against, marginalized or disenfranchised from mainstream society, or exposed to hazardous conditions and polluted environments [1]. Such circumstances are extra challenging for people with diabetes.

Mortality caused by diabetes is estimated at more than 8% of all deaths in the United States and Canada and 13% of deaths in Mexico [2,3]. Vulnerable populations in all three North American nations are affected disproportionately with this disease. Aboriginal populations in Canada have experienced sharp increases in type 2 diabetes over the past 20 years. Compared with other Canadian men and women, prevalence rates for aboriginal men and women were 3.6 and 5.3 times higher, respectively [4]. In the United States, non-Hispanic blacks and Mexican Americans are two times more likely than non-Hispanic whites to have been diagnosed with diabetes. American Indian, Alaska Natives, and Pacific Islanders are even more likely to have diabetes. Rates in Asian Americans also are climbing [5].

Vulnerable populations are also more likely to experience complications from diabetes than the general population. Non-Hispanic blacks are at a 50% greater risk than non-Hispanic whites of developing diabetic

---

* Corresponding author.
E-mail address: agarcia@mail.nur.utexas.edu (A.A. García).

0029-6465/06/$ - see front matter © 2006 Elsevier Inc. All rights reserved.
doi:10.1016/j.cnur.2006.07.005
nursing.theclinics.com

retinopathy; Mexican Americans and American Indians are approximately six times more likely to develop end-stage kidney disease than non-Hispanic whites. Non-Hispanic blacks and Mexican Americans are 1.8 and 2.7 times likely, respectively, to experience a lower-limb amputation than non-Hispanic whites [6].

Nurses have long been concerned for the health of the disadvantaged and underserved in both the United States and internationally. The current trend of increasing attention to the health of minority populations can be traced from the struggle for civil rights of the 1960s, the feminist movement of the 1970s, and the widening income gap during the 1980s. During the 1990s, the political debates over health care and welfare reforms drew attention to the plight of low-income and underinsured patients. In addition, the 1994 mandate from the National Institutes of Health to include women and ethnic minorities in all projects receiving National Institutes of Health funding or communicate a clear justification for their exclusion created a surge of interest in cultural competency and alleviating health disparities [7]. Since 1993, when the *Nursing Clinics of North America* published a comprehensive issue about diabetes, the term "vulnerable," as used in the context of groups of people who are at risk for poor health, has been used with increasing frequency.

In this review of the literature on vulnerable populations with diabetes, trends are identified, major findings are summarized, and strategies to fill gaps in the state of the science are recommended. For the purposes of this article, "vulnerable populations" refers to members of diverse racial and ethnic groups, people of low-income, and those who live in rural and medically underserved areas.

Method

Literature for this article was found using a search of the Medline, CINAHL, Social Science Index, Psychinfo, and PubMed computer databases with the keyword "diabetes" in combination with each of the following terms: "vulnerable," "underserved," "minority," "Hispanics," "African Americans," "black," "Native Americans," "low-income," "disadvantaged," and "rural." The search was limited to English-language articles about North American populations published in peer-reviewed journals from January 1993 to January 2006. Abstracts were searched for evidence of relevance for vulnerable populations related to their diabetes care and self-management. Review articles, essays, and commentaries were excluded.

When studying vulnerable populations it is important to recognize the diversity of members within racial and ethnic groups. For instance, among people classified as Latinos, there are variations in language, dialect, or regional terms used; religious beliefs and practices; nationality; or other socioeconomic characteristics. In addition, terminology to refer to certain populations has shifted, so among the articles reviewed, the populations

under study are referred to as "Hispanic" or "Latino," "African American" or "black," and "American Indian" or "Native American." Some studies refer to particular regions (eg, southern or southwestern) or to subgroups (eg, Mexican American, Puerto Rican, Caribbean, Hmong). When referring to individual articles, the same terms are used as by the study's authors.

Trends

One hundred sixty reports were identified that met the inclusion criteria. There are many ways to categorize the literature. For instance, one could group the studies based on method (qualitative versus quantitative, descriptive versus interventional) or subpopulation (type 1 versus type 2 or by specific racial or ethnic groups, gender, age, geographic location). All the articles cannot be addressed because of space constraints, however, so for this discussion the studies are used to illustrate major trends and topics of general emerging prominence.

Diabetes status

Glycemic control is an indicator of diabetes status and glycosylated hemoglobin A_{1c} levels are recognized as the gold standard of diabetes control measurements [8]. Several researchers have searched for correlates and predictors of hemoglobin A_{1c} levels with mixed results. In general, lower (better) hemoglobin A_{1c} levels have been associated with medication adherence; white race (compared with African Americans); lower intensity of drug therapy [9]; internal locus of control [10]; more diabetes knowledge [11]; and higher acculturation levels [12]. Among African Americans, however, researchers found no relationship among ethnic identity, self-identification, or self-care behaviors and hemoglobin A_{1c} levels [13].

Higher (worse) hemoglobin A_{1c} levels have been linked to not having insurance, having diabetes for longer duration, using insulin or multiple oral medications, having high cholesterol, being of younger age [14], and having less access to medical care [15]. Age, however, may not be a reliable predictor because hemoglobin A_{1c} levels may fluctuate more over time in older participants [14]. The predictors and correlates of hemoglobin A_{1c} are similar across members of various ethnic or racial groups.

Vulnerable populations generally have higher hemoglobin A_{1c} levels than their non-Hispanic white counterparts. For example, the mean hemoglobin A_{1c} level in a sample of African American women was 10.8% [16] and among two Mexican American samples mean hemoglobin A_{1c} levels were over 11% [17,18], all significantly higher than the 7% level recommended by the American Diabetes Association [19].

Another important indicator of diabetes status is quality of life. Among low-income patients with diabetes, having low hemoglobin A_{1c}, cholesterol, and blood pressure predicted higher quality of life scores in physical, mental,

and sexual domains. Those with complaints about legs and feet, low self-rated vision, and higher perceived hassles in self-management tended to have worse quality of life. Overall, minorities have lower quality of life scores compared with the general population [20,21]. Young Hispanic and black adults with diabetes reported that diabetes negatively affected their family lives (eg, difficulty securing child care or securing a job) and affected their personal lives (eg, ability to participate in sports or having difficulty obtaining insurance) [22].

Perceptions and beliefs

Several researchers used focus groups and individual interviews to explore feelings, experiences, or opinions about diabetes held by various vulnerable groups. Mostly women participated in the focus groups, although men and women were more equally represented in studies using individual interviews.

These types of qualitative methods have made a significant contribution to the understanding of patients' explanatory models, or their personal beliefs of illness cause and treatment. They showed participants' belief systems were composed of a blend of biomedical, folk, personal, and cultural beliefs [22–40]. Participants' knowledge of diabetes and its management came largely from interactions with family and friends rather than from the materials provided by health care providers. Even so, they considered the health care provider's attention to their diagnosis and therapy important [27]. Participants' complex explanatory paradigms are also evidenced by their use of alternative therapies, such as herbal remedies, in combination with standard medical therapies, such as medications, to manage type 2 diabetes [28,33,35].

The studies reveal that participants do not entirely embrace medical therapies nor are all health care providers entirely open to their patients' explanatory models of diabetes and its management. In particular, some providers seem unacquainted with the daily contextual realities of living with diabetes. For example, making changes in dietary habits is a major challenge for people with diabetes and is a common point of contention between the patient, family, and health care provider [30,34]. Health care providers viewed nonadherence to standard diabetes dietary guidelines as willful noncompliance or an inability of the patient to exert control of their blood glucose levels [29], whereas African American focus group participants described their frustration with health care providers who did not seem to understand their financial and social constraints to professional care and self-care [39,40].

For African American and Hispanic participants stress was an important aspect of their diabetes. They perceived stress as cause of their diabetes [26,33,36], in response to the diagnosis [36,41], or related to the complex day-to-day management of diabetes [41–43]. Those under stress cited the importance of religious practices or spiritual guidance for coping [36,41–43].

The qualitative studies illustrate the interrelationships of patients' health beliefs, attitudes toward diabetes, and their adherence to diabetes therapy across ethnic and social groups [24,26,30,34,35]. Women were found to have more elaborate and intricate beliefs about diabetes, treatment, and management than men; women's descriptions of diabetes and its progression were detailed and comprehensive [24].

Participants' knowledge about diabetes, its symptoms, therapies, and ways to prevent or mitigate complications varied among the samples. Some had a proficient understanding of diabetes [38], although most others did not clearly understand particular aspects of diabetes management, such as insulin therapy, or the role of lifestyle behaviors in preventing diabetes or attenuating its effects [24,27,31].

Diabetes knowledge has been recognized as an important first step in making recommended behavioral modifications to manage diabetes, although it is generally acknowledged that knowledge alone is not sufficient to inspire behavioral modification [8,44]. None of the studies addressed the prerequisite threshold for diabetes knowledge or specific topics one should have mastery of to self-manage diabetes effectively. Rather, the studies examined correlates of scores on knowledge tests. They found having more education, previous diabetes education, being older [11,45], having a higher income, and being white predicted higher levels of diabetes-related knowledge [46]. Aside from learning in formal diabetes educational settings, African American women were more likely to get diabetes information through religious networks and by the television or radio than white women, who more frequently gained information by informal networks of friends and family [46].

Self-efficacy, or one's level of confidence to carry out a particular behavior, is believed to be an important predictor of diabetes self-management. Only three reports, however, focused on self-efficacy in vulnerable populations with diabetes. Bernal and colleagues [47] found Puerto Ricans on insulin had low to average self-efficacy rating across aspects of diabetes management. Lowest scores were for behaviors that needed problem resolution during evolving circumstances. Speaking English, having had diabetes education, and home visits from nurses were associated with higher self-efficacy, especially for diet and insulin administration. Skelly and coworkers [48] cautioned that self-efficacy levels were not consistent over time for all behaviors, making them an unreliable predictor of behavior. Whittemore and colleagues [49], however, found the perceptions of higher confidence in living with diabetes correlated with lower hemoglobin A_{1c} levels.

Symptoms

Diabetes symptoms, although often vague and attributable to multiple conditions, are an area of growing interest because they correlate with quality of life and hemoglobin A_{1c} levels [50–52]. In two Mexican American samples, most (97%–99%) reported having had symptoms, although most did

not view them as serious or check their glucose level in response to symptoms; women were more apt to report symptoms [50,51].

The number of symptoms reported seems to be a function of the number of symptoms listed on the questionnaire. Samples of Mexican Americans reported having an average of six symptoms (range 0–15) [50] and four symptoms from a shorter list (range 0–10) [51]. A sample of white (29%), Hispanic (47%), and "other" patients reported an average of 5 out of 22 symptoms [52]. African American women reported an average of four symptoms (range from 1–12). Among them the women who experienced symptoms of neuropathy, peripheral vascular disease, or visual changes reported worse general health, mental health role performance, social functioning, and bodily pain [21]. Some participants believed the absence of symptoms meant they were in good control of their disease. Others found some symptoms to be too complicated to construe, especially in the presence of comorbid conditions [38,53].

Skelly and colleagues [54] pilot tested a symptom-focused intervention for African American women in rural North Carolina. In their study 23 women received four home visits from nurses who delivered educational modules that addressed symptom interpretation and management. Women in both intervention and control groups improved their hemoglobin A_{1c} levels from baseline, although the intervention group had lower levels than the controls. The intervention also significantly improved symptom distress, diabetes knowledge, and quality of life suggesting further work in this area is warranted.

Mental health

Few articles address mental health in vulnerable populations with diabetes even though depressive symptoms are associated with increases in diabetes complications. In addition, depressive symptoms are related to poor adherence to diabetes treatment [55]. Approximately 30% of persons with diabetes also experience depression. Having diabetes increases the odds of experiencing depression by more than 50% [56]. There are few published interventions, however, for members of vulnerable populations who have both diabetes and depression. Bell and colleagues [57] noted that rural older adults with diabetes (including African Americans, Native Americans, and whites) are all at risk for depression. In their sample nearly 16% had depressive symptoms. Women, unmarried people, those with less than high school education, those on Medicaid, those with more than five prescription medications, and those with five or more chronic conditions were more likely to report symptoms of depression.

Self-management behaviors

Based on the recognition that all patients, particularly members of vulnerable populations, find diabetes self-management a challenge, researchers

have explored factors that might explain and predict their glucose self-monitoring, diet, physical activity, medications, and stress-management behaviors. Factors that predict rates of self-monitoring of blood glucose in vulnerable populations include being prescribed a diabetes medication regimen, having received instructions from health care providers on how to test and what the results mean, and being told to test glucose. Needing help to test was negatively associated with testing [58]. Rates of self-monitoring of blood glucose increased with income level and insulin use [59–61]. It is unclear if testing rates differ across ethnic groups. Skelly and coworkers [58] reported self-monitoring of blood glucose rates was similar for African Americans and Native Americans, although Miller and coworkers [61] found that African Americans reported more testing than whites.

Comparatively few studies identified in the search addressed correlates of physical activity in vulnerable populations with diabetes. Just over half of Mexican Americans with diabetes in the third National Health and Nutrition Examination Survey said they participated in leisure activities. About one third preferred gardening and walking. More men exercised than women. Almost 40% did not engage in any leisure time physical activity but those who enjoyed three or more leisure activities used only oral medication or none to control diabetes [62].

By contrast, dietary influences were commonly measured. Barriers to following healthy diets for diabetes identified by African Americans were having a low income; time constraints; competing demands; knowledge deficits [63], particularly regarding portion size; and costs [40]. Although many African American women named healthy foods they had eaten during a dietary recall, with prompting they admitted to adding fats after cooking [63]. Eating out of the home is often cited as a barrier; African American women ate mostly at fast food restaurants, consumed mostly high-fat foods, and did not recognize that salads prepared outside the home are often prepared with high-fat dressings [63]. African Americans in Michigan perceived that following a moderate diet was more burdensome than taking oral medications and following a strict diet was as burdensome as being on insulin therapy [40].

Older Hispanic adults perceived fewer barriers to diet self-care if they had family support for the diet [64]. Women, in particular, described difficulties adhering to dietary recommendations when their families preferred other foods [25,27,30,34,36,43,63].

Social support

Vulnerable populations comprise people from collectivist cultures, such as Latinos, African Americans, and Native Americans for whom family ties and social support are believed to be essential for effective diabetes self-management. Researchers of the past 6 years have used descriptive

quantitative methods to explore the role of social support among these groups. For example, Gleeson-Kreig and colleagues [65] found that although Hispanics had large social networks, they reported needing help with transportation, interpretation during interactions with English-speaking health care providers, financial assistance, and personal diabetes care.

Fisher and colleagues [66] explored family characteristics (family structure or organization, family world views, and family emotion management) that might influence disease management among European Americans and Latinos. For both groups sex role was related to diabetes self-management but for European Americans family world view and emotion management were related to disease management and for Latinos family structure was important. In a separate study Fisher and coworkers [67] investigated how Latino and European American couples resolve disagreements about diabetes management to predict how well their diabetes is managed over time. They found Latino couples were significantly closer emotionally and were less avoidant and hostile, and Latino patients were less dominant than European Americans but they achieved less problem resolution and were more often off-task.

Diabetes self-management education

Members of vulnerable populations often do not receive diabetes education, and when they do, they are less likely to benefit from conventional diabetes self-management programs [68]. Several groups have designed and tested culturally specific diabetes self-management interventions aimed at overcoming barriers and improving lifestyle and disease outcomes for Native Americans [69], African Americans [70,71], and Mexican Americans [17,18,72,73]. Culturally specific interventions developed or adapted for vulnerable populations incorporate culturally preferred foods, traditional practices, preferences for learning styles, health beliefs, meaningful symbols and messages, and build on available resources. Focus groups were commonly used to plan, modify, or evaluate interventions and materials [74–77].

Although most educational interventions were conducted at the individual level, a few addressed families and larger communities. Diabetes self-management education programs were delivered in various settings and formats including clinic [78] or community settings (churches, schools, or homes) [17,18,54,77–79]; group or individual sessions, led by nurses, dietitians, or pharmacists [80], some who were certified diabetes educators; or assisted by community health workers (also called lay advisors, peer advisors, or promotoras).

Community health workers are usually volunteers recruited from the target population who live in the same neighborhoods and are trained to increase outreach into the community, provide education, and facilitate access to health services. In typical interventions community health workers make home visits and telephone contacts to increase diabetes awareness,

encourage glucose self-monitoring and behavioral self-management, serve as resource persons, facilitate access to community resources and medical assistance, link participants with providers, measure blood pressures, and do foot examinations [81–83]. Community health workers were effective in keeping participants enrolled in a certified diabetes educators–led educational program [84]. Community health workers were also used to supplement or enhance self-management programs. For instance, in the New Leaf...Choices for Healthy Living with Diabetes program [78], community health workers acted as a resource to program participants, provided social support and feedback, reinforced information, maintained contact with participants, and assisted dietitians to facilitate group educational and support sessions.

One innovative program for African Americans in Detroit offered diabetes self-management education sessions on an ongoing basis. The curriculum was set by the participants. This type of model shows promise for future interventions because it allows the learners to meet their individual learning needs. Few other tailored programs were found for diabetes patients. The program, based on an empowerment model, was effective in decreasing body mass index, lipid levels, and self-care behaviors [85].

Patient-provider interactions

Quality of care for vulnerable populations is typically lower than for mainstream populations. For instance, among patients in Nashville, African Americans had less access to care than whites and were more likely to have hypertension, take insulin, and never have had an eye examination [61].

Health care providers measure hemoglobin A_{1c} levels in underserved populations less frequently than is recommended. Other indicators of diabetes service quality are also lower. For example, fewer African Americans than whites in South Carolina reported receiving recommended hemoglobin A_{1c} tests or nutrition education [86]. In New York, Puerto Ricans were less likely than the general state population with diabetes to have hemoglobin A_{1c} levels tested or receive pneumococcal vaccines even though they were no less likely to see a provider for diabetes monitoring at least four times per year [87]. African Americans in North Carolina were more likely than whites to have a nephropathy assessment; minorities in general were more likely to have a blood pressure test than whites but had worse blood pressures [59]. African Americans were more likely than whites or members of other minority groups to see a foot specialist [88]. Minorities, low-income, and those with complex medical problems were less likely than whites to get lipid levels tested [89].

Patient-provider interactions seem to be an important component of diabetes care that can profoundly influence whether and to what degree patients engage in diabetes self-management. Among medically underserved patients in North Carolina, higher levels of patient trust in doctors were

related to fewer hassles in changing behaviors related to self-management tasks [90]. Studies of patient provider interactions reveal that 14% of diabetes patients (51% were racial and ethnic minorities) reported they had experienced discrimination from their health care providers or their office staff in the prior year because of race or ethnicity, age, sex, or socioeconomic status. Patients who reported discrimination experiences had higher hemoglobin A_{1c} ratings [91]. Piette and coworkers [92] found minority group patients and those of low socioeconomic status rated patient-provider communications as good as or better than other patients. Patients perceived their providers to be good communicators in general but rated them lower on diabetes-specific information related to foot self-care frequency, adherence to diabetes medications, diet, and exercise. Improving patient provider interactions may help patients improve their self-care.

About 12% of Medicaid recipients in New York State were dissatisfied with their diabetes care, information received from their providers, or their health plan. Predictors of their dissatisfaction were being in poor general health, having little patient education, difficulty obtaining diabetes care, and not performing diabetes self-management behaviors [93].

Some service interventions modified the health care infrastructure by practice, such as hiring diabetes educators, gaining support of key administrators, educating staff and patients, purchasing laboratory equipment, implementing reminder call systems or call back systems for missed appointments, using an electronic registry to track changes, and implementing treatment algorithms to guide treatment [94].

Other efforts have focused on making changes in the care delivery. One example is the use of nurses as diabetes nurse case managers in Project Dulce [95,96] with predominantly Hispanic patients in San Diego. The nurse case managers were effective in reducing patients' hemoglobin A_{1c}, blood pressure, and lipid levels without increasing overall health care costs. Another example, Project Sugar, used teams of nurse case managers and community health workers with African Americans in Baltimore with similar results [97].

A recent trend in service delivery is to offer group physician visits. During group visits several patients with similar diagnoses or health issues share an appointment in which they receive physical examinations and group health teaching from a multidisciplinary team. Group visits have been effective in improving standards of care, provider-client relations [98], and mental health but not necessarily clinical outcomes [99].

Advancements of the last decade have increased the availability of technologic resources, such as video-conferencing, for underserved, primarily rural populations. Telemedicine services provide underserved patients access to health examinations and consultation [100]. Piette and colleagues [101,102] evaluated the effectiveness and acceptability of automated telephone calls for diabetes disease management. The biweekly calls requested patients to respond by the telephone touch pad to assessment questions about glucose readings, symptoms, change in health status, and behaviors.

After the assessment patients could elect to hear brief diabetes educational messages. A nurse used reports from the telephone calls to follow-up with patients. Following this intervention participants reported fewer problems with self-monitoring and self-management behaviors, and fewer symptoms. Although not significantly different, hemoglobin A_{1c} levels were lower for intervention participants than controls. These technologic innovations show promise to bring health care expertise to underserved areas.

Research tools and educational materials

Qualitative studies can serve as a good basis for developing surveys and educational materials for use with members of vulnerable populations. Researchers have used focus groups to elicit the way respondents conceptualize and talk about issues and identify phrases and images that are meaningful to those groups [103,104]. Of note is Rosal and colleagues' [105] use of cognitive interviewing, a technique used to evaluate the meaning of survey items and response choices to the participants who complete them. Cognitive interviewing is recommended by the National Center for Health Statistics [106] as part of the development and testing process for all new and modified questionnaires. Rosal and coworkers [105] used cognitive interviewing to ensure literal and conceptual equivalence of a questionnaire modified from English for Spanish speakers.

Developing and disseminating culturally relevant, reliable, and valid instruments for vulnerable populations with diabetes is essential for advancing the knowledge base. Three questionnaires developed or adapted for the Starr County Diabetes Project, the Diabetes Knowledge Questionnaire, the Diabetes Symptom Checklist, and the Diabetes Health Beliefs Questionnaire [45,50,107], were used in the study from 1995 to 2004 and were among the few instruments available for Spanish-speaking populations at the start of the project. Since then, many more instruments have been adapted for Spanish-speakers and tested for evidence of their reliability and validity.

Several surveys and educational materials were adapted for low-literacy groups including English speakers. For instance, the Spoken Knowledge in Low Literacy in Diabetes Scale [108] was developed for oral administration; data collectors code responses to questions addressing basic diabetes self-management based on preset criteria. The Behavioral Checklist [109] is one example of a self-management tool designed for low-literacy English and Spanish speakers.

Intervention planning

Intervention studies can either be clinical research trials that examine whether new behavioral or biomedical interventions are feasible, effective, or acceptable, or they can be nonresearch programs, conducted to improve service delivery. Most clinical trials were initiated by an academic researcher to investigate a new approach to diabetes self-management education. The

authors saw a trend, particularly among the nonresearch programs, for collaboratory projects that emphasize equal participation with the targeted community. These intervention-planning strategies included community organization, development of an advisory board, setting joint priorities and mutual goals, community assessments, data collection and analysis, and program delivery [110,111]. Notable examples include the federally funded projects Border Health ¡Si! [82]; the REACH project 2010 (Racial and Ethnic Approaches to Community Health) [112]; and Project DIRECT (Diabetes Interventions Reaching and Educating Communities Together) [113]. These multifaceted programs aim to increase awareness and screening of diabetes, promote health, and administer diabetes care according to national clinical practice guidelines on a community-wide scale.

Recommendations

Based on the literature on vulnerable populations with diabetes mellitus, it is difficult to determine whether differences in health care attitudes, practices, and status are caused by specific ethnic and cultural priorities or whether they are caused by the effects of low income and social class. Whatever the reason, health care services are likely to be less effective when people feel their circumstances are not understood by those trying to help them. Researchers and clinicians should aim to develop individualized treatment plans for their patients' particular circumstances.

To that end, researchers and intervention providers should continue to monitor the perspective of vulnerable populations using qualitative studies. Findings from qualitative studies serve to remind health care providers of what patients experience and keep research and practice perspectives fresh. Focus groups assist in building communities of research where the participants are treated with deference and are valued for their knowledge. When researchers interact with community members at personal levels, they are able build rapport and gain trust, insight, visibility, and credibility to enhance the validity of research. Clinicians should also elicit the patients' perspectives as a means of gaining trust and building effective care plans. Perhaps health care cultures need to merge clinical expectations with patients' wisdom. For instance, biomedical research on the effects of stress may soon validate the perceptions of many patients who believe their diabetes was caused by susto, a sudden fright, strong emotion, or stress. Perhaps then we can have a health care infrastructure that resonates with those it is trying to assist, and consequently an effective system of care.

Health care providers who view patients from vulnerable populations as necessarily weak tend to reinforce negative stereotypes. When providers unilaterally develop treatment plans, they can contribute to an individual patient's and their vulnerable group's marginalization. Participatory approaches help unite patients and health care providers in common goals. An important strategy is to create more opportunities for members of

vulnerable populations to become health care professionals and researchers who contribute to efforts to bridge communication or cultural gaps. How else can one create interventions that tap into vulnerable populations' strengths, change health care culture, and advance the status of vulnerable populations?

Providers may be disappointed to find using participatory approaches often requires time-intensive and complex solutions. Tensions can rise when providers and patients seem to work at cross-purposes. Providers encourage patients' participation in decision-making hoping that will lead to patients' embracement of and adherence to the providers' treatment recommendations. As one provider remarked, "We struggle with empowering clients who seem to avoid responsibility for their own actions" [114]. Patients may feel so empowered, however, that they choose not adhere to recommended treatments or accept biomedical rationale for treatment. Certainly, patients do not always make wise decisions for themselves. They may misunderstand providers' recommendations, unilaterally decide to modify, or even discontinue important aspects of their treatment. Further work is needed to explore what the goals of participation and empowerment are and how to foster both and attain healthful outcomes.

Other solutions should include family- and community-level interventions to support diabetes self-management behaviors. Diet, exercise, and stress management all affect the family grouping and family members can support or hinder patients' self-care. Community-wide efforts aimed at health promotion facilitate individuals and families' self-management practices. For instance, all members of a community benefit from urban planning that ensures grocery stores with fresh foods are convenient and affordable. Other programs might make human-powered transportation more accessible and acceptable; create and maintain parks for family leisure activities; and establish more convenient health care systems (perhaps open during nontraditional days or hours, sending reminders to patients and providing holistic care). Diabetes self-management strategies should be communicated using a variety of messages by multiple media (eg, printed, Internet, mass communications, television, and radio) to reach the community at large.

Since 1993 several self-management interventions have been effective in changing behaviors and at times lowering hemoglobin A_{1c} levels, although these outcomes are often not sustained over time. Diabetes self-management education must be made available on an ongoing basis to reinforce effective behaviors and to provide updates as new information becomes available. As identified in the literature, multiple interventions have been developed in concert with various communities of vulnerable populations. These interventions must be translated into practice and made available to the most vulnerable groups on a large-scale and long-term basis.

In their 2003 publication Unequal Treatment, The National Academy of Science's Institute of Medicine called attention to health disparities

experienced by minority groups. The publication asserts that long-standing, pervasive, institutionalized practices designed to fit the majority overlook the circumstances of minority and low-income populations and place them at increased risk for poor health. The Institute of Medicine recommended several strategies to improve access and quality of care for vulnerable populations [115], many of which are reflected in the literature on vulnerable populations with diabetes mellitus. Researchers and health care providers must continue their efforts to ensure that all patients receive not merely an equitable share of health care services but that they all receive the best diabetes care possible.

References

[1] Flaskerud JH, Winslow BJ. Conceptualizing vulnerable populations health-related research. Nurs Res 1998;47:69–79.

[2] Roglic G, Unwin N, Bennett PH, et al. The burden of mortality attributable to diabetes: realistic estimates for the year 2000. Diabetes Care 2005;28:2130–5.

[3] Pan American Health Organization. Mexico. Available at: http://www.paho.org/English/sha/prflmex.htm. Accessed February 1, 2006.

[4] Young TK, Reading J, Elias B, et al. Type 2 diabetes mellitus in Canada's First Nations: status of an epidemic in progress. CMAJ 2000;163:561–6.

[5] American Diabetes Association. Diabetes statistics. Available at: http://www.diabetes.org/diabetes-statistics/prevalence.jsp. Accessed February 1, 2006.

[6] American Diabetes Association. Diabetes statistics. Available at: http://www.diabetes.org/diabetes-statistics/complications.jsp. Accessed February 1, 2006.

[7] Flaskerud JH, Lesser J, Dixon E, et al. Health disparities among vulnerable populations: evolution of knowledge over five decades in Nursing Research publications. Nurs Res 2002;51:74–85.

[8] Glasgow RE. Outcomes of and for diabetes education research. Diabetes Educ 1999; 25(6 Suppl):74–88.

[9] Schectman JM, Nadkarni MM, Voss JD. The association between diabetes metabolic control and drug adherence in an indigent population. Diabetes Care 2002;25: 1015–21.

[10] Montague MC, Nichols SA, Dutta AP. Self-management in African American women with diabetes. Diabetes Educ 2005;31:700–11.

[11] Bautista-Martinez S, Alberto C, Aguilar-Salinas CA, et al. Diabetes knowledge and its determinants in a Mexican population. Diabetes Educ 1999;25:374–81.

[12] Brown SA, Harrist R, Villagomez ET, et al. Gender and treatment differences in knowledge, health beliefs, and metabolic control in Mexican Americans with type 2 diabetes. Diabetes Educ 2000;26:425–38.

[13] de Groot M, Buckland GT III, Fergus M, et al. Cultural orientation and diabetes self-care in low-income African Americans with type 2 diabetes mellitus. Ethn Dis 2003;13: 6–14.

[14] Benoit SR, Fleming R, Philis-Tsimikas A, et al. Predictors of glycemic control among patients with type 2 diabetes: a longitudinal study. BMC Public Health [serial online]. April 17, 2005;5:36. Available at: http://www.biomedcentral.com/1471-2458/5/36. Accessed February 6, 2006.

[15] Rhee MK, Cook CB, Dunbar VG, et al. Limited health care access impairs glycemic control in low socioeconomic status urban African Americans with type 2 diabetes. J Health Care Poor Underserved 2003;16:734–46.

[16] Rimmer JH, Silverman K, Braunschweig C, et al. Feasibility of a health promotion program intervention for a group of predominantly African American women with type 2 diabetes. Diabetes Educ 2002;28:571–80.

[17] Brown SA, García AA, Kouzekanani K, et al. Culturally competent diabetes self-management education for Mexican Americans: the Starr County border health initiative. Diabetes Care 2002;25:259–68.

[18] Brown SA, Blozis SA, Kouzekanani KK, et al. Dosage effects of diabetes self-management education for Mexican Americans. Diabetes Care 2005;28:527–32.

[19] American Diabetes Association. Standards of medical care in diabetes: 2006. Diabetes Care 2006;29(Suppl 1):S4–42.

[20] Camacho F, Anderson RT, Bell RA, et al. Investigating correlates of health related quality of life in a low-income sample of patients with diabetes. Qual Life Res 2002;11: 783–96.

[21] Stover JC, Skelly AH, Holditch-Davis D, et al. Perceptions of health and their relationship to symptoms in African American women with type 2 diabetes. Appl Nurs Res 2001;14: 72–80.

[22] Lipton R, Drum M, Burnet D, et al. Self-reported social class, self-management behaviors and the effect of diabetes mellitus in urban, minority young people and their families. Arch Pediatr Adolesc Med 2003;157:919–25.

[23] Alcozer F. Secondary analysis of perceptions and meanings of type 2 diabetes in Mexican American women. Diabetes Educ 2000;26:785–95.

[24] Arcury TA, Skelly AH, Gesler WM, et al. Diabetes beliefs among low-income, white residents of a rural North Carolina community. J Rural Health 2005;21:337–45.

[25] Carter-Edwards L, Skelly AH, Cagle SC, et al. "They care but don't understand": family support of African American women with type 2 diabetes. Diabetes Educ 2004;30: 493–501.

[26] Coronado GD, Thompson B, Tejeda S, et al. Attitudes and beliefs among Mexican Americans about type 2 diabetes. J Health Care Poor Underserved 2004;15:576–88.

[27] Dietrich UC. Factors influencing the attitudes held by women with type II diabetes: a qualitative study. Patient Educ Couns 1996;29:13–23.

[28] Hunt LM, Arar NH, Akana LL. Herbs, prayer and insulin: use of medical and alternative treatments by a group of Mexican American diabetes patients. J Fam Pract 2000;49:216–23.

[29] Hunt LM, Arar NH, Larme AC. Contrasting patient and practitioner perspectives in type 2 diabetes management. West J Nurs Res 1998;20:656–82.

[30] Hunt LM, Pugh J, Valenzuela M. How patients adapt diabetes self-care recommendations in everyday life. J Fam Pract 1998;46:207–15.

[31] Hunt LM, Valenzuela MA, Pugh JA. NIDDM patients' fears and hopes about insulin therapy. Diabetes Care 1997;20:292–8.

[32] Hunt LM, Valenzuela MA, Pugh JA. Porque me toco a mi? Mexican American diabetes patients' causal stories and their relationship to treatment behaviors. Soc Sci Med 1998; 46:959–69.

[33] Jezewski MA, Poss J. Mexican Americans' explanatory models of type 2 diabetes. West J Nurs Res 2002;24:840–58.

[34] Maillet NA, Melkus GD, Spollett G. Using focus groups to characterize the health beliefs and practices of black women with non-insulin-dependent diabetes. Diabetes Educ 1996;22: 39–46.

[35] Poss JE, Jezewski MA, Stuart AG. Home remedies for type 2 diabetes used by Mexican Americans in El Paso, Texas. Clin Nurs Res 2003;12:304–23.

[36] Rivera Adams C. Lessons learned from urban Latinas with type 2 diabetes mellitus. J Transcult Nurs 2003;14:255–65.

[37] Struthers R, Hodge FS, Geishirt-Cantrell B, et al. Participant experiences of talking circles on type 2 diabetes in two Northern Plains American Indian tribes. Qual Health Res 2003; 13:1094–115.

[38] Weller SC, Baer RD, Pachter LM, et al. Latino beliefs about diabetes. Diabetes Care 1999;
     22:722–8.
[39] Wenzel J, Utz SW, Steeves R, et al. "Plenty of sickness": descriptions by African Americans
     living in rural areas with type 2 diabetes. Diabetes Educ 2005;31:98–107.
[40] Vijan S, Stuart NS, Fitzgerald JT, et al. Barriers to following dietary recommendations in
     type 2 diabetes. Diabet Med 2005;22:32–8.
[41] Cagle CS, Appel S, Skelly AH, et al. Mid-life African American women with type 2 diabe-
     tes: influence on work and the multicaregiver role. Ethn Dis 2002;12:555–66.
[42] Egede LE, Bonadonna RJ. Diabetes self-management in African Americans: an explora-
     tion of the role of fatalism. Diabetes Educ 2003;29:105–15.
[43] Samuel-Hodge CD, Headen SW, Skelly AH, et al. Influences on day-to-day self-man-
     agement of type 2 diabetes among African American women. Diabetes Care 2000;23:
     928–33.
[44] Fain JA. Diabetes education outcomes: advancing the role of the diabetes educator. Diabe-
     tes Educ 2000;26:357.
[45] García AA, Villagomez ET, Brown SA, et al. The Starr County Diabetes Education Study:
     development of the Spanish-language diabetes knowledge questionnaire. Diabetes Care
     2001;24:16–21.
[46] Schoenberg NE, Amey CH, Coward RT. Diabetes knowledge and sources of infor-
     mation among African American and white older women. Diabetes Educ 1998;4:
     319–24.
[47] Bernal H, Woolley S, Schensul JJ, et al. Correlates of self-efficacy in diabetes self-care
     among Hispanic adults with diabetes. Diabetes Educ 2000;26:673–80.
[48] Skelly AH, Marshall JR, Haughey BP, et al. Self-efficacy and confidence in outcomes as de-
     terminants of self-care practices in inner-city, African-American women with non-insulin-
     dependent diabetes. Diabetes Educ 1995;21:38–46.
[49] Whittemore R, Melkus GD, Grey M. Metabolic control, self-management and psychoso-
     cial adjustment in women with type 2 diabetes. J Clin Nurs 2005;14:195–203.
[50] Brown SA, Upchurch SA, García AA, et al. Symptom-related self-care of Mexican Amer-
     icans with type 2 diabetes: preliminary finding of the Starr County Diabetes Education
     Study. Diabetes Educ 1998;24:331–9.
[51] García AA. Symptom prevalence and treatments among Mexican Americans with type 2
     diabetes. Diabetes Educ 2005;31:543–54.
[52] Lange LJ, Piette JD. Perceived health status and perceived diabetes control: psychological
     indicators and accuracy. J Psychosom Res 2005;58:129–37.
[53] Phinney A, Wallhagen M. Recognizing and understanding the symptoms of type 2 diabetes.
     Can J Nurs Res 2003;35:108–24.
[54] Skelly AH, Carlson JR, Leeman J, et al. Symptom-focused management for African-Amer-
     ican women with type 2 diabetes: a pilot study. Appl Nurs Res 2005;18:213–20.
[55] Ciechanowski PS, Katon WJ, Russo JE. Depression and diabetes: impact of depressive
     symptoms on adherence, function, and costs. Arch Intern Med 2000;160:3278–85.
[56] Anderson RJ, Freedland KE, Clouse RE, et al. The prevalence of comorbid depression in
     adults with diabetes: a meta-analysis. Diabetes Care 2001;24:1069–78.
[57] Bell RA, Smith SL, Arcury TA, et al. Prevalence and correlates of depression symptoms
     among rural older African Americans, Native Americans, and whites with diabetes. Diabe-
     tes Care 2005;28:823–9.
[58] Skelly AH, Arcury TA, Snively BM, et al. Self-monitoring of blood glucose in a multiethnic
     population of rural older adults with diabetes. Diabetes Educ 2005;31:84–90.
[59] Bell RA, Camacho F, Goonan K, et al. Quality of diabetes care among low-income patients
     in North Carolina. Am J Prev Med 2001;21:124–31.
[60] Lipton R, Losey L, Giachello AL, et al. Factors affecting diabetes treatment and patient
     education among Latinos: results of a preliminary study in Chicago. J Med Syst 1996;20:
     267–76.

[61] Miller ST, Schlundt DG, Larson C, et al. Exploring ethnic disparities in diabetes, diabetes care, and lifestyle behaviors: the Nashville REACH 2010 community baseline survey. Ethn Dis 2004;14:38–44.
[62] Wood FG. Leisure time activity of Mexican Americans with diabetes. J Adv Nurs 2004;45: 190–6.
[63] Gallaso P, Amend A, Melkus GD, et al. Barriers to medical nutrition therapy in black women with type 2 diabetes mellitus. Diabetes Educ 2005;31:719–25.
[64] Wen LK, Parchman ML, Shepherd MD. Family support and diet barriers among older Hispanic adults with type 2 diabetes. Fam Med 2004;36:423–30.
[65] Gleeson-Kreig J, Bernal H, Woolley S. The role of social support in the self-management of diabetes mellitus among a Hispanic population. Public Health Nurs 2002;19:215–22.
[66] Fisher L, Chesla CA, Skaff MA, et al. The family and disease management in Hispanic and European-American patients with type 2 diabetes. Diabetes Care 2000;23: 267–72.
[67] Fisher L, Gudmundsdottir M, Gillis C, et al. Resolving disease management problems in European-American and Latino couples with type 2 diabetes: the effects of ethnicity and patient gender. Fam Process 2000;39:403–16.
[68] Glasgow RE, Hiss RG, Anderson RM, et al. Report of the health care delivery work group: behavioral research related to the establishment of a chronic disease model for diabetes care. Diabetes Care 2001;24:124–30.
[69] Gilliand SS, Azen SP, Perez GE, et al. Strong in body and spirit: lifestyle intervention for Native American adults with diabetes in New Mexico. Diabetes Care 2002;25: 78–83.
[70] Anderson-Loftin W, Barnett S, Sullivan P, et al. Culturally competent dietary education for southern rural African Americans with diabetes. Diabetes Educ 2002;28:245–57.
[71] Anderson-Loftin W, Barnett S, Bunn P, et al. Soul food light: culturally competent diabetes education. Diabetes Educ 2005;31:555–63.
[72] Brown SA, Hanis CL. Culturally competent diabetes education for Mexican Americans: the Starr County study. Diabetes Educ 1999;25:226–36.
[73] Rosal MC, Olendzki B, Reed GW, et al. Diabetes self-management among low-income Spanish-speaking patients: a pilot study. Ann Behav Med 2005;29:225–35.
[74] Anderson RM, Goddard CE, García R, et al. Using focus groups to identify diabetes care and education issues for Latinos with diabetes. Diabetes Educ 1998;24:618–25.
[75] Benavides-Vaello S, García AA, Brown SA, et al. Using focus groups to plan and evaluation diabetes self-management interventions for Mexican Americans. Diabetes Educ 2004; 30:238,242–56.
[76] Blanchard MA, Rose LE, Taylor J, et al. Using a focus group to design a diabetes education program for an African American population. Diabetes Educ 1999;25:917–24.
[77] Rosal MC, Goins KV, Carbone ET, et al. Views and preferences of low-literate Hispanics regarding diabetes education: results of formative research. Health Educ Behav 2004;31: 388–405.
[78] Keyserling TC, Samuel-Hodge CD, Ammerman AS, et al. A randomized trial of an intervention to improve self-care behaviors of African-American women with type 2 diabetes. Diabetes Care 2002;25:1576–83.
[79] Mazzuca KB, Farris NA, Mendenhall J, et al. Demonstrating the added value of community health nursing for clients with insulin-dependent diabetes. J Community Health Nurs 1997;14:211–24.
[80] Rothman RL, Malone R, Bryant B, et al. A randomized trial of a primary care-based disease management program to improve cardiovascular risk factors and glycated hemoglobin levels in patients with diabetes. Am J Med 2005;118:276–84.
[81] Fedder DO, Chang RJ, Curry S, et al. The effectiveness of a community health worker outreach program on healthcare utilization of West Baltimore City Medicaid patients with diabetes, with or without hypertension. Ethn Dis 2003;13:22–7.

[82] Ingram M, Gallegos G, Elenes J. Diabetes is a community issue: the elements of a successful outreach and education model on the US-Mexico border. Prev Chronic Dis [serial online]. January 2005:2. Available at: http://www.cec.gov/pcd/issues/2005/jan/04_0078.htm. Accessed December 9, 2005.

[83] Teufel-Shone NI, Drummond R, Rawiel U. Developing and adapting a family-based diabetes program at the US-Mexico border. Prev Chronic Dis [serial online]. January 2005;2(1). Available at: www.cdc.gov/pcd/issues/2005/jan/04_0083.htm. Accessed December 9, 2005.

[84] Corkery E, Palmer C, Foley ME, et al. Effect of a bicultural community health worker on completion of diabetes education in a Hispanic population. Diabetes Care 1997;20:254–7.

[85] Tang TS, Gillard ML, Funnell MM, et al. Developing a new generation of ongoing diabetes self-management support interventions: a preliminary report. Diabetes Educ 2005;31:91–7.

[86] King MG, Jenkins C, Hossler C, et al. People with diabetes: knowledge, perceptions, and applications of recommendations for diabetes management. Ethn Dis 2004;14:129S–34S.

[87] Hosler AS, Melnik TA. Population-based assessment of diabetes care and self-management among Puerto Rican adults in New York City. Diabetes Educ 2005;31:418–26.

[88] Bell RA, Quandt SA, Arcury TA, et al. Primary and specialty medical care among ethnically diverse, older, rural adults with type 2 diabetes: the ELDER diabetes study. J Rural Health 2005;21:198–205.

[89] Massing MW, Henley NS, Carter-Edwards L, et al. Lipid testing among patients with diabetes who receive diabetes care from primary care physicians. Diabetes Care 2003;26:1369–73.

[90] Bonds DE, Camacho F, Bell RA, et al. The association of patient trust and self-care among patients with diabetes mellitus. BMC Fam Pract [serial online] 2004;5. Available at: http://www.biomedcentral.com/1471-2296/5/26. Accessed January 19, 2006.

[91] Piette JD, Bibbins-Domingo K, Schillinger D. Health care discrimination, processes of care, and diabetes patients' health status. Patient Educ Couns 2006;60:41–8.

[92] Piette JD, Schillinger D, Potter MB, et al. Dimensions of patient-provider communication and diabetes self-care in an ethnically diverse population. J Gen Intern Med 2003;18:624–33.

[93] Pasley B, Roohan PJ, Wagner V, et al. Identifying areas for improvement: results of a Medicaid managed care diabetes survey. J Health Care Poor Underserved 2005;16:691–719.

[94] Johnson EA, Webb WL, McDowall JM, et al. A field-based approach to support improved diabetes care in rural sates. Prev Chronic Dis [serial online] October 2005;2. Available at: http://www.cdc.gov/pcd/issues/2005/oct/05_0012.htm. Accessed December 9, 2005.

[95] Gilmer TP, Tsimikas AP, Walker C. Outcomes of Project Dulce: a culturally specific diabetes management program. Ann Pharmacother 2005;39:817–22.

[96] Philis-Tsimikas A, Walker C, Rivard L, et al. Improvement in diabetes care of underinsured patients enrolled in Project Dulce. Diabetes Care 2004;27:110–5.

[97] Gary TL, Batts-Turner M, Bone LR, et al. A randomized controlled trial of the effects of nurse case manager and community health worker team interventions in urban African Americans with type 2 diabetes. Control Clin Trials 2004;25:53–66.

[98] Clancy DE, Brown SB, Magruder KM, et al. Group visits in medically and economically disadvantaged patients with type 2 diabetes and their relationships to clinical outcomes. Top Health Inf Manage 2003;24:8–14.

[99] Culhane-Pera KA, Peterson KA, Crain AL, et al. Group visits for Hmong adults with type 2 diabetes: a pre-post analysis. J Health Care Poor Underserved 2005;16:315–27.

[100] Shea S, Starren J, Weinstock RS, et al. Columbia University's Informatics for Diabetes Education and Telemedicine (IDEATel) Project: rationale and design. J Am Med Inform Assoc 2002;9:49–62.

[101] Piette JD, McPhee SJ, Weinberger M, et al. Use of automated telephone disease management calls in an ethnically diverse sample of low-income patients with diabetes. Diabetes
Care 1999;22:1302–9.

[102] Piette JD, Weinberger M, McPhee SJ, et al. Do automated calls with nurse follow-up improve self-care and glycemic control among vulnerable patients with diabetes? Am J Med
2000;108:20–7.

[103] Elasy TA, Samuel-Hodge CD, DeVellis RF, et al. Development of a health status measure
for older African-American women with type 2 diabetes. Diabetes Care 2000;23:325–9.

[104] Gilliland SS, Willmer AJ, McCalman R, et al. Adaptation of the Dartmouth COOP charts
for use among American Indian people with diabetes. Diabetes Care 1998;21:770–6.

[105] Rosal MC, Carbone ET, Goins KV. Use of cognitive interviewing to adapt measurement
instruments for low-literate Hispanics. Diabetes Educ 2003;29:1006–17.

[106] Willis GB. Cognitive interviewing and questionnaire design: a training manual. Working
Paper Series No. 7. Atlanta (GA): Centers for Disease Control and Prevention/National
Center for Health Statistics; 1994.

[107] Brown SA, Becker HA, García AA, et al. Measuring health beliefs in Spanish-speaking
Mexican Americans with type 2 diabetes: adapting an existing instrument. Res Nurs Health
2002;25:145–58.

[108] Rothman RL, Malone R, Bryant B, et al. The Spoken Knowledge in Low-Literacy Scale:
a diabetes knowledge scale for vulnerable patients. Diabetes Educ 2005;31:215–24.

[109] García AA, Brown SA, Winchell M, et al. Using the Behavioral Checklist to document diabetes self-management behaviors in the Starr County Diabetes Education Study. Diabetes
Educ 2003;29:758–60, 762, 764, 766.

[110] Balamurugan A, Rivera M, Jack Jr. L, et al. Barriers to diabetes self-management education programs in underserved rural Arkansas: implications for program evaluation. Prev
Chronic Dis [serial online] January 2006;3(1). Available at: http://www.cdc.gov/pcd/
issues/2006/jan/05_0129.htm. Accessed January 31, 2006.

[111] Giachello AL, Arrom JO, Davis M, et al. Reducing diabetes health disparities through
community-based participatory action research: the Chicago Southeast Diabetes Community Action Coalition (CSEDCAC). Public Health Rep 2003;118:309–23.

[112] Schacter KA, Cohen SJ. From research to practice: challenges to implementing national diabetes guidelines with five community health center on the US-Mexico border. Prev
Chronic Dis [serial online] January 2005;2(1). Available at: http://www.cdc.gov/pcd/
issues/2005/jan/04_0079.htm. Accessed December 9, 2005.

[113] Burrus BB, Liburd LC, Burroughs A. Maximizing participation by black Americans in
population-based diabetes research: the project DIRECT pilot experience. J Community
Health 1998;23:15–27.

[114] Harris F, Chamings P, Piper S, et al. Development and initiation of a diabetes self-management program for an underserved population. Diabetes Educ 2000;26:760–7.

[115] Smedley BD, Stith AY, Nelson AR, editors. Unequal treatment: confronting racial and ethnic disparities in healthcare. Washington: The National Academies Press; 2003.

ELSEVIER
SAUNDERS

Nurs Clin N Am 41 (2006) 625–639

NURSING
CLINICS
OF NORTH AMERICA

Interventions for the Family with Diabetes

Irene Cole, RN, MS, CDE,
Catherine A. Chesla, RN, DNSc, FAAN*

*Department of Family Health Care Nursing, University of California San Francisco,
2 Koret Way, San Francisco, CA 94143–0606, USA*

Can families make a difference in diabetes outcomes? Can nurses make a difference in how families organize and interact around the person with diabetes (PWD)? This article demonstrates that the answer to both questions is a resounding yes. This article highlights key findings from the research on families and diabetes across different phases of the lifespan. First examined are families with children with type 1 diabetes. Key findings from the descriptive research on child and family processes in adapting to and managing type 1 diabetes in children and adolescents are reviewed. Some exemplary intervention programs that had as their goal improving family life or diabetes management in families with children with type 1 diabetes are discussed. Next highlighted is what is known about couples and families who are living with type 2 diabetes. Intervention research with type 2 in adult families is not yet developed. The article concludes with recommendations for general practice with families that might be adapted by nurses to different settings in which they care for families with diabetes.

Although diabetes is typically considered an individual problem, some have advocated viewing diabetes through the lens of families and social contexts [1–3]. Multiple arguments can be made for taking the family into account in the clinical management of diabetes. First, families are the primary social context in which PWDs manage their disease, and can have substantial supportive or deleterious effects on their behavior [4]. Second, many aspects of diabetes management require changes in diet and physical activity, activities that are known to be sensitive to family context [5]. Third, diabetes is responsive to social stress and families play an

---

* Corresponding author.
  E-mail address: kit.chesla@nursing.ucsf.edu (C.A. Chesla).

0029-6465/06/$ - see front matter © 2006 Elsevier Inc. All rights reserved.
doi:10.1016/j.cnur.2006.07.001

enormous role in creating or ameliorating personal stress [6]. Finally, families form the basis of many illness beliefs and practices, and families help the PWD interpret symptoms, evaluate change, and decide on action [7].

Family factors in type 1 diabetes: children and adolescents

Children diagnosed with type 1 diabetes have developmentally varied levels of ability and willingness to learn self-management tasks [8] and parental involvement is essential. Mothers caring for small children with a new diagnosis of diabetes have reported feeling overwhelmed and burdened [9]. Some key maternal concerns include fear of hypoglycemic reactions [10,11], sleep deprivation [9], and having to be hypervigilant to the needs and cues of their child, until such time as they feel more competent and skilled in working with the diabetes. Finding adequate resources for childcare is often an additional stressor. Mothers who report coping better with a young child with diabetes tend to have access to a greater number of support resources [11]. Resources reported as being the most helpful to mothers are family and friend support and medical support. Interventions aimed at assisting mothers and families with illness stressors are warranted, but so to is access to consistent advice and support from medical professionals between visits [8].

Adolescence often brings a desire for more independence [8,12]. Diabetes self-management in adolescence is an ongoing process, however, in which responsibility is optimally shared between teenagers and their parents [13]. Disease management involves present-oriented daily responsibilities, such as taking medication daily, and activities that are largely oriented to warding off future complications, such as attempting to keep blood glucose levels near normal. As adolescents develop, they have a greater capacity to understand principles of illness management (eg, being able to circumvent ketoacidosis through frequent blood glucose monitoring and use of an insulin pump on a sick-day). Despite greater intellectual understanding, adolescents' adherence and "buy-in" to treatment goals become more difficult. Concerns about peers, puberty, and personal identity may trump concerns about achieving diabetes self-management goals. This often puts adolescents and their parents at odds [2].

Some of the stressors of diabetes self-management identified by teenagers are care constancy, boredom, rigidity, and guilt [14]. Disease complexity can also be a problem, with teenagers admitting to feeling that diabetes is demanding, constant, and complex. A major theme for teenagers is visibility of their illness; diabetes differentiates them, or makes them stand out from their peers. Adolescents report their proximal relationships with close friends can be stressful, particularly when friends are intrusive about the disease. Relationships with parents can be stressful because parents can nag or over-protect the teenager. Blame is a frequent complaint, especially around

issues of blood glucose monitoring ("bad" glucose results) and dietary choices. Despite these issues, however, teenagers report that parents help and validate their capabilities in times of need. Teenagers desire a complex blend of dependence and independence. They want to contribute more to their care decisions, to not to be blamed and shamed, and to receive help from family in a consistent but not intrusive manner. When this balance is not achieved and family conflict arises, the teenager's quality of life is reduced [15–17].

Despite the challenges to diabetes management that present in adolescence, multiple studies show that teenagers and their parents function relatively well [18]. Many conflicts between teenagers with diabetes and their parents are similar in content to families without diabetes. For instance, conflicts with fathers include getting in trouble in school and making too much noise. Maternal conflicts arise over talking back, lying, and cleaning their rooms. Teenagers with diabetes and their parents often have added conflicts compared with families without diabetes over topics of diabetes management or glucose control. Timing of meals, distractions, such as television watching, and the timing of getting up in the morning are examples. Greater conflict between teenagers and parents is related to worse diabetes outcomes, especially in situations where parents are less active in diabetes care [18,19].

Family characteristics can serve both a risk and a protective function in child and adolescent diabetes. Intensity of family conflict has been found to be related to quality of life in adolescents with type 1 diabetes [15]. Lower family adaptability and cohesion, and less warmth and caring, are associated with greater depression for teenagers with diabetes [20]. Additional family risk factors for diabetes include external family stressors and maternal aloneness [21]. Protective factors are family emotional closeness and parent coping skills, which have been linked to treatment adherence and metabolic control [21]. One interesting point is that a greater degree of parental control can be seen as positive support by teenagers, making them feel cared for and secure [14].

Family interventions for type 1 diabetes in children and adolescents

Interventions with families of children and adolescents with diabetes have demonstrated consistent positive changes in altering difficult or risky family interaction processes; in improving the child's overall well-being; and in a more limited way, improving markers of glucose management. Some interventions appropriately focus directly on easing family suffering and facilitating positive family relations in the face of the demands of diabetes management. Nurses focus holistically on the well-being of PWDs and families and not simply on the control of disease, and these behavioral and relational interventions have great relevance for nursing practice with families.

Four exemplary family intervention programs are reviewed, and the clinically relevant aspects of each program that might be adapted to different settings are highlighted.

Family-to-family network

One community-based family intervention that demonstrated positive results in families with children with type 1 diabetes is the family-to-family network [22,23]. This intervention was designed to include families across a wide range of childhood chronic illnesses: asthma, sickle cell anemia, cystic fibrosis, and type 1 diabetes. The intervention, targeted at parents and children, was designed to improve psychologic adjustment to disease, depression, and anxiety in both parent and child, and improve self-esteem in the child through increased communication and social support. The parent component of the intervention involved establishing a connection between a network mother, who was experienced with one of the chronic childhood diseases, and a mother in the treatment group [22]. During the 15-month intervention the network mother made seven 1- to 1.5-hour visits to her assigned families; made bi-weekly telephone contacts to build support and maintain the relationship; and participated in three special events, such as a bowling party. Network mothers were trained in active listening skills, reflection, and story swapping. Their contacts were designed to provide informational, affirmational, and emotional support.

The children's component of the family-to-family network was implemented by child life specialists who met regularly with the study's pediatrician and social worker [23]. The child life specialists also made visits to families, monthly telephone calls, sent out monthly newsletters, and joined periodic parties. The focus for these specialists, however, was the child. All messages conveyed in their intervention were focused on child-specific objectives, like accepting one's body image.

In a randomized controlled trial, the family-to-family network intervention was compared with usual medical care plus the simple provision of a name of a mother that a parent could call for help. One hundred thirty-six children with diabetes were examined for pediatric outcomes [23], and 193 mothers completed the maternal assessment [22]. At the completion of the intervention, the treatment program demonstrated significant improvements in anxiety in mothers in the treatment versus control group ($P = .03$); no significant effect was noted for maternal depression. Particularly pronounced were anxiety reductions in women with higher anxiety at the beginning of the study. Significant positive effects in child adjustment ($P < .01$) were also noted, with the children in the treatment condition demonstrating improved anxiety-depression and (less) hostility [23]. Children with lower physical self-esteem at the beginning of the study experienced the greatest positive effect overall from the intervention.

Parent-mentor intervention

Sullivan-Bolyai and colleagues [24] adapted the parent-mentor intervention strategy for mothers adapting to a new diagnosis of type 1 diabetes in a young child, 10 years of age or younger. Focus was placed on the mother's social and support needs in the initial phase of the child's diagnosis and treatment. Here, novice mothers were formally connected to an experienced parent mentor. The parent mentor was another mother who had successfully raised a child with type 1 diabetes and could provide informational, affirmational, and emotional support through home visits, telephone calls, and email contact.

A core of discussion objectives and other topics was created by the research team and the parent mentors, to provide structure and consistency to the intervention [24]. Core advice topics, adapted from the Ireys intervention [22], are instructive about the issues faced by parents: (1) helping the child grow and develop, (2) day-to-day management by the caregiver, (3) siblings, (4) behavior management and discipline, (5) dealing with physicians and the medical system, (6) dealing with daycare or school issues, and (7) nonschool issues like babysitting and parties. Additionally, relationship-oriented topics were developed to meet mothers' additional needs. Topics here included dealing with issues that arose in the relationship with the spouse and other family members; problems with the ill child's siblings; and dealing with comments made by friends, family, and strangers [24].

Although this was a feasibility study with a small sample (N = 42), the parent-mentor intervention demonstrated positive results compared with usual care in randomized clinical trial. Over a 6-month study period, mothers in the parent-mentored group as compared with controls had significantly greater reductions in diabetes-related concerns ($P = .02$) and perceptions that the diabetes negatively impacted the family ($P = .05$). Parent-mentored mothers felt encouraged by and believed they had a trusted person to call for details that were inappropriate for physician consultation. They believed they had a supportive person to call when overwhelmed and reported that mentor mothers were particularly of help in crises [24].

Family-focused teamwork

The family-focused teamwork intervention addressed diabetes-specific family conflict, glucose control, and quality of life in youth with type 1 diabetes [25]. In a prospective, randomized-controlled trial, a family teamwork intervention was contrasted with normal interdisciplinary diabetes care. Treatment consisted of a 15- to 20-minute session before or after a regular medical appointment, in which parents and children (ages 8–16) were coached in ways to share diabetes tasks and avoid conflicts about this teamwork. The intervention included short written materials on the scheduled topic, and encouraged family discussion of a responsibility-sharing plan. Topics

included (1) communication around diabetes, (2) meaning of hemoglobin A_{1c} (HbA1c), (3) emotional responses to blood glucose levels and ways to avoid blaming or shaming the child, and (4) sharing the burden of diabetes tasks within the family.

One hundred children and adolescents with type 1 diabetes and their parents enrolled. At the completion of treatment, HbA1c levels in the intervention group were significantly lower than the standard care group ($P < .05$), with multivariate analysis demonstrating that the treatment and blood glucose monitoring were significant predictors of HbA1c. It is noteworthy that for the treatment group, parent involvement was heightened during the intervention year but there was no increase in family conflict or decrease in quality of life for children or parents. More than double the number of families (2.6 times) in the intervention group maintained shared family involvement in the child's diabetes tasks over the year, compared with the standard care group ($P = .05$). This intervention parallels earlier findings [26] and demonstrates that a relatively low-intensity, low-cost, office-based intervention with PWDs and families can target specific family issues that have proved difficult in diabetes management, and effect positive change in both the diabetes outcomes and the family relationship features.

Behavioral family systems therapy for diabetes

Wysocki and colleagues [27] revised a prior family intervention [28,29] to increase treatment effects on diabetes adherence and glycemic control. The prior intervention targeted families with teenagers with type 1 diabetes, where adolescent-parent conflict was severe enough to reduce family diabetes management. Results showed that families in behavioral family systems therapy had a significant change from baseline on overt conflict and skills ($P = .05$) and extreme beliefs ($P = .006$) compared with other study groups. The behavioral therapy group also had significant improvement in the intensity of their family conflict ($P = .022$). There were no significant effects, however, on treatment adherence and glycemic control. The revised intervention, behavioral family systems therapy for diabetes (BFST-D) [30], addressed more specifically the issues of general and diabetes-related conflict between caregiver and adolescent that have direct effects on treatment adherence and glycemic control. The BFST-D was an intensive intervention delivered by a trained therapist in a community setting. The intervention was delivered over a 6-month period and included twice per month sessions that focused on four components: (1) problem-solving training, (2) communication skills training, (3) cognitive restructuring, and (4) functional and structural family therapy. Each family received an individualized treatment plan that reflected their specific needs from the baseline assessment, and observations of family interactions. Behavioral contracts and homework were focused on standard treatment components and family-specific diabetes problems. Advanced diabetes education was provided if needed. An

innovative aspect of the program was that parents simulated living with diabetes for an entire week, giving themselves sterile saline injections, monitoring glucose and carbohydrate intake, and role-playing a hypoglycemic reaction.

The BFST-D group was compared with two other groups, a standard care group and educational support group. Family conflict outcomes were significantly better in the treatment versus comparison groups and this result was most pronounced in families whose adolescents were in worse control (HbA1c>9%) at the start of the study. The intervention group also showed greater effects in treatment adherence ($P < .03$) compared with the other groups after the 6 months of BFST-D. In terms of glycemic control, both the BFST-D group and the educational support group were significantly better than the standard care group at study close ($P < .05$) but not different from each other. The benefits of glycemic control were greatest for those with poorest baseline control (HbA1c $\geq$ 9%) at study initiation [30].

The interventions described here address type 1 diabetes in youth still residing with parents. These interventions assist families in preventing conflicts through agreed-on distribution of diabetes tasks, resolving conflicts through a variety of techniques, providing support for parents and children to reduce anxiety and depression, or providing advanced diabetes education from a diabetes educator or mentored diabetes education from another family with diabetes. The ideal goal is to assist families to reduce the conflicts, anxieties, and burdens, to establish skills in staying engaged and involved in the developmentally appropriate shared care of diabetes, and to assist in careful glycemic control in the youth with diabetes. Some of these studies have not been able to show a significant reduction in HbA1c levels over their study period because of such issues as sample size, length of the study period, or the demographic make-up of their sample. The interventions reviewed, however, have shown improvements in family dynamics, reductions in stress, and greater sense of personal control over diabetes in general. Although the science of family intervention in diabetes is still young, these studies show clinically and statistically meaningful results and provide diabetes practitioners with choices of intervention with families with type 1 diabetes.

Family factors and interventions in type 2 diabetes: adolescents

The most recent estimate of the prevalence of diabetes in the United States is that 20.8 million people, 7% of the population, have diabetes, with 6.2 million of those yet undiagnosed [31]. Type 2 diabetes accounts for approximately 90% to 95% of all diabetes, with some racial groups at higher risk for the disease: African Americans, Latinos, American Indians, some Asian Americans, Native Hawaiians, and other Pacific Islanders.

Type 2 diabetes in children and adolescents is currently a developing science. Published literature is focused on several areas of clinical interest, many of which are reviews of care and clinical treatment of children with type 2 diabetes [32–34] and some that center on prevention of type 2 diabetes in high-risk children [35–38]. One comprehensive article [34] highlights care of type 2 diabetes in children, beginning with primary prevention of high-risk youth, those with a body mass index at or above the 85th percentile. Prevention of type 2 diabetes onset requires lifestyle changes of diet and physical activity for the high-risk individual. This includes education regarding proper nutrition and activity levels, and access to proper foods and areas to exercise. Prevention can include education to make lifestyle changes that address the entire family rather than singling out the high-risk youth.

Early screening by clinicians is an important part of prevention and early treatment [34]. Screening includes assessment of body mass index and skin for acanthosis nigricans, family history of overweight and type 2 diabetes, and blood work to measure circulating insulin levels. Once a diagnosis of type 2 diabetes has been confirmed in a child, treatment appropiately includes the child; the family; and even the community (eg, the school). Clinicians should assess the family and child for readiness and motivation to learn, and set up short- and long-term goals that are mutually beneficial. Parents can help children by using behavioral reward systems, such as sticker charts with prizes earned for completion of tasks. Nutritional goals emphasize glycemic control and maintenance of a desirable body weight or weight loss. Nurses treating and educating children and adolescents with type 2 diabetes can include families in planning recommended dietary and activity changes. Parents can assist by changing family patterns and by being role-models for behavior. As such they can be a positive force in altering the course of type 2 disease for their children.

One study [38] described the family context of meal patterns and eating in a group of adolescents at high risk for type 2 diabetes. Interviews with a subsample of 10 families selected from a larger study [36] revealed four major themes: (1) child and family eating patterns, (2) perspectives on obesity, (3) perspectives on weight control, and (4) health outcomes. The first theme, child and family eating patterns, revealed that daily meal patterns varied widely among the families, with hectic schedules disrupting the possibility of routines. Many children ate meals at school or skipped meals. Structured mealtimes at home occurred during evenings or weekends, but some families had no routines. School meals were often fast-food, such as burgers, pizza, or fried foods. In general, parents reported feeling they had little control over their child's eating. Those who exerted some control did so by rules, such as disallowing snacks before mealtime. The second and third themes, perspectives on obesity and perspectives on weight control, revealed that most overweight children did not believe their weight was a problem. Parents and children believed they had little control over diet, activity, and weight. Regarding the fourth theme, health outcomes, prior attempts

at weight loss were reported as unsuccessful and in some cases contributed to stress in the relationship between parent and adolescent. Several parents reported they had given up on trying to influence their child's weight. The literature on type 2 diabetes in children and adolescents is developing, and family factors are central to its prevention and treatment.

Family factors in type 2 diabetes: adults

It is worth noting that research on families of adult PWDs is limited and no family or couple interventions with type 2 diabetes have been published. Unlike child or adolescent PWDs, adults are developmentally capable of managing the disease independently. The rationale, however, for including families in the care of diabetes is equally relevant to adults. Family interactions have marked influence on health perceptions and actions in PWD and other chronic illnesses [4]. Diet and physical activity are sensitive to family context [5,39]. For example, spouses who support and join in dietary changes rather than resisting or arguing may help the PWD maintain a proper diet. Families create and buffer interpersonal stress [6], a factor known to influence glucose control. Perhaps most importantly, families participate with the patient in interpreting daily changes in well-being and in deciding on actions that might be responsive to those changes [7,40].

Support by family for care of diabetes has been repeatedly examined. Family support positively influences disease management, general health, mental health, and glycemic control [41–43], particularly in situations of high stress [44]. Taking a more refined look at couple "support," Trief and coworkers [6,45] found that overall satisfaction with the couple relationship and level of intimacy in the marriage were related to diabetes quality of life both concurrently and prospectively. She found that couple satisfaction and intimacy predicted less diabetes-related distress and greater satisfaction with a diabetes regimen 2 years hence. Alternatively, conflict has been identified as a risk for diabetes outcomes in adults [46]. These findings parallel a body of research that links emotional family life and chronic illness management [5,47]. Unresolved conflict or negative family emotional tone have proved to be powerful predictors of disease course or mortality in diseases, such as schizophrenia [48], cancer [49], and end-stage renal disease [50]. One problem with family research with adult PWDs is its limited scope; support and conflict have been examined but other family features have received almost no attention.

One team examined family factors in type 2 diabetes in four different ethnic groups: (1) European Americans (N = 113); (2) Latinos (N = 74); (3) African Americans (N = 159); and (4) Chinese Americans (N = 158) [51–53]. Their work is reviewed in some detail, because it illuminates family influences in diabetes in families from ethnic backgrounds in which diabetes is prevalent. A multidimensional view of family life guided these investigations. Three conceptually distinct domains of family life were assessed for their impact on diabetes management: (1) family structure and

organization, (2) world view, and (3) emotion management [51,54]. The studies rely on a theoretical model that posits that families maintain well-being by balancing illness demands with family resources [55]. Family characteristics in each domain are conceptualized as resources for the PWD. Demands include the symptoms of the disease, the requirements for care, and the emotional strain of living with a progressive, life-altering disease.

The first resource, family structure and organization, is the pattern of roles and rules guiding relationships in the family for accomplishing work within and outside the family. Greater organization is marked by clear leadership, roles, and rules for accomplishing tasks. Family organization is a resource because, for example, purchasing proper foods for the diabetic diet and following a predictable meal schedule, which support glucose control, are more likely in organized families. Emotional and quality of life outcomes may also be affected because living in a family with low organization may lead to PWD discouragement, isolation, and lower diabetes quality of life. Slightly different indicators of family structure were used with each ethnicity; family roles (togetherness) were measured for all groups and endorsement of traditional family roles was measured only in Latino and European Americans.

The second domain, family world view, addresses the family's beliefs that guide action and orient the family to its social context. Coherence, a marker of world view, is a family belief that the world is meaningful and manageable. High coherence is thought to support the PWD's continued efforts at self-care, which have ambiguous benefits in the present, but promised long-term health benefits. That is, if the world has order and meaning, then one can trust that self-care efforts taken now may be realized in improved future health. Coherence might also be a resource for helping the PWD cope with the emotional strain of living with a progressive disease.

The third domain of family life, emotion management, includes the family's expression and management of emotions including conflict, intimacy, anger, or loss. Emotional tone and emotion management skills are thought to influence chronic disease directly and indirectly. Family relations marked by conflict or hostility may have a direct negative effect on the PWD's physiology, making endocrine balance and subsequent diabetes control more difficult [47]. Additionally, a hostile or conflicted family environment may impede the PWD's ability to maintain thoughtful, daily self-care practices. Conversely, intimate and caring relations should positively influence a PWD's health by providing emotional support and respite in dealing with disease demands and downturns. In these studies disease management is conceptualized broadly to include indicators of the PWD's well-being, what is termed "morale" (self-perceived general health, depression, and diabetes quality of life); self-care behaviors (physical activity and diet); and subsequent health outcomes (HbA1c).

Significant relationships between family factors and outcomes are displayed in Table 1. Overall, the findings suggest that family context exerts

Table 1
Analyses of the effects of family characteristics on diabetes management in multiethnic families with type 2 diabetes

Dependent variable	Structure organization: togetherness	Structure organization: traditional roles	World view: coherence	Emotion management: unresolved conflict
Morale				
General health		EA[b]	AA[b] EA[c]	LA[c]
Depression			AA[d] EA[c] LA[c]	AA[d] CA[d] EA[c] LA[b]
DQOL: satisfaction	AA[c]	LA[b]	EA[c]	AA[c]
DQOL: low impact			AA[b]	AA[d] CA[d]
Behavior				
Physical activity	LA[c]		AA[c]	
Diet: quality	LA[b]	LA[a]		
Hemoglobin A$_{1c}$			EA[a]	

Abbreviations: AA, African Americans; CA, Chinese Americans; DQOL, diabetes quality of life; EA, European Americans; LA, Latinos.
[a] $P < .10$
[b] $P < .05$
[c] $P < .01$
[d] $P < .001$

a notable influence on disease management among PWDs with type 2 diabetes across all four ethnic groups. The domains of family life that link to disease management vary by ethnicity. Family roles and rules are related to disease management in Latinos, family beliefs are related to management in African and European Americans, and unresolved family conflict relates to disease management in all four ethnic groups. The morale aspects of disease management (emotional responses to the disease, overall sense of one's health, and quality of life related to diabetes) are more closely linked to family context than are behaviors or biologic outcomes of disease. All of these findings are cross-sectional and the direction of the relationship cannot be discerned. In one longitudinal examination, however, family factors predicted disease management, suggesting that family context does exert an influence on future disease management [54].

Factors to consider in family care of diabetes

Multiple suggestions can be made to shape or sensitize clinical practice to be more responsive to the family context of the diabetes. Assessment of child

and family patterns close to the time of diagnosis of type 1 diabetes is warranted. After the first few years after the diagnosis of type 1 diabetes, patient and family patterns of care become established and more difficult to change. Early assessment and intervention in these patterns is warranted [13]. In addition, ongoing assessment of family skills and coping should be performed throughout the disease process [13]. Developmental changes in the child and the family suggest a need for ongoing communication and work with family members.

For families with young children with diabetes and for those with children who are newly diagnosed, support from a multidisciplinary health care team can be meaningfully supplemented by community resources, active linkages with parents in the community who have successfully cared for children with diabetes, and can provide practical and emotional support that may provide significant assistance to parents [22,24]. The role of nurses can include serving as a resource for mentor families, and providing ideas about topics and issues that mentors can address.

Families with adolescents with diabetes are at a critical time in family development. The aim of treatment is the skillful negotiation of engagement between adolescent and parents so that conflict is diminished, roles and responsibilities are negotiated as appropriate to the child's developmental level, and parents remain engaged in supporting and coaching the child's disease management. Sophisticated, well-conceptualized programs have been developed that are readily adaptable to primary care or specialty clinics [25,26]. In addition, intensive therapy programs for adolescents at higher risk have been developed but are likely less adaptable because they require trained therapists for delivery [29,30].

Type 2 diabetes in adult families also warrants family assessment. Key variables that have been identified for these families are the capacity to support disease management, and to avoid conflict, nagging, and disengagement. Although systematic interventions with this population have not been tested, many of the features of office-based interventions for adolescents might well be adapted to adult families [25]. Finding straightforward ways to assist families to communicate with one another about diabetes, to understand the meaning of HbA1c and glucose levels, to anticipate emotional responses to blood glucose levels and dietary transgressions, to avoid blaming or shaming the PWD, and to negotiate sharing of diabetes tasks within the family are all defensible approaches to couples and families living with type 2 diabetes.

Next steps

Clearly, the largest area of need in future work lies with developing interventions targeted toward families and couples with type 2 diabetes. Interventions are particularly warranted for improving diabetes-specific family conflict and maintaining behavioral change over time. The fact that older

Americans have a higher prevalence of diabetes, with 10.3 million (20.9%) over the age of 60 years diagnosed [31], the relative lack of research on older persons with type 2 diabetes and their families is concerning. Additional work must be done to ensure that approaches to diabetes care are ethnically appropriate.

Another obvious gap in research is the near-absence of fathers' perspective in raising children with diabetes and the lack of their presence in interventions. The reasons for this seem to be the perception that mothers continue to be the primary parent caring for a child with diabetes. Despite this, fathers are an important source of support for children, their perspectives and input are largely missing from the current literature, and they have not been included in most interventions.

Finally, as the number of interventions for families with diabetes increases over the years, it is important for the design of these interventions to be accessible for practitioners and PWDs alike. Ideally, interventions should be cost effective, available across a range of settings, and able to be conducted by a broad range of professionals.

References

[1] Anderson BJ. Children with diabetes mellitus and family functioning: translating research into practice. J Pediatr Endocrinol Metab 2001;14(Suppl 1):645–52.

[2] Grey M. Interventions for children with diabetes and their families. Annu Rev Nurs Res 2000;18:149–70.

[3] Fisher L, Chesla CA, Bartz RJ, et al. The family and type 2 diabetes: a framework for intervention. Diabetes Educ 1998;24:599–607.

[4] Fisher L, Weihs KL. Can addressing family relationships improve outcomes in chronic disease? Report of the National Working Group on Family-Based Interventions in Chronic Disease. J Fam Pract 2000;49:561–6.

[5] Campbell TL. The effectiveness of family interventions for physical disorders. J Marital Fam Ther 2003;29:263–81.

[6] Trief PM, Himes CL, Orendorff R, et al. The marital relationship and psychosocial adaptation and glycemic control of individuals with diabetes. Diabetes Care 2001;24:1384–9.

[7] Chesla CA, Skaff MM, Bartz RJ, et al. Differences in personal models among Latinos and European Americans: implications for clinical care. Diabetes Care 2000;23:1780–5.

[8] Curtis JA, Hagerty D. Managing diabetes in childhood and adolescence. Can Fam Physician 2002;48:499–509.

[9] Sullivan-Bolyai S, Deatrick J, Gruppuso P, et al. Constant vigilance: mothers' work parenting young children with type 1 diabetes. J Pediatr Nurs 2003;18:21–9.

[10] Sullivan-Bolyai S, Knafl K, Deatrick J, et al. Maternal management behaviors for young children with type 1 diabetes. MCN Am J Matern Child Nurs 2003;28:160–6.

[11] Sullivan-Bolyai S, Deatrick J, Gruppuso P, et al. Mothers' experiences raising young children with type 1 diabetes. J Spec Pediatr Nurs 2002;7:93–103.

[12] Schilling LS, Grey M, Knafl KA. The concept of self-management of type 1 diabetes in children and adolescents: an evolutionary concept analysis. J Adv Nurs 2002;37:87–99.

[13] Silverstein J, Klingensmith G, Copeland K, et al. Care of children and adolescents with type 1 diabetes: a statement of the American Diabetes Association. Diabetes Care 2005;28:186–212.

[14] Davidson M, Penney ED, Muller B, et al. Stressors and self-care challenges faced by adolescents living with type 1 diabetes. Appl Nurs Res 2004;17:72–80.

[15] Laffel L, Connell A, Vangsness L, et al. General quality of life in youth with type 1 diabetes: relationship to patient management and diabetes-specific family conflict. Diabetes Care 2003;26:3067–73.

[16] Grey M, Lipman T, Cameron ME, et al. Coping behaviors at diagnosis and in adjustment one year later in children with diabetes. Nurs Res 1997;46:312–7.

[17] Grey M, Davidson M, Boland EA, et al. Clinical and psychosocial factors associated with achievement of treatment goals in adolescents with diabetes mellitus. J Adolesc Health 2001;28:377–85.

[18] Viikinsalo MK, Crawford DM, Kimbrel H, et al. Conflicts between young adolescents with type I diabetes and their parents. J Spec Pediatr Nurs 2005;10:69–79 [discussion: 79–80].

[19] Graue M, Wentzel-Larsen T, Bru E, et al. The coping styles of adolescents with type 1 diabetes are associated with degree of metabolic control. Diabetes Care 2004;27:1313–7.

[20] Grey M, Whittemore R, Tamborlane W. Depression in type 1 diabetes in children: natural history and correlates. J Psychosom Res 2002;53:907–11.

[21] Weihs KL, Fisher L, Baird M. Families, health and behavior. Fam Syst Health 2002;20:7–46.

[22] Ireys HT, Chernoff R, DeVet KA, et al. Maternal outcomes of a randomized controlled trial of a community-based support program for families of children with chronic illnesses. Arch Pediatr Adolesc Med 2001;155:771–7.

[23] Chernoff RG, Ireys HT, DeVet KA, et al. A randomized, controlled trial of a community-based support program for families of children with chronic illness: pediatric outcomes. Arch Pediatr Adolesc Med 2002;156:533–9.

[24] Sullivan-Bolyai S, Grey M, Deatrick J, et al. Helping other mothers effectively work at raising young children with type 1 diabetes. Diabetes Educ 2004;30:476–84.

[25] Laffel LM, Vangsness L, Connell A, et al. Impact of ambulatory, family-focused teamwork intervention on glycemic control in youth with type 1 diabetes. J Pediatr 2003;142: 409–16.

[26] Anderson BJ, Brackett J, Ho J, et al. An office-based intervention to maintain parent-adolescent teamwork in diabetes management. Impact on parent involvement, family conflict, and subsequent glycemic control. Diabetes Care 1999;22:713–21.

[27] Wysocki T, Harris MA, Buckloh LM, et al. Self-care autonomy and outcomes of intensive therapy or usual care in youth with type 1 diabetes. J Pediatr Psychol 2005;30:1 10.

[28] Wysocki T, Harris MA, Greco P, et al. Randomized, controlled trial of behavior therapy for families of adolescents with insulin-dependent diabetes mellitus. J Pediatr Psychol 2000;25: 23–33.

[29] Wysocki T, Greco P, Harris MA, et al. Behavior therapy for families of adolescents with diabetes: maintenance of treatment effects. Diabetes Care 2001;24:441–6.

[30] Wysocki T, Harris MA, Buckloh LM, et al. Effects of behavioral family systems therapy for diabetes on adolescents' family relationships, treatment adherence, and metabolic control. J Pediatr Psychol 2006;31:1–11.

[31] Centers for Disease Control and Prevention. National diabetes fact sheet: general information and national estimates on diabetes in the United States, 2005. Washington: US Department of Health and Human Services, Centers for Disease Control and Prevention; 2006.

[32] Loghmani ES. Nutrition therapy for overweight children and adolescents with type 2 diabetes. Curr Diab Rep 2005;5:385–90.

[33] Corrales-Yauckoes KM, Higgins LA. Nutritional management of the overweight child with type 2 diabetes. Pediatr Ann 2005;34:701–9.

[34] McKnight-Menci H, Sababu S, Kelly SD. The care of children and adolescents with type 2 diabetes. J Pediatr Nurs 2005;20:96–106 [quiz: 107–8].

[35] Daniels SR, Arnett DK, Eckel RH, et al. Overweight in children and adolescents: pathophysiology, consequences, prevention, and treatment. Circulation 2005;111:1999–2012.

[36] Grey M, Berry D, Davidson M, et al. Preliminary testing of a program to prevent type 2 diabetes among high risk youth. J Sch Health 2004;74:10–5.

[37] Gahagan S, Silverstein J. Prevention and treatment of type 2 diabetes mellitus in children, with special emphasis on American Indian and Alaska Native children. American Academy of Pediatrics Committee on Native American Child Health. Pediatrics 2003;112:e328.

[38] Seibold ES, Knafl K, Grey M. The family context of an intervention to prevent type 2 diabetes in high-risk teens. Diabetes Educ 2003;29:997–1004.

[39] Trief PM, Ploutz-Snyder R, Britton KD, et al. The relationship between marital quality and adherence to the diabetes care regimen. Ann Behav Med 2004;27:148–54.

[40] Chesla CA, Chun K. Accommodating type 2 diabetes in the Chinese American family. Qual Health Res 2005;15:240–55.

[41] Edelstein J, Linn MW. The influence of the family on control of diabetes. Soc Sci Med 1985; 21:541–4.

[42] Glasgow RE, Toobert DJ. Social environment and regimen adherence among type II diabetic patients. Diabetes Care 1988;11:377–86.

[43] Trief PM, Grant W, Elbert K, et al. Family environment, glycemic control, and the psychosocial adaptation of adults with diabetes. Diabetes Care 1998;21:241–5.

[44] Griffith LS, Field BJ, Lustman PJ. Life stress and social support in diabetes: association with glycemic control. Int J Psychiatry Med 1990;20:365–72.

[45] Trief PM, Wade MJ, Britton KD, et al. A prospective analysis of marital relationship factors and quality of life in diabetes. Diabetes Care 2002;25:1154–8.

[46] Fisher L, Chesla CA, Mullan JT, et al. Contributors to depression in Latino and European-American patients with type 2 diabetes. Diabetes Care 2001;24:1751–7.

[47] Kiecolt-Glaser JK, Newton TL. Marriage and health: his and hers. Psychol Bull 2001;127: 472–503.

[48] Cole RE, Kane CF, Zastowny T, et al. Expressed emotion, communication, and problem solving in the families of chronic schizophrenic young adults. In: Cole RE, Reiss D, editors. How do families cope with chronic illness? Hillsdale (NJ): Lawrence Erlbaum Associates; 1993. p. 141–72.

[49] Weihs KL, Enright TM, Simmens SJ, et al. Negative affectivity, restriction of emotions and site of metastases predict mortality in recurrent breast cancer. J Psychosom Res 2000;49: 59–68.

[50] Kimmel PL, Peterson RA, Weihs KL, et al. Dyadic relationship conflict, gender, and mortality in urban hemodialysis patients. J Am Soc Nephrol 2000;11:1518–25.

[51] Fisher L, Chesla CA, Skaff MM, et al. The family and disease management in Hispanic and European-American patients with type 2 diabetes. Diabetes Care 2000;23:267–72.

[52] Chesla CA, Fisher L, Mullan JT, et al. Family and disease management in African-American patients with type 2 diabetes. Diabetes Care 2004;27:2850–5.

[53] Fisher L, Chesla CA, Chun KM, et al. Patient-appraised couple emotion management and disease management among Chinese American patients with type 2 diabetes. J Fam Psychol 2004;18:302–10.

[54] Chesla CA, Fisher L, Skaff MM, et al. Family predictors of disease management over one year in Latino and European American patients with type 2 diabetes. Fam Process 2003; 42:375–90.

[55] Patterson JM. Families experiencing stress: I. The Family Adjustment and Adaptation Response Model: II. Applying the FAAR Model to health-related issues for intervention and research. Fam Syst Med 1988;6:202–37.

NURSING
CLINICS
OF NORTH AMERICA

ELSEVIER
SAUNDERS

Nurs Clin N Am 41 (2006) 641–654

Behavioral Interventions for Diabetes Self-Management

Robin Whittemore, PhD, APRN

Yale University School of Nursing, 100 Church Street South, PO Box 9740,
New Haven, CT 06536–0740, USA

Type 2 diabetes is emerging as a public health epidemic of the twenty-first century. In the United States, the prevalence of type 2 diabetes increased by 61% from 1990 to 2001, with approximately 15 million persons affected. Ethnic minorities have a disproportionate risk and are twice as likely as non-Hispanic whites of similar age to develop type 2 diabetes [1]. This increasing prevalence of type 2 diabetes is concerning because of the broad spectrum of debilitating complications associated with the disease. Type 2 diabetes is the leading cause of blindness, renal failure, and nontraumatic amputation in adults in the United States. In addition, type 2 diabetes increases the risk of cardiovascular disease and stroke twofold to fourfold [1]. These complications often occur concomitantly and contribute to extensive disability, personal suffering, and significant societal costs. In the United States, the economic costs associated with diabetes in 2002 were estimated to be $132 billion [2].

Intensive glycemic control and cardiovascular risk reduction are the primary objectives of treatment in type 2 diabetes. The United Kingdom Prospective Diabetes Study, a large randomized clinical trial, has established that intensive glycemic control in type 2 diabetes can substantially reduce the development and progression of serious complications. For every percentage point decrease in glycosylated hemoglobin A_{1c} (ie, from 9%–8%) there was a 40% reduction in the risk of complications, such as retinopathy and nephropathy, and a 14% cardiovascular risk reduction [3,4]. Despite the clinical evidence of the benefits of decreasing hemoglobin A_{1c} levels, studies indicate that most patients do not achieve acceptable glycemic control [5,6]. The Third National Health and Nutrition Education Examination Survey reported that only 56% of individuals with type 2 diabetes had hemoglobin A_{1c} values less than 8% and very few individuals sustained hemoglobin A_{1c}

E-mail address: robin.whittemore@yale.edu

0029-6465/06/$ - see front matter © 2006 Elsevier Inc. All rights reserved.
doi:10.1016/j.cnur.2006.07.014   *nursing.theclinics.com*

levels $<7\%$, the targeted goal advocated by the American Diabetes Association [7,8].

Comprehensive treatment of type 2 diabetes consists of (1) quarterly evaluations; (2) pharmacologic management of hyperglycemia, insulin resistance, hypertension, and lipid abnormalities; and (3) dietary and exercise recommendations to improve nutrition, obesity, central adiposity, blood pressure, and lipid profiles [9]. Multifaceted interventions that have included intensified pharmacologic management and dietary and exercise strategies have demonstrated significant improvements in glycemic control, hypertension, hyperlipidemia, cardiovascular events, and progression to nephropathy, retinopathy, and neuropathy [10,11]. Multifaceted interventions without an intensified pharmacologic component have also demonstrated positive outcomes. An intervention that combined diet and exercise strategies significantly improved insulin resistance, body mass index, glycemic control, and cardiovascular risk [12]. Diet and exercise strategies were effective in improving different outcomes, suggesting the benefit of combining diet and exercise strategies in addressing the constellation of metabolic abnormalities associated with diabetes. Yet, it is precisely the dietary and exercise recommendations that are difficult to incorporate into lifestyles with fewer barriers reported following pharmacologic recommendations [13,14].

Dietary and exercise recommendations are aimed at improving hyperglycemia and lipid profiles by reducing carbohydrate, saturated fat, and caloric intake and increasing activity. Dietary management is an essential aspect of diabetes self-management, yet also the most challenging [15,16]. Dietary changes are difficult to sustain and often are abandoned over time. Feeling deprived, resisting temptation, and competing priorities are common barriers that overwhelm the best of intentions [17,18]. The National Health and Nutrition Examination Survey III indicated that of 1480 individuals with diabetes, 62% ate fewer than the recommended five servings of fruits and vegetables per day and 68% consumed more than 30% of their calories from fat [19]. The Diabetes Attitudes, Wishes, and Needs study reported only 28% of adults with diabetes followed their dietary recommendations [20]. In addition to dietary management, exercise is considered to be an important component of successful diabetes self-management. Physical activity increases insulin sensitivity, improves glycogen storage, and allows for more efficient use of glucose in muscles [21]. The strongest argument for inclusion of exercise in type 2 diabetes self-management is to reduce mortality through cardiovascular risk reduction [22]. Unfortunately, exercise is often a neglected aspect of diabetes management. Between 31% and 55% of persons with type 2 diabetes report no regular physical activity or exercise [19,23,24]. Only 26% of adults with diabetes surveyed in the Diabetes Attitudes, Wishes, and Needs study reported that they followed exercise recommendations for diabetes [20]. Moderate-intensity physical activity has demonstrated significant improvement in hyperglycemia and cardiovascular risk reduction in middle-aged adults [12,25].

Behavioral interventions to support diabetes self-management

Dietary and exercise self-management related to diabetes is complex with treatment recommendations difficult to incorporate into existing lifestyles. In addition, self-management of diabetes requires ongoing adjustment because of changing life circumstances that occur over time. Adults living with diabetes report that successful self-management requires considerable experimentation and work, often taking months or years to gain competency [26–28].

Considerable research on interventions to assist individuals with the complex endeavor of diabetes self-management has been undertaken. Early interventions focused on providing didactic education and improved knowledge, yet not necessarily self-management or glycemic control [29]. Knowledge was determined to be a necessary, but insufficient component to diabetes self-management interventions. Educational interventions have been combined with behavioral interventions to help individuals acquire the skills, motivations, and support to change diet and exercise behavior, improving health status. A plethora of research has been undertaken on interventions that combine education with behavioral interventions aimed at improving self-management and glycemic control. Several systematic reviews and meta-analyses report on the combined outcomes of such programs [30–32]. Many of the behavioral interventions developed for diabetes self-management have been derived from behavioral and cognitive theories of psychology and behavioral science (Table 1) [33]. In general, behavioral theories focus on components of specific behaviors and the factors that can be altered to support a new health behavior, and cognitive theories focus on altering thought processes or emotions that may have an influence on a specific health behavior [34].

Table 1
Cognitive and behavioral theories applied to diabetes self-management

Theory	Common factors
Behavior modification theory	Knowledge
Cognitive behavior theory	Skills
Empowerment theory	Values
Health belief model	Beliefs
Health decision model	Attitudes
Motivational interviewing	Intentions
Self-regulation theory	Readiness to change
Social cognitive theory	Self-confidence
Stage of change theory	Coping skills
Stress and coping theory	Barriers to change
Theory of planned behavior	
Theory of reasoned action	

Data from Whittemore R, Bak PS, Melkus GD, et al. Promoting lifestyle change in the Prevention and Management of type 2 diabetes. J Am Acad Nurse Pract 2003;15:341–9.

Many diabetes self-management interventions combine education with several behavioral and cognitive strategies in one intervention or program, recognizing the complexity of the behavioral change process. No single strategy has been identified as superior and most interventions use multiple behavioral and cognitive strategies to affect change. Multifaceted programs are advocated by the American Association of Diabetes Educators and the American Diabetes Association to support diabetes self-management [35,36].

Goal setting, skill practicing, self-monitoring, and problem-solving

The most common strategies used to promote behavior change in diabetes self-management have included progressive goal setting, skill practicing, self-monitoring, and problem-solving. Because of the complexity of diabetes self-management and the multiple skills and behaviors required for optimal self-management, progressive goal setting and skill practicing are often advocated to build self-confidence and support behavior change [37]. Stepwise or incremental goal setting assists individuals to obtain early success, which may enhance self-confidence and ongoing behavior change efforts. Self-monitoring or the systematic self-observation and recording of a target health behavior is another strategy frequently used in diabetes self-management interventions. Self-monitoring has the potential to assist both the individual and the health professional to identify factors that support or pose difficulties to behavior change and has demonstrated efficacy as a strategy to support weight loss [38]. In addition, self–blood glucose monitoring enhances the ability of an individual to observe trends in blood glucose levels and to associate change in blood glucose level with change in diet or activity patterns [27,39]. Self-monitoring of blood glucose levels, dietary intake, and physical activity is often recommended to assist individuals with type 2 diabetes establish diabetes self-management patterns. Lastly, it is well recognized that there are numerous barriers to changing diet and exercise behaviors to support diabetes self-management, so problem-solving is recognized as an additional supportive behavioral strategy. In this approach, individuals are encouraged to identify events or situations that promote unhealthy behaviors, and active problem-solving is used with a professional to identify very specific ways to circumvent the anticipated problem [40].

Patient-centered approaches

More recent interventions aimed at diabetes self-management have combined educational and behavioral strategies with a patient-centered approach. Patient-centered approaches are egalitarian clinical approaches used in professional-patient interactions whereby an individual's lifestyle and meaning of the health experience are explored to determine treatment goals collaboratively [41]. Individuals with a chronic illness have reported

that they are more satisfied, more adherent, and have better health outcomes when health professionals use a patient-centered approach that is less authoritarian and controlling [42]. Common elements to patient-centered approaches include empathetic communication; acknowledgment of the whole person (social context to life); realistic expectations; goal negotiation; guided problem-solving; and individualized strategies. Coping skills training, empowerment training, and nurse-coaching are examples of patient-centered educational and behavioral interventions that have demonstrated positive outcomes with respect to improving self-management behaviors [43], self-confidence [44,45], and glycemic control in individuals with diabetes [44]. Patient-centered approaches have the potential to contribute to behavior change by addressing issues relevant to the individual, negotiating goals, problem-solving personal barriers to behavior change, and identifying realistic strategies.

In addition to providing educational and behavioral strategies, coping skills training, empowerment education, and nurse-coaching begin to address the emotional or affective context of diabetes self-management. Psychosocial distress and depression are more common in adults with type 2 diabetes [46,47] and have the potential to have a detrimental influence on diabetes self-management [48]. Multifaceted interventions that include an affective component explore and address psychosocial challenges in addition to behavioral change challenges associated with diabetes self-management through discussion and problem-solving in a supportive group or individual environment. Experts in diabetes have advocated for the continued development of interventions that include affective strategies in addition to educational and behavioral strategies to support ongoing diabetes self-management [49].

Additional patient-centered approaches that have been recently applied to diabetes self-management have targeted readiness and ambivalence to change. The transtheoretical model or stage of change model postulates that individuals making health behavior change move through predictable stages of change: precontemplation, contemplation, preparation, action, and maintenance [50]. Ongoing research related to the stage of change model supports that individuals in a given stage respond better to specific change strategies. For example, behavioral strategies are most effective when provided to individuals who are in the action stage of change. Assessment of stage of change or readiness to change is advocated, and different strategies are recommended tailored to the specific stage of change. Several studies have demonstrated that diabetes self-management interventions based on stage of change contribute to an increase in participants who advance along the change trajectory to the action stage with respect to diabetes self-management. In addition, participants in the action stage for select diabetes self-management behaviors (ie, blood glucose monitoring, healthy eating, exercise) demonstrate a significant improvement in glycemic control [51–53]. This preliminary research supports that readiness to change may be an important prerequisite to successful behavior change.

Motivational interviewing is another patient-centered behavioral strategy based on readiness and ambivalence to change that has recently been applied to diabetes self-management [54]. This specific counseling approach is primarily aimed at the individual who is not in the action stage of change, but rather who is in the precontemplation or contemplation stage of change. In this approach, open-ended questions, legitimization of individual feelings, and acknowledgment of ambivalence to change are used to promote advancement in the stage of change trajectory. Exploring and resolving ambivalence to change is proposed as a critical part of the change process. Several studies have demonstrated the potential of brief motivational interviewing interventions to improve behavioral outcomes (diet, self–blood glucose monitoring) and weight loss in adults with type 2 diabetes significantly when compared with a standard care control condition. Effect on glycemic control has been variable [55,56]. Because many adults with type 2 diabetes are ambivalent about changing diet and exercise behaviors, enhancing motivation to change seems to be a potentially important strategy to support diabetes self-management.

The patient-centered patient education model

The patient-centered patient education model has been proposed as a way to conceptualize many of the factors that contribute to health behavior change [57,58], which is consistent with the aforementioned research on behavioral interventions for type 2 diabetes. In this model, five levels of the patient education and behavior change process have been identified to facilitate assessment and intervention. These include

1. Cognitive (knowledge and awareness of the health problem, the targeted behavior, and the benefits of change)
2. Attitudinal (beliefs, intentions, and readiness to change)
3. Instrumental (skills necessary to support behavior change, such as performing blood glucose monitoring or measuring portions)
4. Behavioral (goal setting, coping, and problem-solving skills needed to support and maintain change)
5. Social (social support and use of resources)

In this model, assessment involves gathering information about the barriers and facilitators to behavior change. Intervention involves providing individuals with the necessary information, skills, and support to reach diabetes behavior change goals by educating, promoting readiness to change, building confidence in skill acquisition, identifying personally relevant behavioral strategies, assisting with problem-solving, and promoting social support and the use of available resources (Table 2). In light of the research on psychologic issues in type 2 diabetes, emotional assessment and support also seem to be important. Because this model incorporates the principles of

Table 2
The patient-centered patient education model applied to diabetes self-management

Level of education and behavior change	Assessment	Intervention

Cognitive level
  Information
	What do you know about...?	Provide education and
		  information
		Clarify

Attitudinal level
  Values
  Beliefs
  Intentions
  Readiness to change
	What does this mean to you...?
	What do you feel you need
	  to do about...?
	What are you willing
	  to do for...?
		Acknowledge feelings and
		  ambivalence to change
		Build commitment

Instrumental level
  Skills
  Self-confidence
	What are you able to do...?
	How confident are you
	  that you are able to do...?
		Instruct on skills
		Provide opportunity for
		  practice and feedback

Behavioral level
  Goal setting
  Self-monitoring
  Problem solving
	What do you currently do...?
	What are realistic goals...?
	How are you going to
	  implement...?
	What problems might arise...?
		Promote incremental goal setting
		Promote and review
		  self-monitoring
		Assist to problem solve
		  barriers to behavior change
		  and relapse prevention

Social level
  Social support
	What other support do you
	  feel that you need...?
	Who might be able to
	  help you...?
		Identify and assist to mobilize
		  support and resources

Emotional level
  Psychosocial
    adjustment
  Coping skills
	How do you feel about...?
	How does this impact
	  what you do about...?
	How do you cope with...?
		Active listening
		Promote stress management
		  and positive problem-focused
		  coping skills
		Refer for psychologic
		  evaluation as needed

Data from Grueninger UJ, Goldstein MG, Duffy FD. Patient education in hypertension: five essential steps. J Hypertension 1989;7(Suppl 3):S93–9; Goldstein MG, RuggieroL, Guise BJ, et al. Behavioral Medicine strategies for medical patients. In: Stoudemire A, editor. Clinical psychiatry for medical students. 2nd edition. Baltimore: JB Lippincott; 1998. p. 675.

patient-centered care and cognitive and behavioral theories of health behavior change, the model has the potential to provide a framework relevant to behavior change in diabetes self-management.

Current trends in diabetes self-management

Diabetes self-management education programs have become increasingly available in communities during the past decade. Many diabetes self-management education programs are based on the American Diabetes Association standards for care and are aimed at providing educational and

behavioral strategies to support diabetes self-management. Despite the growth of these programs nationally, many adults with type 2 diabetes never receive these services. Approximately 48% of adults with type 2 diabetes reported that they had never attended a diabetes self-management education program [59]. For those who attend diabetes self-management education programs, there is limited fiscal support for follow-up behavioral interventions to assist with the maintenance of behavior change and diabetes self-management. One current trend regarding behavioral interventions to promote diabetes self-management has been to focus on the translation of efficacious behavioral interventions to clinical care to improve access to care or to provide ongoing behavioral change support.

Several studies have examined the effectiveness of educational and behavioral interventions provided within the context of primary care. Many of these interventions aim to support diabetes self-management efforts of individuals with simplified behavioral interventions provided by a known health care professional or within the context of an individual's primary care encounter. These primary care interventions have ranged in scope, intensity, and targeted populations. Interventions have included nurse-physician collaboration models, case management models with a registered nurse or nurse practitioner, or the inclusion of a community health worker. Results have been conflicting. Aubert and colleagues [60] demonstrated a significant improvement in glycemic control with a registered nurse case management approach in a health maintenance organization. In contrast, a collaborative case management approach (registered nurse and physician) for poorly controlled veterans with type 2 diabetes demonstrated no effect on glycemic, lipid, or blood pressure control [61]. Differences in case management approaches, behavioral interventions, the inclusion of participants with more complex comorbidities and social circumstances from a primary care population, suboptimal intervention attendance, and methodologic limitations may contribute to the conflicting and modest findings. For example, frequency of case management contacts has demonstrated a positively significant association with better glycemic control [62]. Further research is indicated.

Another current trend in research on behavioral interventions for diabetes self-management that has the potential to increase access to diabetes self-management education is to provide a behavioral intervention by an interactive computerized program or the internet, capitalizing on the increasing technologic skills of health care consumers. Interactive computer programs emphasizing goal setting and problem-solving, provided within the context of a diabetes-related primary care visit, contributed to significant dietary behavior change in adults with type 2 diabetes [63,64] and a significant decrease in serum cholesterol [64]. No significant effect on glycemic control or body mass index was demonstrated [64]. Computer technology has also been applied to the delivery of an automated telephone disease management intervention. Piette and colleagues [65] demonstrated that participants from a county health system who had access to an automated

self-management assessment and intervention provided by the telephone by a familiar voice had significant improvements in behavioral and psychosocial outcomes compared with participants who received standard care.

Internet interventions that include virtual communication with a health professional have also been developed and evaluated. Short-term efficacy of an internet behavioral intervention for adults with type 2 diabetes that included individualized goal setting and self-monitoring compared with information only has been demonstrated with respect to improving dietary health behaviors [66], yet not physical activity [67]. A steep decline in usage over time was documented in the physical activity study. A subsequent internet behavioral intervention aimed at maintenance of the dietary intervention that also included goal setting, self-monitoring, and peer support resulted in only modest improvements compared with adults who received only the original program [68]. Internet technology has also been used successfully to deliver a behavioral weight loss program to overweight or obese adults without type 2 diabetes. Tate and colleagues [69] demonstrated that participants of a 24-week Internet behavioral program had significant weight loss compared with those who participated in an Internet educational program. Lastly, the Internet has been used to provide supportive virtual communities aimed at enhancing coping with diabetes [70,71]. Clinical trials examining the efficacy of such programs on diabetes self-management have not been undertaken. Computer and Internet technology is emerging as a new modality to provide behavioral interventions supportive of diabetes self-management. Further research is indicated.

Future directions

Considerable research has been undertaken in the past decade on behavioral interventions to promote diabetes self-management. Multifaceted, relatively intensive behavioral interventions provided over time have demonstrated positive outcomes in the short-term. As reported by Gary and colleagues [30] in a review of educational and behavioral interventions for adults with type 2 diabetes, results are "promising, but not compelling." Most interventions support positive outcomes in the short-term, yet long-term benefits in terms of glycemic control, cardiovascular risk reduction, diabetes-related complications, and quality of life have yet to be determined [31]. Behavior change related to diabetes self-management is complex, difficult to initiate, and difficult to maintain over time. With longer follow-up, interventions that provided regular reinforcement have demonstrated better outcomes [32]. Yet, maintenance of behavior change over time is difficult to achieve. Benefits of behavioral change interventions often decline approximately 1 to 3 months after an intervention terminates without ongoing supportive contact [32]. Difficulty with maintaining health behaviors over time and experiencing relapse are now considered part of the process of health

behavior change [50]. Interventions that focus on the maintenance of behavior change and the prevention and treatment of relapse are imperative for research advancement in diabetes self-management.

Developing cost-effective and clinically efficacious behavioral interventions that can be translated into current systems of care and community settings are additional priorities that have the potential to support diabetes self-management and improve outcomes. Institutional and community support for behavioral interventions has the potential to allow for ongoing follow-up to promote the maintenance of behavior change over time. In addition, widespread translation and dissemination of behavioral interventions for diabetes self-management into current systems of care and community settings has the potential to increase the reach and availability of interventions to the greater population of adults with type 2 diabetes, particularly those of lower socioeconomic status and diverse race and ethnicity who carry an increased burden of prevalence, morbidity, and mortality associated with type 2 diabetes [72].

Although many self-management interventions have demonstrated significant improvements in health behaviors, readiness to change, self-efficacy, and psychosocial outcomes, the modest or variable effect on important physiologic outcomes (ie, weight, glycemic control) remains a considerable challenge. Improvement in glycosylated hemoglobin averaged only 0.26% and 0.43% in two meta-analyses of self-management interventions for adults with diabetes [30,32]. In a meta-analysis of diabetes self-management interventions aimed at weight loss, the pooled weight loss was 1.7 kg or 3.1% of baseline body weight [73]. Norris and colleagues [31] advocate for the need to define better the relationship between intermediate outcomes, such as self-efficacy, problem solving, coping skills, and behavior change, glycemic control, and diabetes-related complications to advance understanding of self-management interventions in type 2 diabetes.

In addition, interventions focused primarily on the individual with type 2 diabetes may also have the potential for a limited effect on producing substantial behavior change that improves physiologic outcomes. Concern has been raised by public health advocates about the limited focus on social and environmental factors in programs or interventions aimed at health behavior change [74]. Multilevel interventions consisting of individual, social, and environmental resources may be necessary to address more comprehensively the complexities inherent in individual behavior change. Modern technology and contemporary culture have fostered sedentary lifestyles amid an environment that promotes high fat, high calorie, and nonnutritious foods [75]. Low-income communities are particularly vulnerable to these societal trends [76]. There is emerging consensus that behavioral interventions recognize that people live in social, economic, and political systems that shape behaviors and access to resources needed to maintain good health [77]. Glasgow and colleagues [78] advocate for a broadened scope of diabetes self-management interventions to include individual, social, cultural, and

environmental factors to support and maintain behavior change adequately. Individual-focused interventions to modify health behavior may need to be integrated with environmental and societal-focused efforts to enhance physical and social surroundings, which in turn supports individual behavior change [79].

Summary

Many interventions to support behavioral change in diabetes self-management have been developed. Research supports that interventions that are multifaceted, tailored to the individual, and provided 6 months or longer demonstrate modest effects in improving diabetes-related outcomes. Improving access to diabetes self-management education or behavioral interventions, maintaining the effects of behavioral interventions, and addressing the more complex social and environmental factors that contribute to behavior change are current challenges in diabetes self-management that warrant further attention and research.

References

[1] Centers for Disease Control and Prevention. National Diabetes Fact Sheet 2005. Available at: www.cdc.gov/diabetes/pubs/estimates05.htm. Accessed January 31, 2006.

[2] American Diabetes Association. Economic costs of diabetes in the United States in 2002. Diabetes Care 2003;26:917–32.

[3] Turner R, Cull C, Holman R. United Kingdom Prospective Diabetes Study 17: a 9-year update of a randomized, controlled trial on the effect of improved metabolic control on complications in non-insulin-dependent diabetes mellitus. Ann Intern Med 1996;124(1 Pt 2): 136–45.

[4] UK Prospective Diabetes Study Group. Intensive blood-glucose control with sulphonylureas or insulin compared with conventional treatment and risk of complications in patients with type 2 diabetes (UKPDS 33). Lancet 1998;35:837–53.

[5] Gilmer TP, O'Connor PJ, Manning WG, et al. The cost to health plans of poor glycemic control. Diabetes Care 1997;20:1847–53.

[6] Harris MI. Medical care for patients with diabetes: epidemiologic aspects. Ann Intern Med 1996;1(1 Pt 2):117–22.

[7] Saaddine JB, Engelgau MM, Beckles GL, et al. A diabetes report card for the United States: quality of care in the 1990s. Ann Intern Med 2002;136:565–74.

[8] Koro CE, Bowlin SJ, Bourgeois N, et al. Glycemic control from 1988 to 2000 among US adults diagnosed with type 2 diabetes: a preliminary report. Diabetes Care 2004;27:17–20.

[9] American Diabetes Association. Clinical practice recommendations: standards of medical care. Diabetes Care 2006;29(Suppl 1):S4–42.

[10] Gaede P, Vedel P, Larsen N, et al. Multifactorial intervention and cardiovascular disease in patients with type 2 diabetes. N Engl J Med 2003;348:383–93.

[11] Gaede P, Vedel P, Parving HH, et al. Intensified multifactorial intervention in patients with type 2 diabetes mellitus and microalbuminuria: the Steno type 2 randomized study. Lancet 1999;353:617–22.

[12] Torjesen PA, Birkeland KI, Anderssen SA, et al. Lifestyle change may reverse development of the insulin resistance syndrome: the Oslo diet and exercise study. A randomized trial-Diabetes Care 1997;20:26–31.

[13] Ruggiero L, Glasgow R, Dryfoos JM, et al. Diabetes self-management: self-reported recommendations and patterns in a large population. Diabetes Care 1997;20:568–76.

[14] Sullivan ED, Joseph DH. Struggling with behavior changes: a special case for clients with diabetes. Diabetes Educ 1998;24:72–7.

[15] Glasgow RE, Fisher EB, Anderson BJ, et al. Behavioral science in diabetes: contributions and opportunities. Diabetes Care 1999;22:832–43.

[16] Swift CS, et al. Dietary habits and barriers among exercising and non-exercising persons with NIDDM. Topics Clin Nutr 1997;12:45–52.

[17] Hall RF, Joseph DH, Schwartz-Barcott D. Overcoming obstacles to behavior change in diabetes self-management. Diabetes Educ 2003;29:303–11.

[18] Schlundt DG, Rea MR, Kline SS, et al. Situational obstacles to dietary adherence for adults with diabetes. J Am Diet Assoc 1994;94:874–6, 879.

[19] Nelson KM, Reiber G, Boyko EJ. Diet and exercise among adults with type 2 diabetes: findings from the third national health and nutrition examination survey (NHANES III). Diabetes Care 2002;25:1722–8.

[20] Rubin RR, Peyrot M. Patients' and providers perspectives on diabetes care: results of the Diabetes Attitudes, Wishes and Needs (DAWN) study. Practical Diabetology 2005;24:6–13.

[21] Wallberg-Henriksson H. Exercise and diabetes mellitus. Exerc Sport Sci Rev 1992;20:339–68.

[22] Christakos CN, Fields KB. Exercise in diabetes: minimize the risks and gain the benefits. J Musculoskeletal Med 1995;12:16–25.

[23] Hays LM, Clark DO. Correlates of physical activity in a sample of older adults with type 2 diabetes. Diabetes Care 1999;22:706–12.

[24] Krug LM, Haire-Joshu D, Heady SA. Exercise habits and exercise relapse in persons with non–insulin-dependent diabetes mellitus. Diabetes Educ 1991;17:185–8.

[25] Guthrie JR, Dudley EC, Dennerstein L, et al. Changes in physical activity and health outcomes in a population-based cohort of mid-life Australian-born women. Aust N Z Public Health 1997;21:682–7.

[26] Ellison GC, Rayman KM. Exemplars' experience of self-managing type 2 diabetes. Diabetes Educ 1998;24:325–30.

[27] Price MJ. An experiential model of learning diabetes self-management. Qual Health Res 1993;3:29–54.

[28] Wierenga ME, Browning JM, Mahn JL. A descriptive study of how clients make life-style changes. Diabetes Educ 1990;16:469–73.

[29] Padgett D, Mumford E, Hynes M, et al. Meta-analysis of the effects of educational and psychosocial interventions on management of diabetes mellitus. J Clin Epidemiol 1988;41:1007–30.

[30] Gary TL, Genkinger JM, Guallar E, et al. Meta-analysis of randomized educational and behavioral interventions in type 2 diabetes. Diabetes Educ 2003;29:488–501.

[31] Norris SL, Engelgau MM, Narayan KM. Effectiveness of self-management training in type 2 diabetes: a systematic review of randomized controlled trials. Diabetes Care 2001;24:561–87.

[32] Norris SL, Lau J, Smith SJ, et al. Self-management education for adults with type 2 diabetes: a meta-analysis of the effect on glycemic control. Diabetes Care 2002;25:1159–71.

[33] Whittemore R, Bak PS, Melkus GD, et al. Promoting lifestyle change in the prevention and management of type 2 diabetes. J Am Acad Nurse Pract 2003;15:341–9.

[34] Dubbart DM, Stetson BA. Cognitive and behavioral approaches to enhancing exercise participation. In: Rippe JM, editor. Lifestyle medicine. London: Blackwell Science; 1999. p. 511–9.

[35] American Association of Diabetes Educators. The 1999 scope of practice for diabetes educators and the standards of practice for diabetes educators. Available at: www.aadenet.org/AboutUs/99ScopeStandards.shtml. Accessed January 31, 2006.

[36] American Diabetes Association. Clinical practice recommendations: national standards for diabetes self-management education. Diabetes Care 2006;29(Suppl 1):S78–85.

[37] Krichbaum K, Aarestad V, Buethe M. Exploring the connection between self-efficacy and effective diabetes self-management. Diabetes Educ 2003;29:653–62.

[38] Wing RR. Behavioral aspects of obesity. In: Bray GA, Bouchard C, James WPT, editors. Handbook of obesity. New York: Marcel Dekker; 1998. p. 855–73.

[39] Cox DJ, Gonder-Frederick L, Julian DM, et al. Long-term follow-up evaluation of blood glucose awareness training. Diabetes Care 1994;17:1–5.

[40] Steed L, Lankester J, Barnard M, et al. Evaluation of the UCL diabetes self-management programme (UCL-DSMP): a randomized controlled trial. J Health Psychol 2005;10: 261–76.

[41] Shumaker SA, Schron E, Ockene JK, editors. The handbook of health behavior change: models for provider-patient interaction. New York: Springer Publishing Company; 1998.

[42] Street RL Jr, Piziak VK, Carpentier WS, et al. Provider-patient communication and metabolic control. Diabetes Care 1993;16:714–21.

[43] Whittemore R, Melkus GD, Sullivan A, et al. A nurse-coaching intervention for women with type 2 diabetes. Diabetes Educ 2004;30:795–804.

[44] Anderson RM, Funnell MM, Butler PM, et al. Patient empowerment: results of a randomized controlled trial. Diabetes Care 1995;18:943–9.

[45] Rubin RR, Peyrot M, Saudek C. The effect of a diabetes education program incorporating coping skills training on emotional well-being and diabetes self-efficacy. Diabetes Educ 1993;19:210–4.

[46] Anderson RJ, Freedland KE, Clouse RE, et al. The prevalence of comorbid depression in adults with diabetes: a meta-analysis. Diabetes Care 2001;24:1069–78.

[47] Gary TL, Crum RM, Cooper-Patrick L, et al. Depressive symptoms and metabolic control in African-Americans with type 2 diabetes. Diabetes Care 2000;23:23–9.

[48] Ciechanowski PS, Katon WJ, Russo JE. Depression and diabetes: impact of depressive symptoms on adherence, function, and costs. Arch Intern Med 2000;160:3278–85.

[49] Weissberg-Benchell J, Pichert JW. Counseling techniques for clinicians and educators. Diabetes Spectrum 1999;12:103–7.

[50] Prochaska JO, DiClemente CC, Norcross JC. In search of how people change: applications to addictive behaviors. Am Psychol 1992;47:1102–14.

[51] Jones H, Edwards L, Vallis TM, et al. Changes in diabetes self-care behaviors make a difference in glycemic control: the Diabetes Stages of Change (DiSC) study. Diabetes Care 2003; 26:732–7.

[52] Kim CJ, Hwang AR, Yoo JS. The impact of a stage-matched intervention to promote exercise behavior in participants with type 2 diabetes. Int J Nurs Stud 2004;41:833–41.

[53] Parchman ML, Arambula-Solomon TG, Noel PH, et al. Stage of change advancement for diabetes self-management behaviors and glucose control. Diabetes Educ 2003;29:128–34.

[54] Miller WR, Rollnick S. Motivational interviewing: preparing people to change addictive behavior. New York: Guilford Press; 1991.

[55] Clark M, Hampson SE, Avery L, et al. Effects of a tailored lifestyle self-management intervention in patients with type 2 diabetes. Br J Health Psychol 2004;9:365–79.

[56] Smith DE, Heckemeyer CM, Kratt PP, et al. Motivational interviewing to improve adherence to a behavioral weight-control program for older obese women with NIDDM: a pilot study. Diabetes Care 1997;20:52–4.

[57] Grueninger UJ, Goldstein MG, Duffy FD. Patient education in hypertension: five essential steps. J Hypertens 1989;7(Suppl 3):S93–9.

[58] Goldstein MG, Ruggiero L, Guise BJ, et al. Behavioral medicine strategies for medical patients. In: Stoudemire A, editor. Clinical psychiatry for medical students. 2nd edition. Baltimore: JB Lippincott Company; 1998. p. 675.

[59] Strine TW, Okoro CA, Chapman DP, et al. The impact of formal diabetes education on the preventive health practices and behaviors of persons with type 2 diabetes. Prev Med 2005;41:79–84.

[60] Aubert RE, Herman WH, Waters J, et al. Nurse case management to improve glycemic control in diabetic patients in a health maintenance organization: a randomized, controlled trial. Ann Intern Med 1998;129:605–12.

[61] Weinberger M, Kirkman MS, Samsa GP, et al. A nurse-coordinated intervention for primary care patients with non–insulin-dependent diabetes mellitus: impact on glycemic control and health-related quality of life. J Gen Intern Med 1995;10:59–66.

[62] Polonsky WH, Earles J, Smith S, et al. Integrating medical management with diabetes self-management training: a randomized control trial of the Diabetes Outpatient Intensive Treatment program. Diabetes Care 2003;26:3048–53.

[63] Estabrooks PA, Nelson CC, Xu S, et al. The frequency and behavioral outcomes of goal choices in the self-management of diabetes. Diabetes Educ 2005;31:391–400.

[64] Glasgow RE, LaChance PA, Toobert DJ, et al. Long term effects and costs of brief behavioural dietary intervention for patients with diabetes delivered from the medical office. Patient Educ Couns 1997;32:175–84.

[65] Piette JD, Weinberger M, McPhee SJ. The effect of automated calls with telephone nurse follow-up on patient-centered outcomes of diabetes care: a randomized, controlled trial. Med Care 2000;38:218–30.

[66] McKay HG, Glasgow RE, Feil EG, et al. Internet-based diabetes self-management and support: initial outcomes from the Diabetes Network Project. Rehabil Psychol 2002;47:31–48.

[67] McKay HG, King D, Eakin EG, et al. The diabetes network Internet-based physical activity intervention: a randomized pilot study. Diabetes Care 2001;24:1328–34.

[68] Glasgow RE, Boles SM, McKay HG, et al. The D-Net diabetes self-management program: long-term implementation, outcomes, and generalization results. Prev Med 2003;36:410–9.

[69] Tate DF, Jackvony EH, Wing RR. Effects of Internet behavioral counseling on weight loss in adults at risk for type 2 diabetes: a randomized trial. JAMA 2003;289:1833–6.

[70] Barrera M, Glasgow RE, McKay HG, et al. Do Internet-based support interventions change perceptions of social support? An experimental trial of approaches for supporting diabetes self-management. Am J Community Psychol 2002;30:637–54.

[71] Zrebiec JF. Internet communities: do they improve coping with diabetes? Diabetes Educ 2005;31:825–8.

[72] Glasgow RE, Vogt TM, Boles SM. Evaluating the public health impact of health promotion interventions: the RE-AIM framework. Am J Public Health 1999;89:1322–7.

[73] Norris SL, Zhang X, Avenell A, et al. Long-term effectiveness of lifestyle and behavioral weight loss interventions in adults with type 2 diabetes: a meta-analysis. Am J Med 2004; 117:762–74.

[74] Emmons KE. Health behaviors in a social context. In: Berkman LF, Kawachi I, editors. Social epidemiology. Oxford: Oxford University Press; 2000. p. 242–66.

[75] Jeffrey RW. Prevention of obesity. In: Bray GA, Bouchard C, James WPT, editors. Handbook of obesity. New York: Dekker; 1998. p. 819–29.

[76] Kaplan GA, Everson SA, Lynch JW. The contribution of social and behavioral research to an understanding of the distribution of disease in a multi-level approach. In: Berkman LF, Kawachi I, editors. Social epidemiology. Oxford: Oxford University Press; 2000. p. 32–80.

[77] Pellmar TC, Brandt EN Jr, Baird MA. Health and behavior: the interplay of biological, behavioral, and social influences. Summary of an Institute of Medicine report. Am J Health Prom 2002;16:206–19.

[78] Glasgow RE, Strycker LA, Toobert DJ, et al. A social-ecologic approach to assessing support for disease self-management: the Chronic Illness Resources Survey. J Behav Med 2000; 23:559–83.

[79] Stokols D. Translating social ecological theory into guidelines for community health promotion. Am J Health Promot 1996;10:282–98.

ELSEVIER
SAUNDERS

Nurs Clin N Am 41 (2006) 655–666

NURSING
CLINICS
OF NORTH AMERICA

Diabetes Self-Management Education

David K. Miller, RN, MSEd, BSN, BC, CDE[a],*,
James A. Fain, PhD, RN, BC-ADM, FAAN[b]

[a]Health Education and Life Promotion, 16122 NE Lakeshore Drive S,
Suite 200, Hope, IN 47246, USA
[b]College of Nursing, University of Massachusetts Dartmouth,
285 Old Westport Road, North Dartmouth, MA 02747–2300, USA

Diabetes self-management education (DSME) is an essential component of diabetes care for all individuals and families with diabetes. Individuals with diabetes make many day-to-day decisions relating to behavior, such as what and when to eat, whether or not to take medications, and whether or not to engage in physical activity. It is imperative for individuals with diabetes to learn self-management skills to manage their chronic disease effectively and avoid or delay the onset of diabetes-related complications. The goal of DSME is to optimize glycemic control by providing individuals with knowledge, information, self-care practices, positive attitudes, and coping skills for the effective management of their diabetes [1].

This article provides a definition of diabetes education along with a review of the national standards for DSME, including a discussion of relevant content areas that promote behavior change rather than simply imparting knowledge. Outcomes measurement of DSME is reviewed, and information is provided on self-care behaviors as defined by the American Association of Diabetes Educators (AADE). A review of newly defined standards for outcomes measurement of DSME that are practical, feasible, and consistent across DSME programs is likewise provided.

Defining diabetes education

The process of diabetes education has evolved over time, from the traditional inpatient classes where a nurse or dietitian co-taught specific skills

* Corresponding author.
 E-mail address: david@help-stat.com (D.K. Miller).

0029-6465/06/$ - see front matter © 2006 Elsevier Inc. All rights reserved.
doi:10.1016/j.cnur.2006.07.010
nursing.theclinics.com

and provided information to the present where self-management education is a critical component of comprehensive care for individuals with diabetes. Diabetes education is the foundation of diabetes self-management and central to achieving improved outcomes of care. Educational techniques and approaches have likewise evolved with a shift from didactic presentations to interventions where individuals with diabetes are completely responsible for the self-management of their disease [2].

In 1998, the American Diabetes Association, with representatives from the AADE, charged a task force to answer the question, "Who, when, where, and how should DSME be provided"? When task force members began their work, it became apparent that to complete the charge a definition of diabetes education was needed. Although members of the task force acknowledged that a consensus definition of diabetes education did not exist, the following definition was recognized as beginning to capture the wide variety of settings and delivery methods of diabetes education. DSME is an interactive, collaborative, ongoing process involving the person with diabetes and the educator. The process includes the following: (1) assessing the individual's specific education needs, (2) identifying the individual's specific self-management goals, (3) education and behavioral intervention directed toward helping the individual achieve identified self-management goals, and (4) evaluating the individual's attainment of identified self-management goals [2].

This definition of DSME refers to a collaborative approach whereby educators are responsible "to" individuals with diabetes rather than responsible "for" them. The traditional approach or what was referred to as the "compliance-based approach" [3,4] to diabetes education intended individuals to be passively cared for by educators and not part of the decision-making process. The "empowerment approach" [5–7] to DSME is based on an understanding that diabetes and its self-management belongs to the individual. DSME must be developed cooperatively and be consistent with the individual's needs, resources, and goals. The empowerment approach to DSME provides information, resources, and support to individuals so they can make informed, meaningful, and realistic self-management decisions.

The foundation of DSME is essential to the development and implementation of national standards for DSME. The push to revise the national standards began in 1998, when several major organizations with significant interest in the provision of diabetes care, federal agencies, and federally funded programs convened to review and revise the current standards.

National standards for diabetes self-management education

The national standards for DSME are designed to define quality DSME that can be implemented in diverse settings and facilitate improvement in health care outcomes. A systematic review of the literature for each standard has been conducted that provides a benchmark for quality assessment of DSME. The national standards for DSME are reviewed every 5 years if

research findings suggest a need for significant changes to support evidence-based practice.

The task force convened in 1998 to review and revise the national standards for DSME, with the final set of standards being published in the spring of 2000. The 10 standards by which DSME should be delivered are outlined in Box 1.

Major components of DSME, including self-care behaviors, are outlined specifically in Standard 7. Standard 7 refers to a written curriculum (10 relevant content areas) with criteria identified for successful learning outcomes. Individuals with diabetes need the knowledge and skills to make informed choices to facilitate self-directed behavior change and ultimately reduce the risk of diabetes-related complications. The 10 relevant content areas that have been identified in Standard 7 are listed next.

Disease process

This component of self-management education provides individuals with in-depth information about diabetes (or prediabetes) including signs, symptoms, and metabolic effects. Individuals should have an understanding of diagnostic criteria, types of diabetes, and risk factors with an emphasis on modifiable risk factors.

Nutritional management

Medical nutrition therapy is essential for successful diabetes management. It is imperative that all individuals with diabetes receive education related to nutrition therapy and an individualized meal plan appropriate for caloric needs, likes, dislikes, lifestyle, and treatment goals. The meal plan and treatment goals need to be reviewed regularly and modified as needed throughout the course of treatment.

The goals of medical nutrition therapy are to help the individual improve their nutritional status, including normal growth and development for children and pregnant women, and attain normal lipid and blood glucose levels.

There are several different methods for teaching meal planning. No single method works for every individual. Some methods teach basic nutrition and diabetes nutrition guidelines, whereas others are more in-depth. Sample methods include *Month of Meals,* plate method, exchange list, and carbohydrate counting.

A *Month of Meals* is a booklet that contains 28 days of complete menus for breakfast, lunch, dinner, and snacks. Menus are written for a meal plan of 1500 kcal/day with instructions to adjust the calorie level up or down.

The plate method is a way to plan meals with no measuring. One fills their plate to match the amount of vegetables, starch, and meat. Then a piece of fruit or a glass of milk is added. The plate is divided into fourths. One fourth of the plate is for starches, one fourth of the plate is for meat, with the remaining one half of the plate for vegetables.

Box 1. National standards for DSME

Standard 1: The DSME entity will have documentation of its
   organizational structure, mission statement, and goals, and
   will recognize and support quality DSME as an integral
   component of diabetes care.
Standard 2: The DSME entity will determine its target population,
   assess educational needs, and identify the resources
   necessary to meet the self-management educational needs of
   the target population.
Standard 3: An established system (committee, governing board,
   advisory board) involving professional staff and other
   stakeholders will participate annually in a planning and review
   process that includes data analysis and outcome
   measurements, and addresses community concerns.
Standard 4: The DSME entity will designate a coordinator with
   academic or experiential preparation in program management
   and the care of individuals with chronic disease. The
   coordinator will oversee the planning, implementation, and
   evaluation of the DSME entity.
Standard 5: DSME will involve the interaction of the individual
   with diabetes with a multifaceted education, instructional
   team, which may include a behaviorist, exercise physiologist,
   ophthalmologist, optometrist, pharmacist, physician,
   podiatrist, registered dietitian, registered nurse, other health
   care professionals, and paraprofessionals. DSME instructors
   are collectively qualified to teach the content areas. The
   instructional team must consist of at least a registered dietitian
   and a registered nurse. Instructional staff must be certified
   diabetes educators or have didactic and experiential
   preparation in education and diabetes management.
Standard 6: DSME instructors will obtain regular continuing
   education in the areas of diabetes management, behavioral
   interventions, teaching and learning skills, and counseling
   skills.
Standard 7: A written curriculum, with criteria for successful
   learning outcomes, shall be available. Assessed needs of the
   individual will determine which content areas are delivered.
   Content areas include describing the disease process,
   nutritional management, physical activity, medications,
   monitoring blood glucose, acute complications, risk reduction,
   goal setting, psychosocial adjustment, preconception care,
   and gestational diabetes.

Standard 8: An individualized assessment, development of an educational plan, and periodic reassessment between participant and instructors will direct the selection of appropriate educational materials and interventions.

Standard 9: There shall be documentation of the individual's assessment, education plan, intervention, evaluation, and follow-up in the permanent confidential education record. Documentation also will provide evidence of collaboration among instructional staff, providers, and referral sources.

Standard 10: The DSME entity will use a continuous quality improvement process to evaluate the effectiveness of the education experience provided, and determine opportunities for improvement.

Use of an exchange list to teach meal planning ensures a variety foods while maintaining a proper mix of calories, carbohydrates, and other nutrients. In the exchange system, foods are grouped into basic types: starches, fruits, milk and milk products, meat and meat substitutes, and so forth. Foods in each list can be traded or exchanged with other foods in the same list. The diabetes educator must evaluate and determine how many exchanges from each food group an individual must eat at each meal or snack.

Carbohydrate counting offers increased flexibility in food choices but requires more self-monitoring of blood glucose. The educator should emphasize the total amount of carbohydrate rather than the type. The diabetes educator must also consider other nutrients, such as fats and proteins, because of their potential for weight gain. Several variations of carbohydrate counting exist. They include counting carbohydrate serving choices, counting carbohydrate grams, and carbohydrate-to-insulin ratios.

Physical activity

Benefits of increased physical activity include lowering of blood pressure and lipid levels, weight loss, relaxation, lowering of blood glucose, and reduction of hemoglobin A_{1C}. There are two types of exercise: aerobic and anaerobic. Aerobic exercise uses oxygen to help release energy from fat cells. Anaerobic exercise does not use oxygen to burn fuel. To obtain substantial health benefits it is recommended to accumulate a total of 30 minutes of moderately intense aerobic exercise, stretching, and weight-bearing activity each day. Diabetes educators should assist individuals in finding a type of physical activity they enjoy participating in along with identifying barriers to an exercise program.

The level of exercise is described as light, moderate, or strenuous. Light exercise does not make one breathe heavily but the pulse rate may increase

slightly. Moderate exercise involves noticeably heavier breathing, with a pulse rate increase to more than 100 beats per minute. Strenuous exercise involves rapid breathing with a pulse rate between 125 and 160 beats per minute. Individuals should gradually decrease their intensity and finish with about 5 minutes of stretching exercises. This is called a "cool down." A cool down helps prevent later muscle cramping.

Exercised-induced hypoglycemia is a major concern for people with diabetes. Individuals need to be familiar with general guidelines that can decrease the risk of hypoglycemia, like knowing the signs and symptoms of hypoglycemia; checking pre-exercise and postexercise blood glucose monitoring; carrying a source of carbohydrate to treat low blood glucose; and reducing the amount of insulin or a pre-exercise snack. Special considerations should be taken for individuals who are elderly, obese, or who have complications associated with diabetes. These individuals should consult their health care provider before participating in an exercise program.

Medication taking

Approximately 90% of people with diabetes require a pharmacologic intervention to control their blood glucose. These interventions include a variety of oral medications or insulin to assist the individual with achieving their glucose goals. In addition to these interventions, it is important the educator include other medications used to treat the associated comorbid conditions or complications of diabetes, such as high cholesterol and hypertension.

Oral agents may be used as a monotherapy for individuals with type 2 diabetes or in combination with insulin. Generally, a reduction of 0.5% to 1.5% in the patient's hemoglobin A_{1C} is seen with oral agents. When using combination therapy an additive effect is seen as demonstrated by a further decrease in hemoglobin A_{1C}.

The diabetes educator should discuss the actions, pharmacokinetics, contraindications, precautions, and adverse effects of all medications. Individuals should understand when and how to take the prescribed medications. Certain medications have a potential interaction with blood glucose levels. These interactions may include drug-disease interaction, drug-drug interaction, or drug-food interaction. Drug-disease interaction is defined as a desirable or undesirable alteration of blood glucose level by a drug prescribed for a purpose other than its glycemic effect. A drug-drug interaction is defined as a desirable or undesirable effect of a drug on the efficacy or toxicity on the antidiabetes drug. A drug-food interaction is defined as a desirable or undesirable effect of food on the efficacy of the antidiabetes drugs.

Monitoring

Individuals must understand that monitoring their blood glucose levels provides them with information about their diabetes and the effects of

meal patterns, food intake, medications, activity, stress, and illness. Monitoring by individuals includes self-monitoring of blood glucose and urine ketones. Monitoring by the health care team includes hemoglobin A_{1C}, reviewing blood glucose patterns, patterns of weight change, and monitoring development and progression of long-term complications.

Self-monitoring of blood glucose is an integral part of the treatment plan for individuals with diabetes because it provides immediate feedback. The feedback assists individuals in achieving and maintaining specific glucose goals and preventing and detecting hypoglycemia.

The frequency of self-monitoring of blood glucose is determined by the educator and the individual with diabetes. Monitoring schedules are based on individuals' needs, desires, and the use of data. More frequent monitoring is beneficial during insulin dose adjustments or the use of insulin pumps.

The diabetes educator should demonstrate the proper technique to check blood glucose using control solution first and then using the individual's blood. After performing the demonstration the diabetes educator should ask the person to return the demonstration. It is important the educator discuss the proper technique to dispose of lancets.

Urine ketones appear in the blood and urine when the cells do not have enough glucose to use for energy. A buildup of ketones upsets the body's balance and ketoacidosis results. Urine ketone tests reflect the amount of ketones in the blood during the time the urine was made by the kidneys.

Acute complications

Hypoglycemia is a serious concern for individuals using insulin therapy, especially those with type 1 diabetes. Persons with type 2 diabetes using insulin or sulfonylurea are also at risk for hypoglycemia. Hypoglycemia tends to occur suddenly and almost always requires treatment to prevent blood glucose levels from continuing to fall to a dangerously low level.

The negative consequences associated with hypoglycemia include unpleasant physical symptoms, impaired cognitive function, embarrassment, emotional trauma, accidents, and bodily injury including death. Some individuals do not have any signs or symptoms with their hypoglycemia. They may remain alert, whereas others become stuporous at the same glucose level. It is important that people with diabetes carry a carbohydrate source with them at all times. Factors that increase the risk of hypoglycemia in patients with type 2 diabetes are advanced age, poor nutrition, and hepatic or renal disease.

Glucagon is a hormone that helps the liver release its store of glucose into the bloodstream. Glucagon is given as an injection to raise blood glucose levels. It should be given when someone is unable to swallow or is at risk for choking. A prescription is needed to buy glucagon.

It is important to record the time of day, blood glucose level, participating causes, and treatment of the hypoglycemia. Patients who have more than

one unexplained reaction a week should consult their health care team. It is very important to wear identification that states one has diabetes.

Hyperglycemia is another acute complication for patients with diabetes. A major cause of hyperglycemia is illness. During an illness the body releases a stress hormone that opposes the actions of insulin and contributes to hyperglycemia. It is important for the educator to discuss sick-day management.

Sick-day management includes increasing the frequency of blood glucose monitoring. Monitoring may need to be increased to every 2 to 4 hours depending on the individual. Insulin and oral medications are still needed during illness even when the individual is unable to eat. It is important that the person with diabetes maintain adequate hydration. Individuals should be instructed to drink at least 8 ounces (240 mL) of calorie-free fluids every hour while they are awake.

The person with diabetes should be instructed to contact their health care professional if they have persistent vomiting or an inability to tolerate fluids by mouth, persistent diarrhea, difficulty breathing, rapid or labored respirations, or change in mental status.

Risk reduction

The person with diabetes has many options to decrease diabetes-related complications. Among these are smoking cessation and immunization. Smoking is a risk factor for many diseases that are complicated by diabetes.

Cigarette smoking is the avoidable cause of mortality in the United States. Cigarette smoking accounts for 400,000 deaths annually. Smoking cessation is one of the few interventions that can be recommended to all individuals. The diabetes educator should ask individuals if they smoke. If the person is currently smoking, the diabetes educator should provide information regarding smoking cessation. The diabetes educator should discuss risks associated with individuals who smoke, smoking cessation strategies, alternative nicotine options, and referrals or support groups to assist in stopping. Nicotine-replacement therapies include gums, patches, inhalers, and spray. These may be used in conjunction with antidepressants. The health care team must be supportive of all individuals who smoke. Despite demonstrated cost-effectiveness, smoking cessation has not received the priority it deserves from health care providers.

Pneumonia and influenza take a high toll on people with chronic diseases, such as diabetes, particularly among the elderly. The diabetes educator should emphasis the importance of immunization for individuals with diabetes and ascertain if they have been received.

Goal setting and problem solving

The individual with diabetes may be overwhelmed with all the information obtained from the diabetes educator. Often problems that seem enormous

can be solved one step at a time. The educator should work with individuals to identify goals along with implementing a step-by-step approach to achieving those goals.

In order for the person with diabetes to live well they must possess problem-solving skills. Living with diabetes makes life more complicated. People with diabetes have more decisions to make and problems to solve on a daily basis than people who do not have diabetes. Individuals learn problem-solving skills through trial and error and practice. The diabetes educator is responsible for facilitating these problem-solving skills.

Psychosocial adjustment

The prevalence of depression among people with diabetes is estimated to affect one of every five people. People with diabetes are about three times more likely to experience depression than the general public.

The feelings of helplessness and hopelessness often hamper the management of diabetes. Depression has been associated with hyperglycemia, diabetes-related complications, and perceived functional limitations of diabetes. Signs and symptoms of depression include depressed mood most of the day, significant weight loss, trouble sleeping or sleeping too much, feeling agitated, fatigue, loss of energy, diminished ability to think, diminished interest in pleasure, and recurrent thoughts of death.

Depression is unrecognized and untreated in most individuals. Treatment for depression in the context of diabetes should be managed by a mental health professional (psychiatrist, psychologist). These professionals should be in constant contact with the physician providing the diabetes care. There are many different treatment options for depression.

Treatment options include psychotherapy or counseling or antidepressants. If antidepressant medication is needed, it is important to discuss the drug interactions and side effects, including how it might affect blood sugars and sexual dysfunction. The diabetes educator should also be aware that many people use herbal supplements to treat depression. Ask individuals if they are currently using any herbal supplements for depression. The most common herbal supplement is St. John's wort. It is sold over-the-counter but can have harmful interactions with other medications.

It is important to note that recovery is different for every individual. Recovery from depression takes time. Some medications take several weeks to start having therapeutic effects. Prescriptions and dosing may need to be adjusted.

Preconception care, pregnancy, and gestational diabetes management

One of the most commonly occurring complications of pregnancy is diabetes mellitus. Diabetes affects 130,000 pregnancies in the United States annually. Improvements in self-monitoring blood glucose and intensive insulin

therapy have improved the care for women and their children affected by diabetes.

There are two groups of women that diabetes affects during pregnancy. These two groups are women with pre-existing diabetes (either type 1 or type 2 before pregnancy) and women who develop diabetes during pregnancy (gestational diabetes). The later group may actually include women who have diabetes but are undiagnosed. Gestational diabetes is usually diagnosed between 24 and 28 weeks gestation when insulin resistance of pregnancy increases. Diagnosis is made with an oral glucose tolerance test.

Despite modern advances in treatment women with diabetes and their infants remain at a greater risk of complications. First-trimester complications consist of congenital malformations and spontaneous abortions. These are usually seen with women with pre-existing diabetes. Second- and third-trimester complications include macrosomia, increased childhood obesity, and respiratory distress syndrome. These complications can be seen in infants whose mothers have pre-existing diabetes or developed gestational diabetes mellitus. Euglycemia is the most important key to preventing these malformations. Euglycemia must begin with preconception and continue through delivery.

Preconception counseling is an important first step in preventing complications. Unfortunately, preconception counseling in the United States is not used. Preconception counseling should consist of an assessment to detect vascular complications, dietary counseling, assessment of self-management skills, achieving a hemoglobin A_{1C} level of near normal, and starting folic acid supplements. Contraception methods should be continued until glucose goals are obtained.

Care and education during pregnancy are focused on maintaining blood glucose levels to ensure a positive outcome. Dietary guidelines should be reviewed at this time. Special consideration should be given to caloric requirement, protein intake, and calcium intake. Options for morning sickness should be discussed if this becomes an issue. It is likewise important for women with gestational diabetes to have a postpartum follow-up because of their increased risk of subsequent diabetes. The initial evaluation should be completed at the first 6- to 8-week postpartum check.

Outcomes Task Force

In 1977, the AADE convened an Outcomes Task Force to help diabetes educators identify, measure, monitor, and evaluate outcomes. The need for standards for diabetes outcome measurements became evident because there was an absence of outcomes measures related to diabetes education.

In 2002, AADE approved and published the Standards for Outcome Measurement of Diabetes Self-Management Education [8]. At the same time, AADE published a technical review paper that further defined the seven diabetes self-care behavior measures with detailed guidelines for

measuring, monitoring, and evaluating these behaviors [9]. The seven diabetes self-care behaviors are as follows:

1. Healthy eating
2. Being active (physical activity)
3. Monitoring of blood glucose
4. Medication taking
5. Problem solving
6. Reducing risks associated with diabetic complications
7. Healthy coping skills

It is important to understand that the 10 relevant content areas as defined in the national standards (Standard 7) are not the seven diabetes self-care behaviors as defined by AADE. One does not replace the other. Although the relevant content areas list the topics a person with diabetes needs to know, the seven diabetes self-care behaviors focus specifically on those areas that have behaviors that must be learned or changed for effective diabetes care.

The Standards for Outcome Measurement of DSME complement the 2000 National Standards and provide a benchmark for quality assessment of DSME. Continuous quality improvement is an effective method to ensure quality DSME. Through the use of continuous quality improvement, the diabetes educator is able to determine the effectiveness of individuals and populations and compare their performance with benchmarks. The need to monitor outcomes has been mandated from the Center for Medicare

---

Box 2. Standards for outcomes measurement of DSME

1. Behavior change is the unique outcome measurement of DSME.
2. Seven diabetes self-care behavior measures determine the effectiveness of DSME at individual, participant, and population levels.
3. Diabetes self-care behaviors should be evaluated at baseline and then at regular intervals after the education program.
4. The continuum of outcomes, including learning, behavioral, clinical, and health status, should be assessed to demonstrate the interrelationship between DSME and behavior change in the care of individuals with diabetes.
5. Individual patient outcomes are used to guide the intervention and improve care for that patient. Aggregate population outcomes are used to guide programmatic services and for continuous quality improvement activities for the DSME and the population it serves.

and Medicaid Services and other regulatory accrediting agencies. AADE has developed standards for outcomes measurement of DSME that are displayed in Box 2.

Summary

DSME is a vital and integral part of treating people diagnosed with diabetes. Because diabetes is a chronic disease, DSME is an ongoing process that must be evaluated on a periodic basis. The national standards of DSME are based on scientific evidence and best practice and serve as a benchmark for quality assessment of DSME. Ten relevant content areas have been identified, providing a list of topics that are significant to the development and implementation of a diabetes education curriculum. By identifying the knowledge and skills needed for individuals with diabetes to make informed choices, behavior change is the unique outcome measurement for DSME. Seven diabetes self-care behaviors have been identified within the Standards for Outcomes Measurement as being central to diabetes education.

References

[1] Clement S. Diabetes self-management education. Diabetes Care 1995;18:1204–14.
[2] Report of the Task Force on the Delivery of Diabetes Self-Management Education and Medical Nutrition Therapy. Diabetes Spectrum 1999;12:44–7.
[3] Raymond MW. Teaching toward compliance: a patient's perspective. Diabetes Educ 1984;10: 42–4.
[4] Resler MM. Teaching strategies that promote adherence. Nurs Clin North Am 1983;18: 799–811.
[5] Feste C, Anderson RM. Empowerment: from philosophy to practice. Patient Educ Couns 1995;26:139–44.
[6] Funnell MM, Anderson RM, Arnold MS. Empowerment: an idea whose time has come in diabetes education. Diabetes Educ 1991;17:37–41.
[7] Mensing CR, Boucher J, Cypress M, et al. National standards for diabetes self-management. Diabetes Care 2006;29(Suppl 1):S78–85.
[8] American Association of Diabetes Educators (Position Statement). Standards for outcomes measurement of diabetes self-management education. Diabetes Educ 2003;29:804–16.
[9] Mulchay K, Maryniuk M, Peeples M, et al. Diabetes self-management education core outcomes measures. Diabetes Educ 2003;29:768–803.

ELSEVIER
SAUNDERS

NURSING
CLINICS
OF NORTH AMERICA

Nurs Clin N Am 41 (2006) 667–680

Psychosocial and Psychiatric Challenges of Diabetes Mellitus

Katie Weinger, EdD, RN[a,b,*], Jarim Lee, BA[a]

[a]Section on Behavioral and Mental Health Research, Joslin Diabetes Center,
1 Joslin Place, Boston, MA 02115, USA
[b]Department of Psychiatry, Harvard Medical School, Boston, MA, USA

Diabetes is a demanding chronic illness that places a large burden of care on the individual person and family. The impact of diabetes extends beyond physical well-being; it impacts psychosocial and emotional well-being and quality of life. Because humans are social beings, the burden of diabetes is shared with, and sometimes compounded by, family members and others. The complexity of diabetes management along with the risk of severe complications and serious comorbidities place the person with diabetes at risk for psychologic and psychiatric complications. Health care professionals caring for those with diabetes must be aware of strategies to minimize these mental health complications. This article examines mental health implications of living with diabetes, first at diagnosis and then as a part of everyday life. Discussed are typical stressors that individuals with this chronic illness may face. Briefly reviewed are mental health conditions that are commonly associated with diabetes. These include depressive and anxiety disorders, disordered eating, schizophrenia, and cognitive disorders.

Psychosocial issues for adults living with diabetes

Diabetes influences the psychosocial well-being of individuals and their families, and their psychosocial status can, in turn, influence their ability to care for their diabetes and to live full and healthy lives. Three categories of psychosocial factors that impact how an individual adapts to diabetes are (1) stress, (2) coping ability, and (3) social and family environment [1].

This work was supported by National Institutes of Health grant R01 DK60115 (KW) and the Diabetes and Endocrinology Research Core NIH P30 DK36836.
* Corresponding author.
E-mail address: katie.weinger@joslin.harvard.edu (K. Weinger).

Although individuals differ in their ability to cope and respond to stress, many face similar issues relating to diabetes diagnosis and treatment. Moreover, culture and ethnicity may influence the person's and family's response to diabetes, disease management, and treatment [2–5].

Diagnosis of diabetes

Type 1 diabetes can be diagnosed at any age; however, it most commonly is diagnosed during adolescence (age 10–19 years) and from age 40 to 70 years [6]. Diagnosis is typically an acute event that may involve diabetic ketoacidosis and hospitalization, which can be traumatic for both the person with diabetes and the family [7]. The person with sudden-onset of diabetes has to accept and adjust to a new identity as someone with a chronic illness that requires frequent monitoring of blood glucose levels, insulin injections or wearing an insulin delivery device, and lifestyle requirement changes around food and physical activity [8]. Diagnosis of diabetes may be accompanied by feelings of upheaval, loss of identity and health, worries about the future and the development of serious complications, and concerns about one's ability to live successfully and to achieve prior life goals [8,9].

Family members undergo similar feelings of loss and fear as the person with diabetes. Successful adjustment to the sudden onset of diabetes often mirrors the effectiveness of the family's communication style and ability to cope with other disruptions or crises [8,10]. Individuals and families who rarely discuss feelings or emotional responses may experience a more difficult time adjusting to the diagnosis of diabetes.

The diagnosis of type 2 diabetes may be less threatening for older individuals or people with family history of diabetes who have anticipated the onset. Some may view diabetes as a typical consequence of aging. People recently diagnosed with type 2 diabetes may experience similar feelings of loss as those with type 1, however, particularly as the American population becomes more overweight and obese and the onset of type 2 diabetes occurs at younger ages [6,11]. Health care professionals serve an important role in providing concrete information about living with diabetes and listening to patient and family concerns. Encouraging family discussion around the diagnosis of diabetes can help establish communication patterns that serve the family well in the future.

Stress and diabetes

Some evidence suggests that stress may play a role in the onset of both type 1 and type 2 diabetes [12–15], yet this idea remains controversial [1,16]. Although many studies have methodologic issues that temper the interpretation of results [16], the impact of stress on glucose levels in established diabetes is less controversial than the impact of stress on the onset of diabetes. The physiologic response to stress involves stimulation of hormone levels, such as epinephrine, norepinephrine, cortisol, and growth

hormone, all of which can act to increase blood glucose levels [1]. These same hormones are secreted to raise blood glucose levels as the first line of defense against hypoglycemia in long-duration type 1 diabetes [17].

The study of stress in diabetes presents important methodologic challenges. One issue is the definition of stress. Is stress the response to major life crises or is it the response to everyday irritations and hassles? Individuals differ in their experience of and response to stress. What is stressful for one person may be an exciting challenge for another. Further, the response to laboratory-induced stress may not reflect the response to real life stress [16]. Certain life crises are stressful for most people. Based on this assumption, Lloyd and colleagues [18] found that people with type 1 diabetes who improved glycemic control during the prior month had only positive stressors (eg, birth, engagement), whereas those whose glycemic control was poor or deteriorated in the prior month experienced more negative stressors (eg, conflict, death) than positive stressors. Stress can also be a consequence of living with a chronic illness, such as diabetes.

Coping ability

In groundbreaking work on coping processes, Lazarus and Folkman [19] examined differences in how individuals appraise stressful situations and in the cognitive and behavioral approaches used under stressful conditions. They theorize that individuals cope with stress in one of two general ways: they try to remove the stress by changing the stressful situation, resolving the issue, or reducing the stress (problem-focused coping); or they try to control their emotional response to the situation through avoidance, denial, or distraction (emotion-based coping). Peyrot and colleagues [20,21] have examined coping styles among people with diabetes and found that emotion-focused coping is associated with poorer glycemic control.

Diabetes-specific stress and distress

The rigorous lifestyle demands associated with diabetes, in conjunction with the risk of hypoglycemia and severe hyperglycemia, creates more stress in already stressful lives. Both the person and the family can be affected by the diabetes-specific stressors. Polonsky and colleagues [22–24] developed a clinical assessment tool that has also proved to be a useful research tool to measure diabetes-related emotional distress. Some areas of distress include feeling overwhelmed by diabetes and its care, feeling discouraged with the treatment plan, and feeling afraid of the future and of living with diabetes. High levels of diabetes-related distress are associated with poor glycemic control and poor self-reported quality of life [25].

The impact that diabetes has on the person and family is particularly important, and family members may be frightened by the possibility of serious

acute and chronic complications of diabetes. Family members often recognize when the person with diabetes does not follow the rigorous self-care recommendations, but they may not know how to help. Anderson and Coyne [26] describe the phenomenon of "miscarried helping" in which misdirected families may turn adherence to diabetes self-care recommendations into autonomy issues. Family members may resort to nagging; doing too much for the person with diabetes; and if the person is an adolescent, not letting the person with diabetes learn how to care for his or her self, or if an adult, treating the person like a child. Polonksy [27] uses the term "diabetes police" to describe this concept in adults. Family members, through their concern for their loved one, become a police force that watches and critiques every move of the person with diabetes, particularly if the person is not caring for his or her diabetes according to rigid standards. These conditions place significant strain on family relationships that may require thoughtful counseling to resolve.

Psychologic insulin resistance

Insulin can be an important tool in the treatment of type 2 diabetes to achieve optimal glycemic levels. Those with type 2 diabetes may have to use insulin temporarily to reach target glucose levels. Some people with type 2 diabetes, however, are reluctant to use insulin as a treatment. Psychologic insulin resistance may be learned from health providers who worry about complicating patients' lives and withhold insulin until the pancreas completely fails.

Rubin and Peyrot [28] identify several issues that may interfere with one's acceptance of insulin as a needed treatment for diabetes. Although some issues may be misconceptions, these concerns are real and may be based on the experience of family and friends. These issues can be significant barriers to receiving needed treatment. They include

Taking insulin hurts
Insulin makes life more complicated
Taking insulin is a sign that one's diabetes is getting worse
Requiring insulin is a sign of failure in controlling diabetes
Insulin is associated with hypoglycemia
Insulin causes complications
People who take insulin are treated differently by others

New delivery systems, such as inhaled insulin, may help reduce the fear of injections; however, more discussion around insulin as an important tool to reach glycemic targets is also necessary to overcome psychologic insulin resistance. Researchers have begun to examine this issue recently to understand better its complexities and to develop solutions to this problem.

Fear of hypoglycemia

People often associate hypoglycemia with unpleasant or embarrassing symptoms and consequences. As blood glucose levels fall, a person may experience tremors, profuse sweating, cognitive dysfunction, and irritability [29]. If the blood glucose drops to dangerously low levels, loss of consciousness and seizures can occur. Many people try to avoid hypoglycemia at all costs, and some even prefer to keep blood glucose at high levels to avoid hypoglycemic episodes. Fear of hypoglycemia is especially prevalent in people with past hypoglycemic experiences and adverse outcomes related to it [30,31]. Adolescents are especially vulnerable to the possible embarrassment associated with hypoglycemic episodes and may keep their glucose levels higher, although their parents may be more worried about high glucose levels [32].

Fear of high blood glucose and complications

Improved glycemic control is often associated with an increased incidence of hypoglycemia. For others, fear of serious diabetes complications may be a driving force to maintain blood glucose at extremely low levels, increasing the risk of severe hypoglycemic episodes. Frequent hypoglycemia, even at mild levels, causes a defect in the body's usual defense against low glucose levels for people with diabetes (ie, the secretion of epinephrine and norepinephrine and other counterregulatory hormones) [17]. These hormones help the glucose levels to increase and are responsible for many of the unpleasant symptoms of hypoglycemia. Frequent hypoglycemia may cause a person to be unaware of low glucose levels, greatly increasing the risk of loss of consciousness and seizures placing the person at risk of injury to self and others. Those who have developed neuropathy may not be trying to avoid high glucose levels but have become less sensitive to hypoglycemic symptoms. The inability to detect hypoglycemia, termed "hypoglycemia unawareness," places the person at increased risk of severe hypoglycemia and accidental injury. Many can regain their ability to feel symptoms through strict avoidance of any, even mild, hypoglycemia [33]. Blood Glucose Awareness Training is a psychoeducational training program that helps individuals learn how to detect fluctuations in glucose levels [34,35].

Psychiatric comorbidities

Depression

People with diabetes are at increased risk for developing depressive disorders, as much as two or three times that of people without diabetes [36,37]. About 15% to 20% of diabetic patients suffer from depression, and close to 40% experience depressive symptoms [36]. This high prevalence of depression in diabetic patients does not imply that diabetes causes depression or that depression causes diabetes, but highlights complex reciprocal

interaction between diabetes and depression. Some reports suggest depression may precede the onset of type 2 diabetes, whereas initial diagnosis of type 1 diabetes tends to be associated with increased rate of major depressive episodes [37,38]. Although biochemical and psychosocial aspects of having diabetes contribute to the increased risk for depression, presence of depression can also lead to poorer diabetes self-management, disrupted adherence to treatment prescriptions, and outcomes in diabetes.

Diabetes is also associated with higher recurrence rates and longer duration of depressive disorders, indicating that coexistence of depression and diabetes has the potential for impacting patients' diabetes self-management throughout their lives, and ultimately their health and quality of life [38]. Even subclinical depression, such as decreased motivation, lack of energy, and hopelessness, interferes with the ability to perform demanding diabetes self-management tasks [39]. Depressed individuals with diabetes tend to be less physically active, eat less healthy diets, and be nonadherent to oral hypoglycemic medicine prescriptions [40–42]. In addition, depression in diabetes is linked to higher body mass indexes, smoking, and higher health care costs [40,41]. Although causal links between depression and diabetes are not yet established, the complexity of genetic, biologic, and psychosocial factors associated with both conditions negatively impacts the lives of people with diabetes.

Depressive symptoms are associated with poor glycemic control [43–45]. Depression may affect patients' glycemic control through decreased quality and frequency of self-care behaviors, counterregulatory hormones, or another, unknown mechanism. The Diabetes Control and Complications Trial [46] and the UK Prospective Diabetes Study [47] definitively established that poor glycemic control is associated with the onset and exacerbation of diabetes complications. Depression is associated with increased rates and severity of diabetes complications, such as retinopathy, neuropathy, nephropathy, sexual dysfunction, and macrovascular complications [39,40]. Moreover, people with diabetes and depression have increased mortality rates compared with people with diabetes alone or people without diabetes [48–50].

Health care professionals need to pay attention to depressive symptomatology, especially in patients with worsening glycemic control. Symptoms of depression include loss of interest or energy, significant weight loss or gain, fatigue, and feelings of worthlessness or guilt [51]. Major depression should be considered if a patient experiences depressed mood or loss of interest in usually pleasurable activities and at least four other symptoms listed in Box 1 for more than 2 weeks [51]. Asking simple questions, such as "Have you been bothered by feeling down, depressed, or hopeless during the past month"? and "Have you been bothered by little interest or pleasure in doing things during the past month"? is a validated, practical approach to screening for depression that can easily be used in clinical settings [52].

Several other depressive disorders, such as dysthymia and bipolar disorders, can affect self-care behaviors of patients. Symptoms of dysthymic

---

Box 1. Symptoms of depression

Depressed mood
Fatigue, loss of energy
Loss of interest or pleasure
Significant weight (appetite) loss or weight gain*
Insomnia or hypersomnia*
Psychomotor agitation
Psychomotor retardation*
Irritability*
Decreased concentration*
Decreased recent memory*
Crying spells
Feelings of worthlessness or guilt
Thoughts or attempts of suicide
Social withdrawal
Pessimism

---

* Symptoms may also be signs of poorly controlled diabetes or hypoglycemia.

---

disorder, a chronic depressive disorder with less severity than major depression, are characterized by prolonged depressed moods for at least 2 years without any major depressive episode. Bipolar disorder is characterized by alternating periods of low and high moods, where the severe mood swings can cause significant impairment in normal life activities. Depression in patients with diabetes is both underrecognized and undertreated, and changes in mood with worsening glycemic control should trigger immediate assessment and referral to a mental health professional.

Treatment of depression can improve adherence to diabetes self-care recommendations and treatment prescriptions and ultimately overall quality of life for patients with diabetes [44,45,48]. Depression is very responsive to pharmacotherapy, and many medication choices exist. Some medications may impact important aspects of diabetes treatment, however, and must be used with caution in people with diabetes. Some tricyclic and selective serotonin reuptake inhibitor antidepressants have been associated with changes in blood glucose levels resulting in hyperglycemia or hypoglycemia, and changes in appetite and weight [53]. Other possible side effects for people with diabetes include sexual dysfunction, aggravated gastroparetic symptoms, and increased risk for arrhythmia [53].

Lustman and colleagues [54,55] demonstrated that cognitive behavior therapy is an effective treatment that produces remission of depression and improves glycemic control in patients with diabetes. Combination of

cognitive behavior therapy and supportive diabetes education, and pharmacologic interventions, are available for successful treatment of depression.

Anxiety disorders

People with diabetes have a higher rate of anxiety disorders than the general population [56,57]. People with chronic illness may be exposed to a prolonged period of anxiety, living under constant stress. Higher psychologic distress is associated with poorer glycemic control, and the distress can cause further anxiety regarding complications and other health outcomes [18,43]. Anxiety disorder diagnoses include generalized anxiety disorder, panic disorder, obsessive-compulsive disorder, and phobia. Common anxiety in people with diabetes includes fear of complications and fear of extreme blood glucose levels.

Anxiety can interfere with diabetes management adherence and glycemic control, such as phobic avoidances of blood glucose checking or insulin injection [43]. A considerable percentage of people with type 1 diabetes have a fear of hypoglycemia and generalized anxiety about diabetes management [58]. Experiences of hypoglycemic episodes can be aversive or even frightening to patients with diabetes, and the resulting fear of hypoglycemia and related avoidant behaviors can turn into further anxiety provoking stressors [30,31,59]. Although little is known about treatment of anxiety disorders in people with diabetes, behavioral and cognitive therapies and pharmacologic interventions similar to those used in the treatment of depression may be effective for treating anxiety symptoms [28]. Family involvement and support is also crucial in relieving anxiety symptoms.

Disordered eating

Diabetes increases the likelihood of developing eating disorders [60,61]. Young women with diabetes are twice as likely to have an eating disorder that meets Diagnostic and Statistic Manual-IV criteria and twice as likely to have subclinical eating disorders [60]. Consistent with the findings in the overall population, disordered eating is markedly more prevalent in younger women with diabetes than men. Women with diabetes and eating disorders have poorer glycemic control and higher hemoglobin A_{1c} than diabetic women without an eating disorder, which contributes to an increased risk of microvascular complications, such as diabetic retinopathy [60,62–66]. They are also at high risk for comorbid anxiety, panic attacks, and alcohol disorders compared with women without diabetes and with women with diabetes but without an eating disorder [61].

Type 1 diabetes is associated with a higher prevalence of bulimia nervosa in women [67]. Bulimia nervosa is characterized by a distorted sense of self influenced by body weight and efforts to compensate through binge eating followed by self-induced vomiting, misuse of medications, or extreme fasting or exercise [66]. Bulimia nervosa can appear in the form of insulin omission

in patients with type 1 diabetes, also known as "insulin purging," where one takes less than the needed dose of insulin to lose weight. When an individual takes less insulin than needed to match carbohydrate intake, hyperglycemia and glycosuria results. Fat and muscle stores in the body are broken down to meet the body's requirement for energy, inducing weight loss. Insulin omission is the most common weight loss method next to dieting in adolescent girls with type 1 diabetes [60].

Women with type 1 diabetes and eating disorders involving insulin omission are at higher risk for comorbid psychopathology than those who do not omit insulin for weight loss, because coexistence of diabetes and eating disorders increases risk of physical and psychologic morbidities, and ultimately mortality [68]. Women who intentionally omit insulin tend to have poorer regimen adherence, poorer glycemic control, greater psychologic distress over hypoglycemia, and higher rates of retinopathy and neuropathy [62].

Whereas bulimia nervosa is prevalent in type 1 diabetes, binge eating is the most predominant eating disorder in type 2 diabetes. About 25% of people with type 2 diabetes have binge eating disorder, which is strongly associated with increased body mass index and higher rates of anxiety disorders [11,69].

Although patient education is the primary tool for improving patients' self-care skills, it may be unsuited for the uniqueness of disordered eating in diabetes. Emphasis on negative consequences, such as complications, may do little to transform the distorted sense of self in women with diabetes. A multidisciplinary team approach is necessary for treatment of eating disorders in diabetic patients, which includes an endocrinologist, nurse educator, and nutritionist with diabetes and eating disorder training, and a psychologist or a psychiatrist to provide psychotherapy and possibly psychopharmacologic treatment [66,70].

Schizophrenia

The association between schizophrenia and type 2 diabetes has been controversial, although a growing number of studies report that patients with schizophrenia are at increased risk for developing type 2 diabetes compared with the general population [71–74]. Although the specific mechanisms involved are not understood, recent literature indicates that the antipsychotic medications used to treat schizophrenia, such as clozapine or olanzapine, may play a role in increasing the risk for diabetes [73,75–78]. Weight gain and obesity associated with schizophrenia treatment may contribute to the prevalence of type 2 diabetes in schizophrenic patients [74,78]. Moreover, some antipsychotic medications are also associated with increased plasma glucose and cholesterol level, which may be a factor in the link between diabetes and schizophrenia [75]. Although the link between schizophrenia and onset of diabetes is unclear at this point, caution must be used when selecting treatment options for people with schizophrenia who may be at predisposed risks for type 2 diabetes.

Cognitive deficits

Recent studies have shown that diabetes is associated with cognitive impairments leading to a higher incidence of dementia and Alzheimer's disease. The increased risk of dementia in the diabetes population has been documented by several studies, however, specific risk factors involved are not known [79,80].

Although acute hypoglycemia is associated with cognitive dysfunction [81,82], recurrent hypoglycemia may not have a lasting effect on cognitive functioning in adults [83,84]. Studies have shown, however, that diabetes onset early in life (before age 6) may lead to cognitive difficulties throughout childhood and adolescence [85–87]. Further, diabetes may exacerbate memory changes associated with the normal aging process [88]. Further research is needed to understand more fully cognitive function implications of long-term diabetes, particularly the impact of chronic hypoglycemia on memory and executive functioning.

Summary

The person with diabetes is at increased risk of both psychologic and psychiatric challenges that require support, counseling, and sometimes pharmacotherapy. Health care professionals have an important role in helping the person with diabetes and the family adapt to this demanding chronic illness. Knowledge of the problems commonly faced by those living with diabetes, the ability to assess these issues, and the identification of mental health professionals who are familiar with the treatment of diabetes are important skills for nurses working in most aspects of health care delivery. To be treated successfully, diabetes requires a multidisciplinary team with the patient at the forefront.

References

[1] Anderson BJ, Goebel-Fabbri AE, Jacobson AM. Behavioral research and psychological issues in diabetes: progress and prospects. In: Kahn CR, King GL, Moses AC, et al, editors. Joslin's diabetes mellitus. 14th edition. Philadelphia: Lippincott, Williams & Wilkins; 2005. p. 633–48.

[2] Chesla CA, Fisher L, Mullan JT, et al. Family and disease management in African-American patients with type 2 diabetes. Diabetes Care 2004;27:2850–5.

[3] Chesla CA, Fisher L, Skaff MM, et al. Family predictors of disease management over one year in Latino and European American patients with type 2 diabetes. Fam Process 2003; 42:375–90.

[4] Chesla CA, Skaff MM, Bartz RJ, et al. Differences in personal models among Latinos and European Americans: implications for clinical care. Diabetes Care 2000;23:1780–5.

[5] Fisher L, Chesla CA, Skaff MM, et al. The family and disease management in Hispanic and European-American patients with type 2 diabetes. Diabetes Care 2000;23:267–72.

[6] Warram JH, Krolewski AS. Epidemiology of Diabetes Mellitus. In: Kahn CR, King GL, Moses AC, et al, editors. Joslin's Diabetes Mellitus. 14th ed. Philadelphia: Lippincott, Williams & Wilkins; 2005. p. 341–54.
[7] Hamburg BA, Inoff GE. Coping with predictable crises of diabetes. Diabetes Care 1983;6: 409–16.
[8] Jacobson AM, Weinger K. Psychosocial complications in diabetes. In: Leahy J, Clark N, Cefalu W, editors. Medical management of diabetes. New York: Marcel Dekker; 2000. p. 559–72.
[9] Jacobson AM. The psychological care of patients with insulin-dependent diabetes mellitus. N Engl J Med 1996;334:1249–53.
[10] Lyons RF, Sullivan MJL, Ritvo PG, et al. Relationships in chronic illness and disability. Thousand Oaks (CA): SAGE Publications; 1995.
[11] Papelbaum M, Appolinario JC, Moreira O, et al. Prevalence of eating disorders and psychiatric comorbidity in a clinical sample of type 2 diabetes mellitus patients. Rev Bras Psiquiatr 2005;27:135–8.
[12] Mooy JM, de Vries H, Grootenhuis PA, et al. Major stressful life events in relation to prevalence of undetected type 2 diabetes: the Hoorn Study. Diabetes Care 2000;23:197–201.
[13] Thernlund GM, Dahlquist G, Hansson K, et al. Psychological stress and the onset of IDDM in children. Diabetes Care 1995;18:1323–9.
[14] Surwit RS, McCubbin JA, Livingston EG, et al. Classically conditioned hyperglycemia in the obese mouse. Psychosom Med 1985;47:565–8.
[15] Stein SP, Charles ES. Emotional factors in juvenile diabetes mellitus: a study of the early life experiences of eight diabetic children. Psychosom Med 1975;37:237–44.
[16] Lloyd CE, Smith J, Weinger K. Stress and diabetes: a review of the links. Diabetes Spectrum 2005;18:121–7.
[17] Cryer PE, Davis SN, Shamoon H. Hypoglycemia in diabetes. Diabetes Care 2003;26: 1902–12.
[18] Lloyd CE, Dyer PH, Lancashire RJ, et al. Association between stress and glycemic control in adults with type 1 (insulin-dependent) diabetes. Diabetes Care 1999;22:1278–83.
[19] Lazarus RS, Folkman S. Stress, appraisal and coping. New York: Springer Publishing Company; 1984.
[20] Peyrot M, McMurry JF Jr, Kruger DF. A biopsychosocial model of glycemic control in diabetes: stress, coping and regimen adherence. J Health Soc Behav 1999;40:141–58.
[21] Peyrot MF, McMurry JF Jr. Stress buffering and glycemic control: the role of coping styles. Diabetes Care 1992;15:842–6.
[22] Polonsky WH, Anderson BJ, Lohrer PA, et al. Assessment of diabetes-related distress. Diabetes Care 1995;18:754–60.
[23] Welch G, Weinger K, Anderson B, et al. Responsiveness of the Problem Areas In Diabetes (PAID) questionnaire. Diabet Med 2003;20:69–72.
[24] Welch GW, Jacobson AM, Polonsky WH. The Problem Areas in Diabetes Scale: an evaluation of its clinical utility. Diabetes Care 1997;20:760–6.
[25] Weinger K, Jacobson AM. Psychosocial and quality of life correlates of glycemic control during intensive treatment of type 1 diabetes. Patient Educ Couns 2001;42:123–31.
[26] Anderson BJ, Coyne JC. Miscarried helping in the interactions between chronically ill children and their parents. In: Johnson JH, Johnson SB, editors. Advances in child health psychology. Gainesville (FL): University of Florida Press; 1991. p. 167–77.
[27] Polonsky WH. Diabetes burnout. Alexandria (VA): American Diabetes Association; 1999.
[28] Rubin RR, Peyrot M. Psychological issues and treatment for people with diabetes. J Clin Psychol 2001;57:457–78.
[29] Weinger K, Jacobson AM, Draelos MT, et al. Blood glucose estimation and symptoms during hyperglycemia and hypoglycemia in patients with insulin-dependent diabetes mellitus. Am J Med 1995;98:22–31.

[30] Green L, Feher M, Catalan J. Fears and phobias in people with diabetes. Diabetes Metab Res Rev 2000;16:287–93.

[31] Polonsky WH, Davis CL, Jacobson AM, et al. Correlates of hypoglycemic fear in type I and type II diabetes mellitus. Health Psychol 1992;11:199–202.

[32] Weinger K, O'Donnell KA, Ritholz MD. Adolescent views of diabetes-related parent conflict and support: a focus group analysis. J Adolesc Health 2001;29:330–6.

[33] Fanelli CG, Pampanelli S, Porcellati F, et al. Shift of glycaemic thresholds for cognitive function in hypoglycaemia unawareness in humans. Diabetologia 1998;41:720–3.

[34] Cox D, Gonder-Frederick L, Polonsky W, et al. A multicenter evaluation of blood glucose awareness training-II. Diabetes Care 1995;18:523–8.

[35] Cox DJ, Gonder-Frederick L, Julian D, et al. Intensive versus standard blood glucose awareness training (BGAT) with insulin-dependent diabetes: mechanisms and ancillary effects. Psychosom Med 1991;53:453–62.

[36] Anderson RJ, Freedland KE, Clouse RE, et al. The prevalence of comorbid depression in adults with diabetes: a meta-analysis. Diabetes Care 2001;24:1069–78.

[37] Petrak F, Hardt J, Wittchen HU, et al. Prevalence of psychiatric disorders in an onset cohort of adults with type 1 diabetes. Diabetes Metab Res Rev 2003;19:216–22.

[38] Talbot F, Nouwen A. A review of the relationship between depression and diabetes in adults: is there a link? Diabetes Care 2000;23:1556–62.

[39] de Groot M, Anderson R, Freedland KE, et al. Association of depression and diabetes complications: a meta-analysis. Psychosom Med 2001;63:619–30.

[40] Katon W, von Korff M, Ciechanowski P, et al. Behavioral and clinical factors associated with depression among individuals with diabetes. Diabetes Care 2004;27:914–20.

[41] Ciechanowski PS, Katon WJ, Russo JE. Depression and diabetes: impact of depressive symptoms on adherence, function, and costs. Arch Intern Med 2000;160:3278–85.

[42] Lin EH, Katon W, Von Korff M, et al. Relationship of depression and diabetes self-care, medication adherence, and preventive care. Diabetes Care 2004;27:2154–60.

[43] Berlin I, Bisserbe JC, Eiber R, et al. Phobic symptoms, particularly the fear of blood and injury, are associated with poor glycemic control in type I diabetic adults. Diabetes Care 1997; 20:176–8.

[44] Van Tilburg MA, McCaskill CC, Lane JD, et al. Depressed mood is a factor in glycemic control in type 1 diabetes. Psychosom Med 2001;63:551–5.

[45] Lustman PJ, Anderson RJ, Freedland KE, et al. Depression and poor glycemic control: a meta-analytic review of the literature. Diabetes Care 2000;23:934–42.

[46] The Diabetes Control and Complications Trial Research Group. The effect of intensive treatment of diabetes on the development and progression of long-term complications in insulin-dependent diabetes mellitus. N Engl J Med 1993;329:977–86.

[47] UK Prospective Diabetes Study (UKPDS) Group. Intensive blood-glucose control with sulphonylureas or insulin compared with conventional treatment and risk of complications in patients with type 2 diabetes (UKPDS 33). Lancet 1998;352:837–53.

[48] Egede LE, Nietert PJ, Zheng D. Depression and all-cause and coronary heart disease mortality among adults with and without diabetes. Diabetes Care 2005;28:1339–45.

[49] Zhang X, Norris SL, Gregg EW, et al. Depressive symptoms and mortality among persons with and without diabetes. Am J Epidemiol 2005;161:652–60.

[50] Katon WJ, Rutter C, Simon G, et al. The association of comorbid depression with mortality in patients with type 2 diabetes. Diabetes Care 2005;28:2668–72.

[51] American Psychiatric Association. Diagnostic and Statistical Manual of Mental Disorders, Fourth Edition Test Revision. Washington (DC): American Psychiatric Association; 2000. p. 349–97.

[52] Whooley MA, Avins AL, Miranda J, et al. Case-finding instruments for depression: two questions are as good as many. J Gen Intern Med 1997;12:439–45.

[53] Weinger K, Welch G, Jacobson A. Psychological and psychiatric issues in diabetes mellitus. In: Poretsky L, editor. Principles of diabetes mellitus. Norwell (MA): Kluwer Academic Publishers; 2002. p. 639–54.

[54] Lustman PJ, Griffith LS, Freedland KE, et al. Cognitive behavior therapy for depression in type 2 diabetes mellitus: a randomized, controlled trial. Ann Intern Med 1998;129: 613–21.

[55] Lustman PJ, Freedland KE, Griffith LS, et al. Predicting response to cognitive behavior therapy of depression in type 2 diabetes. Gen Hosp Psychiatry 1998;20:302–6.

[56] Lloyd CE, Dyer PH, Barnett AH. Prevalence of symptoms of depression and anxiety in a diabetes clinic population. Diabet Med 2000;17:198–202.

[57] Grigsby AB, Anderson RJ, Freedland KE, et al. Prevalence of anxiety in adults with diabetes: a systematic review. J Psychosom Res 2002;53:1053–60.

[58] Zambanini A, Newson RB, Maisey M, et al. Injection related anxiety in insulin-treated diabetes. Diabetes Res Clin Pract 1999;46:239–46.

[59] Deary IJ. Symptoms of hypoglycemia and effects on mental performance and emotions. In: Frier BM, Fisher BM, editors. Hypoglycemia and clinical diabetes. Chichester: Wiley; 1999. p. 29–54.

[60] Jones JM, Lawson ML, Daneman D, et al. Eating disorders in adolescent females with and without type 1 diabetes: cross sectional study. BMJ 2000;320:1563–6.

[61] Goodwin RD, Hoven CW, Spitzer RL. Diabetes and eating disorders in primary care. Int J Eat Disord 2003;33:85–91.

[62] Polonsky WH, Anderson BJ, Lohrer PA, et al. Insulin omission in women with IDDM. Diabetes Care 1994;17:1178–85.

[63] Rydall AC, Rodin GM, Olmsted MP, et al. Disordered eating behavior and microvascular complications in young women with insulin-dependent diabetes mellitus. N Engl J Med 1997;336:1849–54.

[64] Affenito SG, Adams CH. Are eating disorders more prevalent in females with type 1 diabetes mellitus when the impact of insulin omission is considered? Nutr Rev 2001;59:179–82.

[65] Affenito SG, Backstrand JR, Welch GW, et al. Subclinical and clinical eating disorders in IDDM negatively affect metabolic control. Diabetes Care 1997;20:182–4.

[66] Goebel-Fabbri AE, Fikkan J, Connell A, et al. Identification and treatment of eating disorders in women with type 1 diabetes mellitus. Treat Endocrinol 2002;1:155–62.

[67] Mannucci E, Rotella F, Ricca V, et al. Eating disorders in patients with type 1 diabetes: a meta-analysis. J Endocrinol Invest 2005;28:417–9.

[68] Peveler RC, Bryden KS, Neil HA, et al. The relationship of disordered eating habits and attitudes to clinical outcomes in young adult females with type 1 diabetes. Diabetes Care 2005; 28:84–8.

[69] Crow S, Kendall D, Praus B, et al. Binge eating and other psychopathology in patients with type II diabetes mellitus. Int J Eat Disord 2001;30:222–6.

[70] Crow SJ, Keel PK, Kendall D. Eating disorders and insulin-dependent diabetes mellitus. Psychosomatics 1998;39:233–43.

[71] Dixon L, Weiden P, Delahanty J, et al. Prevalence and correlates of diabetes in national schizophrenia samples. Schizophr Bull 2001;26:903–12.

[72] Kornegay CJ, Vasilakis-Scaramozza C, Jick H. Incident diabetes associated with antipsychotic use in the United Kingdom general practice research database. J Clin Psychiatry 2002;63:758–62.

[73] Buse JB, Cavazzoni P, Hornbuckle K, et al. A retrospective cohort study of diabetes mellitus and antipsychotic treatment in the United States. J Clin Epidemiol 2003;56:164–70.

[74] Cohen D, Dekker JJ, Peen J, et al. Prevalence of diabetes mellitus in chronic schizophrenic inpatients in relation to long-term antipsychotic treatment. Eur Neuropsychopharmacol 2006;16:487–94.

[75] Lindenmayer JP, Czobor P, Volavka J, et al. Changes in glucose and cholesterol levels in patients with schizophrenia treated with typical or atypical antipsychotics. Am J Psychiatry 2003;160:290–6.

[76] Holt RI, Peveler RC. Association between antipsychotic drugs and diabetes. Diabetes Obes Metab 2006;8:125–35.

[77] Henderson DC, Cagliero E, Copeland PM, et al. Glucose metabolism in patients with schizophrenia treated with atypical antipsychotic agents: a frequently sampled intravenous glucose tolerance test and minimal model analysis. Arch Gen Psychiatry 2005;62:19–28.

[78] Henderson DC, Cagliero E, Gray C, et al. Clozapine, diabetes mellitus, weight gain, and lipid abnormalities: a five-year naturalistic study. Am J Psychiatry 2000;157:975–81.

[79] Bruce DG, Harrington N, Davis WA, et al. Dementia and its associations in type 2 diabetes mellitus: the Fremantle Diabetes Study. Diabetes Res Clin Pract 2001;53:165–72.

[80] Biessels GJ, Staekenborg S, Brunner E, et al. Risk of dementia in diabetes mellitus: a systematic review. Lancet Neurol 2006;5:64–74.

[81] Draelos MT, Jacobson AM, Weinger K, et al. Cognitive function in patients with insulin-dependent diabetes mellitus during hyperglycemia and hypoglycemia. Am J Med 1995;98:135–44.

[82] Weinger K, Jacobson AM. Cognitive impairment in patients with type 1 (insulin dependent) diabetes mellitus: incidence, mechanisms and therapeutic implications. CNS Drugs 1998;9:233–52.

[83] Austin EJ, Deary IJ. Effects of repeated hypoglycemia on cognitive function: a psychometrically validated reanalysis of the Diabetes Control and Complications Trial data. Diabetes Care 1999;22:1273–7.

[84] The Diabetes Control and Complications Trial. Effects of intensive diabetes therapy on neuropsychological function in adults. Ann Intern Med 1996;124:379–88.

[85] Rovet JF, Ehrlich RM, Hoppe M. Intellectual deficits associated with early onset of insulin-dependent diabetes mellitus in children. Diabetes Care 1987;10:510–5.

[86] Rovet JF, Ehrlich RM, Hoppe M. Specific intellectual deficits in children with early onset diabetes mellitus. Child Dev 1988;59:226–34.

[87] Bjorgaas M, Gimse R, Vik T, et al. Cognitive function in type 1 diabetic children with and without episodes of severe hypoglycaemia. Acta Paediatr 1997;86:148–53.

[88] Ryan CM, Geckle M. Why is learning and memory dysfunction in type 2 diabetes limited to older adults? Diabetes Metab Res Rev 2000;16:308–15.

NURSING
CLINICS
OF NORTH AMERICA

Nurs Clin N Am 41 (2006) 681–695

Diabetes Mellitus and Cardiovascular Disease

Deborah A. Chyun, PhD, RN, FAHA[a],*,
Lawrence H. Young, MD, FACC, FAHA[b]

[a]Yale University School of Nursing, 100 Church Street South, PO Box 9740,
New Haven, CT 06536–0740, USA
[b]Section of Cardiovascular Disease, Department of Internal Medicine, Yale University School
of Medicine, FMP3, 333 Cedar Street, New Haven, CT 06520, USA

Cardiovascular diseases (CVD) include hypertension, coronary heart disease (CHD), acute myocardial infarction (MI), heart failure (HF), sudden death, peripheral vascular disease, and stroke. The high risk of CVD in individuals with diabetes mellitus (DM) was recognized more than 30 years ago in the Framingham Study [1], and since then other large epidemiologic trials have confirmed these findings [2,3]. In the United Kingdom Prospective Diabetes Study, 20% of the individuals with type 2 DM developed CVD over 10 years of follow-up [4].

The pathophysiologic mechanisms responsible for CVD in individuals with DM are complex and multifactorial. Increasing attention is being focused on the constellation of risk factors (dyslipidemia, elevated blood pressure and blood glucose, and obesity) known as the "metabolic syndrome," because these factors predict not only the development of CVD, but also type 2 DM [5]. Diabetes is associated with the presence of oxidized, small dense low-density lipoprotein cholesterol, which is atherogenic, and reduced high-density lipoprotein cholesterol and increased triglyceride levels. Although traditional risk factors play a role, other factors, such as microalbuminuria, elevated levels of homocysteine, vascular inflammation, and hemostatic abnormalities, also have an important contribution to the development of CVD in individuals with DM [6].

Hypertension is seen in most individuals with type 2 DM and contributes to the risk of CHD, stroke, and HF. Chronic HF causes substantial morbidity in individuals with DM, including both exertional limitation and

* Corresponding author.
  E-mail address: deborah.chyun@yale.edu (D.A. Chyun).

recurrent hospitalizations. Women, older individuals, and those treated with insulin are at increased risk of HF [7]. Individuals with hypertension and DM often develop HF despite normal systolic function, sometimes referred to as "diastolic heart failure" [8]. The importance of blood pressure control in preventing CVD in individuals with DM was clearly demonstrated in the United Kingdom Prospective Diabetes Study [9].

Elevated blood glucose levels have long been theorized to contribute to CVD and recent evidence in younger individuals with type 1 DM has shown this to be true [10]. Appreciation of the multiple risk factors and complex pathophysiologic process responsible for CVD in individuals with both type 1 and type 2 DM is critical for the prevention, early detection, and management of CVD in this population. The focus of this article is on the acute and chronic manifestations of CHD. Stroke, however, which is not discussed, is another important cause of morbidity and mortality in the population with DM.

Prevention of coronary heart disease

The prevention of both CHD and the microvascular complications of DM is critical. The presence of underlying retinopathy, nephropathy, and neuropathy place the individual at higher risk for the development of CHD, and in addition, indicate a poorer prognosis after a CHD event. Prevention of both macrovascular CHD and microvascular complications requires risk reduction aimed at modifying the multiple factors that contribute to CHD (Table 1) [11,12]. Lifestyle recommendations should include intensive dietary management, weight control, regular physical activity, moderation in alcohol and sodium intake, and smoking cessation when indicated. Hypertension and dyslipidemia should be aggressively treated. All individuals with DM should strive to maintain optimal glycemic control with target glycosylated hemoglobin A_{1c} <7% and most should be taking daily aspirin. Blood pressure should be lowered to below 130/80 mm Hg.

Regular physical activity is vital in the management of both type 1 and type 2 DM, having beneficial effects on glycemic control, lipids, weight, and blood pressure. Many older individuals with type 2 DM are deconditioned, however, and find activity difficult because of the presence of osteoarthritis, obesity, and peripheral or autonomic neuropathy. In addition, a goal of 30 minutes of activity during one session may not be achievable and may deter these individuals from any participation. Shorter, more frequent periods of activity may be better tolerated. This approach, in combination with resistance exercise, may allow many individuals gradually to increase their level of endurance. Sedentary individuals should always initiate exercise programs at a low level and gradually increase the intensity of exercise. Because of the possibility of unrecognized CHD, individuals with type 2 DM should generally engage in moderate-intensity exercise regimens. Walking, however, is safe and should be encouraged. Individualized

Table 1
Prevention, early detection, and management of cardiovascular disease

Goal	Strategies
Blood pressure	
<130/80 mm Hg	Measured at each visit; ensure proper cuff size
	Educate regarding lifestyle modification (weight control, physical activity, moderate alcohol and sodium intake)
	Medication: monitor adherence and assess for side effects
Lipids	
LDL-C <100 mg/dL[a]	Tested annually or every 2 y if low-risk
HDL-C >40 mg/dL in men; >50 mg/dL in women	Educate regarding lifestyle modification (as above plus reduction in saturated fat and cholesterol)
Triglycerides <150 mg/dL	Daily fat intake: <7%–10% saturated fat and <200–300 mg cholesterol
	Regular physical activity
	Weight and glycemic control
	Medication: monitor adherence and assess for side effects
Hemoglobin A1c	
<7%	Tested two to three times annually if meeting goal; four times annually if above goal or therapy changed
	Medical nutrition therapy
	Weight control
	Regular physical activity
	Self-monitoring of blood glucose
	Education in self-management and problem solving
Physical activity	
150 min/wk of moderate-intensity aerobic activity	Routinely assess physical activity and exercise status
	Encourage moderate aerobic regimen and increase in daily activities
Resistance exercise 3 times/wk	Activity over at least 3 days with no more than two consecutive days without activity
	Individualization of activity prescription
	Resistance exercise should target all major muscle groups and progress to 8–10 repetitions
	Caution with peripheral or cardiac autonomic neuropathy, proliferative retinopathy, or microalbuminuria and nephropathy
	Educate regarding typical and atypical signs and symptoms of myocardial ischemia and how to respond
Weight	
Body mass index 21–25 kg/m^2	Height, weight, body mass index calculation, and waist circumference at each visit

(*continued on next page*)

Table 1 (*continued*)

Goal	Strategies
Waist circumference <102 cm in men and <88 cm in women	Weight control Regular physical activity
Smoking	
Complete cessation	Assess smoking status Provide counseling, problem-solving, or coping skills training, and pharmacotherapy
Antiplatelet therapy	
Consider enteric-coated aspirin 75–162 mg/d	Consider if age 30–40 y and additional cardiac risk factors
Use enteric-coated aspirin 75–162 mg/d	Known CVD or type 1 or 2 diabetes mellitus with family history CVD, hypertension, smoking, dyslipidemia, or albuminuria

Abbreviations: CVD, cardiovascular disease; HDL-C, high-density lipoproteins; LDL-C, low-density lipoproteins.

[a] With known CVD, LDL-C <70 mg/dL may be appropriate [11].

Data from American Diabetes Association. Standards of medical care in diabetes. Diabetes Care 2005;28:S4–36; Grundy SM, Howard B, Smith S, et al. Prevention Conference VI: Diabetes and cardiovascular disease. Circulation 2002;105:2231–9.

exercise recommendations are required in individuals with peripheral or cardiovascular autonomic neuropathy (CAN), severe retinopathy, or known CHD as discussed later, as is the use of stress testing in high-risk individuals. Education regarding symptoms of myocardial ischemia and instructions about reporting them to their health care provider should be stressed. All individuals with DM should have their CHD risk factor status assessed yearly.

Detection of coronary heart disease

Coronary atherosclerosis is typically more diffuse, more widespread, and more severe in individuals with DM than in those without DM. The atherosclerotic process results in plaque build up that may result in plaque rupture leading to acute coronary syndromes (ACS), unstable angina, and acute MI. Advanced atherosclerosis may significantly narrow the vessel lumen and restrict blood flow, leading to myocardial ischemia during exercise or emotional stress. In addition, CHD and hypertension also contribute to the development of HF, with atherosclerotic CHD being the most common cause of HF in the United States, and in individuals with DM.

Frequently, individuals with and without DM experience exertional or stress-induced angina as the first manifestation of underlying CHD. Ischemia may result in pressure, squeezing, fullness, or pain in the center of the chest; pain or discomfort in one or both arms, back, neck, jaw, or abdomen; feeling out of breath with or before the chest discomfort; breaking out into a cold sweat; feeling sick to the stomach; or lightheadedness. In these individuals, the electrocardiogram (ECG) may reveal ST-segment depression,

significant Q waves, deep T-wave inversions, left bundle branch block, ventricular arrhythmias, or heart block. The diagnosis of CHD is relatively straightforward in individuals with chronic stable angina or ACS and is confirmed by coronary angiography or exercise or pharmacologic stress testing with ECG, myocardial perfusion imaging, or echocardiography.

More problematic is the fact that CHD may go unrecognized until advanced, placing the individual at high risk of ACS and sudden death. Ischemia and accompanying anginal symptoms may not be provoked in the presence of mild underlying CHD or at low levels of physical activity, often found in individuals with DM. An important problem in DM is that even with severe underlying CHD, however, many individuals may have atypical symptoms or be totally asymptomatic, referred to as "silent" or "asymptomatic" myocardial ischemia.

Asymptomatic myocardial ischemia is often associated with CAN that affects the parasympathetic and sympathetic innervation of the heart and peripheral vasculature. CAN leads to a variety of manifestations including a slightly increased resting heart rate; severe orthostatic hypotension with recurrent lightheadedness, unsteadiness, or even frank syncope; impaired exercise tolerance; QT interval prolongation and increased QT dispersion on the ECG; and arrhythmias. Although symptoms of CAN may appear late in the disease course, some individuals with type 2 DM already have CAN at the time of initial DM diagnosis [13].

CAN is often associated with poor glycemic and lipid control. It develops in as many as one quarter of individuals with DM and is associated with a high risk of death [14]. CAN should be considered in patients with DM who have peripheral neuropathy or other forms of autonomic neuropathy, such as erectile dysfunction or gastroparesis. Testing, however, which typically includes changes in heart rate during deep breathing (the expiratory/inspiratory ratio), standing, and Valsalva maneuvers, along with blood pressure responses to hand grip and standing, is required to diagnose CAN. Standard cutpoints for diagnosing abnormal tests are available [15,16] and newer, automated systems simplify testing and diagnosis. Participant co-operation and correct performance of the tests are essential to obtain accurate results [17].

Analysis of heart rate variability through measuring instantaneous heart rate (R-R) intervals, assessed by either statistical analysis of R-R interval changes (time-domain) or power spectral analysis of successive R-R intervals (frequency-domain) [18], can also identify CAN. Variations that occur in the high-frequency range (0.15–0.40 Hz) reflect parasympathetic activity, whereas low-frequency (0.04–0.15 Hz) variability is modulated primarily by sympathetic activity. The ECG can also be used to determine general evidence of CAN, which can then be further quantified by standard heart rate and blood pressure–based means or heart rate variability methods. An ECG rhythm strip, which shows obvious sinus arrhythmia, generally indicates that cardiac autonomic function is healthy, whereas rapid, fixed heart rates may indicate CAN. A drop in the orthostatic systolic pressure > 15 mm Hg in the absence

of acute hypovolemia or diuretic use is suggestive and >20 mm Hg is fairly diagnostic of advanced autonomic dysfunction [6,17].

CAN may not only contribute to exercise intolerance, but it may identify patients at high risk of asymptomatic myocardial ischemia and underlying CHD [19]. As many as 22% of older adults with type 2 DM have evidence of ischemia in the absence of symptoms [20]. Recent recommendations are that all patients with type 2 DM be screened for CAN at the time of diagnosis and those with type 1 be screened 5 years after diagnosis [21]. If screening is negative, it should be repeated yearly.

The presence of CAN should alert providers to the possibility of asymptomatic CHD. This requires examination of the ECG for abnormalities suggestive of prior MI or ischemia, and potentially stress testing using either exercise or pharmacologic stress. Stress testing is also indicated when symptoms suggestive of CHD are present; when the individual wants to engage in high-intensity exercise; or in those with a long duration of DM, multiple CHD risk factors, or known DM-related complications [22].

Nursing has an important role in the detection of CHD, and the prevention, detection, and management of CAN. Many individuals with DM are unaware of the problem of autonomic neuropathy, having heard more about retinopathy, nephropathy, or painful peripheral neuropathy. Education regarding the signs or symptoms of other forms of autonomic neuropathy and CAN should be provided, along with stressing the importance of glucose and CHD risk factor control, as a means to prevent these complications [23]. If CAN is present, caution to prevent hypoglycemia is required because many of these individuals experience hypoglycemia unawareness. Peripheral neuropathy and CAN mandate special exercise precautions, such as increased vigilance for foot trauma and avoidance of postural hypotension and dehydration. These individuals should generally engage in moderate-intensity exercise regimens. Interventions used for prevention and management of CHD (improving nutritional intake, decreasing alcohol intake, and cessation of smoking) are also likely to benefit CAN and these should be encouraged.

Individuals with DM should also be aware that they are at an increased risk of developing CVD and should be alerted to typical and atypical symptoms of CHD. They should understand the fact that women and older individuals and people with DM tend to present atypically. They should also be instructed to seek help if symptoms do not resolve on their own or rapidly with nitroglycerin. Importantly, nurses in all settings should be vigilant for the presence of asymptomatic CHD in individuals with DM.

Acute manifestations of coronary heart disease: medical and surgical interventions

Early and appropriate management of the ACS is critical to limit myocardial damage and prevent complications. In the presence of ST-segment

elevation MI (STEMI) this can be accomplished with either thrombolytic therapy or percutaneous interventions (PCI). Individuals with DM, however, tend to present with non-STEMI more frequently than STEMI. Although these individuals tend to have a less complicated in-hospital course, they remain at extremely high risk for subsequent events including death, progression to acute STEMI, and subsequent readmission for unstable angina within the next year, unless appropriately evaluated and treated.

Individuals with and without DM in the setting of ACS require aspirin, β-blockers, and nitrates to prevent ischemia [24–26]. In addition, clopidogrel, heparin, or glycoprotein IIb-IIIa inhibitors may be used if additional interventions are planned. In the presence of STEMI individuals with DM who are within 12 hours of the onset of symptoms usually are treated with primary PCI with stent placement, particularly if there is evidence of HF or hemodynamic instability. Although the use of drug-eluting stents has significantly reduced the risk of restenosis in the presence of DM, long-term risks of restenosis, subsequent revascularization, and mortality remain elevated, with older individuals, women, and insulin-using individuals being at highest risk [24,27]. Importantly, following the acute event, the underlying hemostatic abnormalities frequently found in individuals with DM and the predilection of drug-eluting stents to thrombosis require ongoing, aggressive antithrombotic treatment with aspirin and clopidogrel to prevent reocclusion [24]. Aspirin and clopidogrel are continued for a minimum of 6 to 12 months and then aspirin therapy indefinitely.

In addition to standard nursing care delivered to all individuals with ACS, including those undergoing thrombolytic therapy and PCI, the presence of comorbid disease and poorer cardiac function, often found in DM, indicates a higher risk during hospitalization, requiring increased vigilance for complications. Renal function should be closely monitored, as should serum potassium levels. Individuals with DM are also at increased risk for contrast nephropathy, underscoring the importance of adequate hydration, careful assessment of renal function, and strict adherence to protocols used to prevent contrast-induced nephropathy.

Because individuals with DM frequently have a previous history of hypertension and stroke, the use of thrombolytics and PCI demands careful baseline and ongoing assessment of neurologic status. Changes in neurologic status should be conveyed immediately so that fibrinolytic, antiplatelet, and anticoagulant therapy can be discontinued. More extensive vascular disease in DM also increases the risk of stroke or peripheral embolization with PCI. An important part of the baseline medication history includes use of antihypertensives, agents to manage DM and other comorbidities, all over-the-counter medication and herbal preparation use, existing aspirin or antiplatelet therapy, and use of phosphodiesterase inhibitors for erectile dysfunction. The presence of erectile dysfunction or other evidence of autonomic neuropathy may place the individual at higher risk for adverse outcomes following ACS.

HF develops more commonly in DM, even though the index MIs are no larger than in those individuals without DM. Coexistent hypertension and renal disease, commonly found in DM, may further promote the development of symptomatic HF. Individuals with CAN or IIF may have an increased heart rate contributing to increased myocardial oxygen demands, underscoring the importance of ongoing monitoring for continued ischemia. There is also evidence that individuals with DM and acute MI may have an increase risk of heart block (atrioventricular, fascicular, and bundle branch blocks); atrial arrhythmias; renal insufficiency; and cardiogenic shock [6]. These complications should be closely monitored during hospitalization.

Following stabilization with medical therapy, individuals with DM may be further evaluated with angiography and possible revascularization. Nonurgent PCI is usually reserved for those individuals with DM who have single-vessel disease. Concerns regarding the use of multivessel PCI in individuals with DM were first raised in the late 1980s, and whereas more recent data suggest that the risk associated with multivessel PCI is now lower [28], many individuals with DM and advanced multivessel CHD still require surgical revascularization.

Although mortality associated with coronary artery bypass graft (CABG) surgery in individuals with DM in the current era is less than 5%, long-term patency of saphenous vein grafts remains problematic. The use of an internal mammary artery graft is especially important in individuals with DM because of its superior long-term patency. Individuals with DM are at risk for a number of postoperative complications, however, including angina and HF as a result of less complete revascularization, graft occlusion, and accelerated native disease progression.

Post-CABG nursing care is based on the recognition that individuals with diabetes are at increased risk of a number of cardiac and noncardiac complications, requiring careful assessment so that they can be promptly treated. The most concerning complications are postoperative MI, stroke, renal failure, mediastinitis, sternal wound infection, and sepsis [29], with women, older individuals, and those with a history of prior stroke or renal insufficiency being at high risk. The risk of sternal wound infection may also be increased when preoperative blood glucose is suboptimal. Additionally, poor glycemic control has been linked to postoperative MI and stroke [29]. Intensive control of blood glucose with intravenous insulin during and following CABG is advocated, because it has been shown to improve metabolic and hemodynamic parameters; decrease the risk of immediate postoperative complications (need for pacing, atrial fibrillation, and infection); shorten the length of stay; and reduce the long-term risk of death [30].

Aggressive management of hyperglycemia in the acute care setting has received increased attention over the past decade, with improved short and long-tem outcomes following ACS being demonstrated with lowering of the blood glucose levels in individuals with and those without DM [31].

Current guidelines call for the use of an insulin infusion to normalize blood glucose in all individuals with STEMI with complicated courses, and this strategy being considered in all individuals, even in the absence of complications [26]. The transition to subcutaneous insulin or other oral agents should be made after the acute phase [32] and oral agents should not be used to control blood glucose in critically ill individuals. Importantly, metformin should be stopped because of the risk of lactic acidosis. In critically ill individuals blood glucose levels should be kept as close to 110 mg/dL as possible and under 180 mg/dL [21]. Although in noncritically ill individuals subcutaneous insulin may be used, this method of administration is more likely to lead to both hyperglycemia and hypoglycemia. Hypoglycemia must be carefully assessed for because it may trigger myocardial ischemia in individuals with DM. Insulin infusion protocols have been shown to reduce these risks [33].

The goal after discharge is to maintain hemoglobin A_{1c} levels <7%, and this may be accomplished with a variety of agents. Recent evidence suggests that use of insulin-sensitizing thiazolidinediones, such as rosiglitazone and pioglitazone, may contribute to lower restenosis rates following PCI [34], and improved outcomes following ACS in individuals treated with glycoprotein IIb-IIIa inhibitors [35]. These agents not only have beneficial effects on blood pressure and lipids, but directly affect vascular inflammation and other mechanisms responsible for atherosclerosis, thereby slowing the atherosclerotic process.

Because individuals with DM have several factors that may lead to less than optimal thrombolysis and predispose to reocclusion after PCI or CABG, careful ongoing assessment must also be made for adequacy of reperfusion and evidence of recurrent ischemia. Nurses in all settings should maintain a high index of suspicion for myocardial ischemia because of the presence of atypical symptoms in individuals with DM. Importantly, patient teaching should stress the importance of recognizing ischemic symptoms, both in the hospital and following discharge, and the need for CHD risk-reduction efforts discussed later. Following PCI and stent placement, the importance of not discontinuing antiplatelet therapy without medical supervision should be stressed because of the high risk for reocclusion.

Management of chronic coronary heart disease

Long-term management of CHD is aimed at preventing new or recurrent MI, HF, and death. Following ACS, PCI, or CABG, or in individuals with chronic stable angina or asymptomatic CHD, an intensive effort is required to modify CHD risk factors and optimize glucose control. Because CVD is the result of numerous factors in the presence of DM, secondary and tertiary prevention require a multifaceted approach. Although this requires intensive and often expensive treatments, along with lifestyle modification, recent

evidence emphasizes that comprehensive reduction of multiple CHD risk factors along with glucose control prevents cardiac events in individuals with type 2 DM [23]. Aggressive treatment of dyslipidemia and hypertension, prevention of thrombosis with aspirin, and medications to reduce the occurrence of myocardial ischemia should be instituted. Intensive therapy should be aimed at decreasing the likelihood of subsequent cardiac events and death, slowing the progression of coronary atherosclerosis, and preventing ischemic symptoms.

Specific therapy for angina should include β-blockers, which prevent ischemia and improve exercise tolerance, reducing the risk of recurrent events. β-Blockers are used if the risk of ischemia is high or following MI. Their use necessitates assessment for worsening lipid and glycemic control, masking of hypoglycemia, and caution in the presence of CAN because of the risk of orthostatic hypotension. Angiotensin-converting enzyme inhibitors have an important role in the treatment of CHD in individuals with DM, particularly in the presence of HF, decreased left ventricular function, and hypertension. In addition, they may also have a more generalized benefit, stabilizing coronary plaques and preventing ACS, thereby preventing cardiac events in individuals with DM and CHD [36].

Nitrates are useful for the symptomatic relief and prevention of angina, but need to be used with caution in individuals with autonomic neuropathy because hypotension may result. Use of a phosphodiesterase inhibitor for erectile dysfunction within the previous 24 hours is a contraindication for nitrate use and individuals using both types of agents should be appropriately instructed. Calcium-channel blockers have an important role in controlling blood pressure when hypertension is present and are also helpful in the treatment of angina. Nondihydropyridines are contraindicated when HF caused by systolic dysfunction is present, however, in which case dihydropyridines may be used for hypertension.

Adequate control of blood pressure and treatment of lipid abnormalities are critically important. Lipid-lowering medications require that liver function be monitored. Education regarding rhabdomyolysis, particularly with concomitant fibrate therapy, should be provided. In addition, the mild hyperglycemic effects of niacin should be recognized, along with the need to monitor liver functions tests and creatine phosphokinase levels when niacin and statins are used in combination. Improved glucose control and avoiding alcohol may assist in lowering elevated triglyceride levels, whereas increasing the level of physical activity may have beneficial effects on raising high-density lipoprotein cholesterol levels. Individualized recommendations for regular exercise should be reinforced with limitations placed on strenuous activity that might place the individual at risk for a cardiac event. Importantly, the individual should understand how to manage angina and should be able to recognize when prolonged symptoms may signal ACS and how to respond. Asymptomatic CHD poses additional challenges, because the individual may not recognize the presence of ischemia and react

appropriately. Anginal equivalents or atypical symptoms should be recognized to prevent delay in seeking treatment.

Despite the increased platelet reactivity that occurs with DM, cardiac events are generally reduced by relatively low doses of aspirin through its effect on prevention of coronary thrombus formation. Thienopyridine agents, such as clopidogrel, block the platelet activation pathway and are effective in inhibiting platelet aggregation. Clopidogrel is used routinely following coronary stent placement and in chronic CHD in individuals allergic to or unable to take aspirin. All individuals with DM, however, following ACS, should be taking daily aspirin unless there is a contraindication, in which case clopidogrel or warfarin should be used. Clopidogrel, however, is more expensive than aspirin and although rare, granulocytopenia and thrombotic thrombocytopenic purpura may result. The combination of aspirin and clopidogrel may have a small benefit over aspirin alone; however, combination use may increase the risk of bleeding [37].

After CABG, individuals with DM should still be considered to have ongoing cardiovascular risk, with less favorable long-term outcomes, including lower survival than those individuals without diabetes. This reflects, in part, both their more advanced cardiac disease and comorbidity at the time of surgery, particularly peripheral vascular disease and renal insufficiency. Predictors of worse outcomes following CABG include preoperative stroke, hypertension, HF, high glucose levels, proteinuria, multivessel disease, male gender, left ventricular dysfunction, and surgery with less than three grafts [6]. Careful, ongoing assessment should be made for graft occlusion and progression of CHD, and for the development of HF.

The prevention and treatment of HF in the presence of DM requires optimal management of coexistent hypertension, CHD, and left ventricular dysfunction. Although other conditions may cause HF, if the individual with DM is not known to have underlying CHD, further testing is initiated to assess for occult CHD, because revascularization or anti-ischemic medications (eg, nitrates and β-blockers) may improve cardiac function.

HF is frequently seen in individuals with DM with acute MI, and during long-term follow-up after ACS. Lower socioeconomic status, older age, female gender, longer diabetes duration, insulin use, poorer glycemic control, higher body mass index, higher serum creatinine, and the presence of DM-related comorbidities, particularly nephropathy, have been linked with an increased risk of HF in individuals with diabetes [7,38,39]. The association with glycemic control is not only strong, but shows that the level of risk increases as the level of hemoglobin A_{1c} rises above $>7\%$.

In individuals with DM, the prevention and management of HF follows standard recommendations, including intensive treatment of coexistent hypertension, CHD, renal disease, and hyperglycemia [40]. Because HF is extremely common in the elderly with DM [8], however, comorbidities, such as chronic renal insufficiency, may complicate treatment. Optimal treatment of

hypertension is critical to both the prevention and treatment of HF in individuals with DM. Blood pressure should be below 130/80 mm Hg and angiotensin-converting enzyme inhibitors are the cornerstone of prevention and treatment of HF [36]. Angiotensin-receptor blockers are also used widely for the prevention and treatment of HF, particularly when individuals are unable to use angiotensin-converting enzyme inhibitors because of the development of cough [41]. Renal function and hyperkalemia should be assessed, especially in the presence of underlying renal dysfunction. Although there is sometimes reluctance to use β-blockers in the presence of DM and symptomatic HF, because of concerns for worsening insulin resistance, masking hypoglycemia, or aggravating orthostatic hypotension, these agents have been shown to contribute to improved outcomes [42]. Careful monitoring and treatment for these effects, however, is required. When diuretics are used serum potassium levels should be monitored because of an increased risk of hyperkalemia with potassium-sparing agents and of hypokalemia with loop diuretics.

The treatment of individuals with diabetes and HF caused by diastolic dysfunction poses additional challenges. Poorly controlled hypertension, tachycardia, atrial fibrillation, active myocardial ischemia, and volume over load can all potentially exacerbate HF in these individuals and should be avoided [8,43]. Aggressive blood pressure control, sodium restriction, and diuretics are important in symptomatic individuals [8]. The primary approaches to treat HF caused by diastolic dysfunction include intensive treatment of hypertension to reduce afterload and left ventricular mass and diuretics to prevent volume overload.

Cardiac transplantation has been successfully used in younger individuals with DM who are unresponsive to medical therapy. Following transplantation, DM management may be complicated by the use of corticosteroids for immunosuppression, necessitating high doses of insulin or oral agents. Infection is another concern, as is posttransplant vasculopathy, with insulin resistance and dyslipidemia increasing that risk. Aggressive control of blood glucose and lipid-lowering with statins are important to reduce the development of posttransplant vasculopathy.

The presence of HF also affects the choice of medications used to treat type 2 DM. Metformin and thiazolidinediones are not recommended in individuals with moderate-to-severe HF, although recent observational data suggest that use of these agents was associated with a lower risk of death [44]. Decreased clearance of metformin in individuals with HF caused by hypoperfusion or renal insufficiency can lead to potentially dangerous lactic acidosis. Thiazolidinediones are sometimes associated with fluid retention, pedal edema, and weight gain, particularly when used in conjunction with insulin, and occasionally contributes to HF [45]. Careful clinical assessment before initiation of thiazolidinediones, lower doses with slow dose escalation, and careful ongoing monitoring should be implemented when these drugs are used in the presence of known structural heart disease or a prior

history of HF. Insulin and insulin secretagogues are considered safe for use in individuals with HF.

Summary

Although short- and long-term outcomes in individuals with DM following ACS, PCI, and CABG have improved over the past decade, CVD continues to be an important cause of morbidity and mortality in this population. Nursing has a critical role in the prevention of CVD, and in the early detection of symptomatic and asymptomatic CHD. Following ACS, PCI, or CABG, ongoing assessment for new ischemia, HF, or renal insufficiency, and specific complications of ACS or revascularization is crucial. Long-term prevention of recurrent ischemia, ACS, HF, and death necessitates multifactorial CHD risk factor reduction, along with aggressive glucose control, in all individuals with DM.

References

[1] Kannel WB, McGee DL. Diabetes and cardiovascular risk factors: the Framingham Study. Circulation 1979;2:8–13.

[2] Fox S, Coady S, Sorlie PD, et al. Trends in cardiovascular complications of diabetes. JAMA 2004;292:2495–9.

[3] Hu FB, Stampfer MJ, Solomon CG, et al. The impact of diabetes mellitus on mortality from all causes and coronary heart disease in women. Arch Intern Med 2001;161:1721–3.

[4] United Kingdom Prospective Diabetes (UKPDS) Group. Intensive blood-glucose control with sulfonylureas or insulin compared with conventional treatment and risk of complications in patients with type 2 diabetes (UKPDS 33). Lancet 1998;352:837–53.

[5] Grundy SM, Cleeman JI, Daniels SR, et al. Diagnosis and management of the metabolic syndrome. Circulation 2005;112:2735–52.

[6] Young LH, Chyun DA. Heart disease in patients with diabetes. In: Porte D, Baron A, Sherwin RS, editors. Ellenberg and Rifkin's diabetes mellitus: theory and practice. 6th edition. New York: McGraw-Hill; 2002. p. 823–44.

[7] Bertoni AG, Bonds DE, Hundley WG, et al. Heart failure prevalence, incidence, and mortality in the elderly with diabetes. Diabetes Care 2004;27:699–703.

[8] Piccini JP, Klein L, Gheorghiade M, et al. New insights into diastolic heart failure: role of diabetes mellitus. Am J Med 2004;116(Suppl 5A):64S–75.

[9] The UKPDS Group. Tight blood pressure control and risk of macrovascular and microvascular complications in type 2 diabetes: UKPDS 38. BMJ 1998;317:703–13.

[10] Diabetes Control and Complications Trial/Epidemiology of Diabetes Interventions and Complications (DCCT/EDIC) Study Research Group. Intensive diabetes treatment and cardiovascular disease in patients with type 1 diabetes. N Engl J Med 2005;353:2643–53.

[11] American Diabetes Association. Standards of medical care in diabetes. Diabetes Care 2005; 28:S4–36.

[12] Grundy SM, Howard B, Smith S, et al. Prevention conference VI: Diabetes and cardiovascular disease. Circulation 2002;105:2231–9.

[13] Low PA, Benrud-Larson LM, Sletten DM, et al. Autonomic symptoms and diabetic neuropathy. Diabetes Care 2004;27:2942–7.

[14] Maser RE, Vinik AI, Mitchell BD, et al. The association between cardiovascular autonomic neuropathy and mortality in individuals with diabetes. Diabetes Care 2003;26:1895–901.

[15] Ewing DJ, Borsey DQ, Bellavere F, et al. Cardiac autonomic neuropathy in diabetes: comparison of measures of R-R interval variation. Diabetologia 1981;21:18–24.

[16] O'Brien IA, O'Hare P, Corrall RJM. Heart rate variability in healthy subjects: effects of age and the derivation of normal ranges for tests of autonomic function. Br Heart J 1986;55: 348–54.

[17] Herzog R, Chyun DA, Young LH. Cardiovascular autonomic neuropathy. Practical Diabet, in press.

[18] Task Force of the European Society of Cardiology and the North American Society of Pacing and Electrophysiology. Heart rate variability: standards of measurement, physiological interpretation, and clinical use. Circulation 1996;93:1043–65.

[19] Vinik AI, Mitchell BD, Maser RE, et al. Diabetic autonomic neuropathy. Diabetes Care 2003;26:1895–901.

[20] Wackers FJTH, Young LH, Inzucchi SE, et al. Detection of silent myocardial ischemia in asymptomatic diabetic subjects: the DIAD Study. Diabetes Care 2004;27:1954–61.

[21] Boulton AJM, Vinik AI, Arezzo JC, et al. Diabetic neuropathies: a statement by the American Diabetes Association. Diabetes Care 2005;28:956–62.

[22] American Diabetes Association. Consensus development conference on the diagnosis of coronary heart disease in people with diabetes. Diabetes Care 1998;21:1551–9.

[23] Gaede P, Vedel P, Larsen N, et al. Multifactorial intervention and cardiovascular disease in patients with type 2 diabetes. N Engl J Med 2003;348:383–93.

[24] Roffi M, Topol EJ. Percutaneous coronary intervention in diabetes patients with non–ST-segment elevation acute coronary syndromes. Eur Heart J 2004;25:190–8.

[25] Braunwald E, Antman EM, Beasley JW, et al. ACC/AHA 2002 guideline update for the management of patients with unstable angina and non-ST-segment elevation myocardial infarction – summary article: a report of the American College of Cardiology/American Heart Association task force on practice guidelines (committee on the management of patients with unstable angina). J Am Coll Cardiol 2002;40:1366–74.

[26] Antman EM, Anbe DT, Armstrong PW, et al. ACC/AHA Guidelines for the management of patients with ST-elevation myocardial infarction: executive summary. Circulation 2004;110: 588–636.

[27] Gilbert J, Raboud J, Zinman B. Meta-analysis of the effect of diabetes on restenosis rates among patients receiving coronary angioplasty stenting. Diabetes Care 2004;27: 990–4.

[28] Abizaid A, Costa MA, Centemero M, et al. Clinical and economic impact of diabetes mellitus on percutaneous and surgical treatment of multivessel coronary disease patients: insights for the Arterial Revascularization Therapy Study (ARTS) Trial. Circulation 2001;104: 533–40.

[29] McAlister FA, Man J, Bistritz L, et al. Diabetes and coronary artery bypass surgery. Diabetes Care 2003;26:1518–24.

[30] Lazar HL, Chipkin SR, Fitzgerald CA, et al. Tight glycemic control in diabetic coronary artery bypass graft patients improves perioperative outcomes and decreases recurrent ischemic events. Circulation 2004;109:1497–502.

[31] Stranders I, Diamant M, van Gelder RE, et al. Admission blood glucose level as risk indicator of death after myocardial infarction in patients with and without diabetes. Arch Intern Med 2004;164:982–8.

[32] Clement S, Braithwaite SS, Magee MF, et al. Management of diabetes and hyperglycemia in hospitals. Diabetes Care 2004;27:553–91.

[33] Goldberg PA, Siegel MD, Sherwin RS, et al. Implementation of a safe and effective insulin infusion protocol in a medical intensive care unit. Diabetes Care 2004;27:461–7.

[34] Choi D, Kim SK, Choi SH, et al. Preventive effects of rosiglitazone on restenosis after coronary stent implantation in patients with type 2 diabetes. Diabetes Care 2004;27: 2654–60.

[35] McGuire DK, Newby LK, Bhapkar MV, et al. Association of diabetes mellitus and glycemic control strategies with clinical outcomes after acute coronary syndromes. Am Heart J 2004; 147:246–52.

[36] Heart Outcomes Prevention Evaluation (HOPE) Study Investigators. Effects of ramipril on cardiovascular and microvascular outcomes in people with diabetes mellitus: results of the HOPE study and MICRO-HOPE substudy. Lancet 2000;355:253–9.

[37] Bhatt DL, Fox KAA, Hacke W, et al. Clopidogrel and aspirin versus aspirin alone for prevention of atherothrombotic events. N Engl J Med 2006;354:1706–17.

[38] Iribarren C, Karter AJ, Go AS, et al. Glycemic control and heart failure among adult patients with diabetes. Circulation 2001;103:2668–73.

[39] Bibbins-Domingo K, Lin F, Vittinghoff E, et al. Predictors of heart failure among women with coronary disease. Circulation 2004;110:1424–30.

[40] Hunt SA, Abraham WT, Chin MH, et al. American College of Cardiology/American Heart Association 2005 Guideline update for the diagnosis and management of chronic heart failure in the adult – summary article: a report of the ACC/AHA Task Force on Practice Guidelines. Circulation 2005;112:1825–52.

[41] Barnett A, Bain S, Bouter C, et al. Angiotensin-receptor blockade versus converting-enzyme inhibition in type 2 diabetes and nephropathy. N Engl J Med 2004;351:1952–61.

[42] Haas SJ, Vos T, Gilbert RE, et al. Are beta-blockers as efficacious in patients with diabetes mellitus as in patients without diabetes mellitus who have chronic heart failure? A meta-analysis of large-scale clinical trials. Am Heart J 2003;146:848–53.

[43] Zile MR, Brutsaert DL. New concepts in diastolic dysfunction and diastolic heart failure: Part II: causal mechanisms and treatment. Circulation 2002;105:1503–8.

[44] Masoudi FA, Inzucchi SE, Wang Y, et al. Thiazolidinediones, metformin, and outcomes in older patients with diabetes and heart failure. Circulation 2005;111:583–90.

[45] Nesto RW, LeWinter M, Bell D, et al. Thiazolidinedione use, fluid retention, and congestive heart failure. Diabetes Care 2004;27:256–63.

NURSING
CLINICS
OF NORTH AMERICA

ELSEVIER
SAUNDERS

Nurs Clin N Am 41 (2006) 697–717

Diabetic Neuropathies: Diagnosis and Treatment

Geralyn R. Spollett, MSN, ANP, CDE

*Yale Diabetes Center, Yale University School of Medicine, 333 Cedar Street, PO Box 208020,
New Haven, CT 06520–8020, USA*

Diabetic neuropathy is the most common neuropathy in the Western world [1]. Among the population of patients with diabetes, it is the most frequently occurring chronic complication affecting at least 50% or more, and increases with age and duration of disease [2]. Approximately 7% of newly diagnosed patients already have neuropathy [3]. It is difficult to accurately approximate the incidence and prevalence of this complication, however, because the definition and diagnostic criteria for neuropathy vary. There is a lack of consensus regarding clinical criteria for the diagnosis of early neuropathy and variable guidelines for use and interpretation of electrodiagnosis in subclinical neuropathy [4]. Although prevalence rates have varied from 5% to 100%, epidemiologic studies suggest that the incidence of diabetes in hospitalized patients is 30% and 20% in community patients [5].

Pathophysiology

Just as there are many manifestations of diabetic neuropathy, multiple theories exist to explain the pathophysiologic changes. Metabolic alterations, microvascular changes, and inflammation may all contribute in some way to the pathology of diabetic neuropathy. As with the other microvascular complications, retinopathy and nephropathy, poor glycemic control, specifically hyperglycemia, plays a central role in the development of neuropathy.

In the first theory, high blood glucose levels that enter the peripheral nerve independent of insulin accumulate leading to high nerve glucose concentrations. Glucose converts to sorbitol by the polyol pathway through a series of reactions catalyzed by aldose reductase [4]. The increase in

E-mail address: geralyn.spollett@yale.edu

sorbitol leads to a decrease in myoinositol levels causing interference with sodium pump and sodium-potassium ATPase activity. The activation of aldose reductase causes decreased levels of nitric oxide and glutathione. Without these, oxidative injury occurs. A decreased level of nitric oxide also inhibits vascular relaxation, which can result in ischemia [6].

The microvasculature of diabetic nerves is altered in neuropathy. Capillary basement membrane thickening, endothelial cell hyperplasia, and neuronal ischemia and infarction all lead to nerve dysfunction. Increased oxidative stress may decrease nerve blood flow by disruption in the signal transduction pathways in the vascular endothelium. Reduced nerve blood supply and endoneurial hypoxia damage nerve tissue [7]. In addition, chronic intracellular hyperglycemia contributes to the formation of advanced glycosylation end products that interfere with axonal transport and slow nerve conduction velocity. Advanced glycosylation end products can reduce NADPH leading to hydrogen peroxide formulation and further oxidative stress [4].

An inflammatory vascular process may cause certain asymmetric neuropathies, such as amyotrophy and mononeuritis multiplex. Diabetic nerves seem to have an increased susceptibility to cellular and humoral immune factors [4]. The development of nonsystemic vasculitis is restricted to the peripheral nerves. An inflammatory vasculopathy with multifocal axon loss may be the underlying cause of mononeuritis multiplex [8].

Classification of neuropathies

Every organ system of the body that relies on innervation for function can be affected by neuropathy associated with diabetes. Because the neuropathies are heterogeneous, presenting with diverse clinical manifestations and requiring body-specific treatment, various classification systems have been used. An American Diabetes Association Consensus Conference classified diabetic neuropathy into groups determined by neurologic disturbance: subclinical neuropathy, diffuse clinical neuropathy with distal symmetric sensorimotor and autonomic syndromes, and focal syndromes [9].

Three components make up the basis for the diagnosis of subclinical neuropathy: (1) abnormal electrodiagnostic tests with decreased nerve conduction velocity or decreased amplitude; (2) abnormal quantitative sensory tests for vibration, tactile, thermal warming, and cooling thresholds; and (3) quantitative autonomic function tests revealing diminished heart rate variation with deep breathing, Valsalva's maneuver, and postural testing [10].

In subclinical neuropathy, the damage to the nerve may be progressing but the patient is asymptomatic in this early stage. For patients with newly diagnosed type 2 diabetes, it is not unusual to see clinical signs of an asymptomatic neuropathy. The insidious onset of type 2 diabetes makes it difficult to estimate duration of disease and it is possible that the patient has had diabetes for 7 to 12 years before the actual diagnosis during which time nerve

damage occurred. The most rapid deterioration of nerve function, however, occurs soon after the onset of type 1 diabetes. Within 2 to 3 years the progression slows, moving at a reduced rate toward dysfunction [10].

Vinik [11] describes three proposed stages of neuropathy:

1. Functional neuropathy: No pathology but biochemical alteration in nerve function is present; it is reversible.
2. Structural neuropathy: Loss of structural change in nerve fibers; may be reversible.
3. Nerve death: Critical decrease in nerve fiber density and neuronal death; it is irreversible.

Because there is a distal-to-proximal gradient in nerve fiber loss in diabetic neuropathy, it is likely that the potential for reversibility is in a proximal-to-distal direction. Distal nerves are at greater risk for structural damage than proximal nerves.

Understanding the clinical presentation of neuropathy

There are a number of ways to discuss diabetic neuropathy: focal versus diffuse, proximal versus distal, and large fiber versus small fiber. Each of these descriptions helps to characterize the neuropathy and gives the clinician a way systematically to refine the clinical picture.

The definition of diabetic peripheral neuropathy is "the presence of symptoms or signs of peripheral nerve dysfunction in people with diabetes after the exclusion of other causes" [10]. Diabetic neuropathy is a diagnosis of exclusion; there are many causes for neuropathy and its signs and symptoms that are not related to diabetes. Because treatment is available for many of the diseases or syndromes that cause neuropathic dysfunction and pain, a thorough clinical examination with the appropriate diagnostic testing should be done before the decision to label the cause as diabetes-related. A discussion of the differential diagnoses for the generalized symmetric polyneuropathies and the focal and multifocal neuropathies is included in the diagnosis and treatment for each category.

Sensory neuropathies

The most common of the neuropathies is distal symmetric peripheral polyneuropathy (DSPN). The Centers for Disease Control and Prevention estimates that approximately 12% of patients have this condition at diagnosis and nearly 60% have it after 25 years of diabetes [12]. The pathogenesis seems to be related to abnormal neural metabolism and neural ischemia but the understanding of its etiology is incomplete. The onset may be insidious with the initial changes occurring in the most distal areas of the body in a symmetric fashion. As the disease progresses, it has a stocking-glove distribution, first affecting the lower extremities, progressing to mid-calf, and

then developing at the tips of the fingers and advancing to the wrists. Initially, the patient may notice a change in sensation in their great toes or report no altered sensations only to have signs of DSPN present on physical examination. Small nerve fiber dysfunction usually occurs early in the disease process and can be present without symptoms or changes on electrophysiologic testing [13]. Research studies indicate that the cutaneous nerve fibers or C-fibers are damaged in this early stage [14]. Most patients, however, experience symptoms as the disease progresses. Burning, electrical or stabbing sensations, paresthesias, and deep aching pain often accompany DSPN. Typically, the pain worsens at night.

Unlike chronic peripheral neuropathy, acute sensory neuropathy develops without other significant neurologic impairment. This "insulin neuritis" can occur late or early in the course of disease and may be associated with the initiation of insulin therapy, significant weight loss, or with wide fluctuations of glucose levels [15]. The symptoms tend to worsen at night. Patients may describe the pain as burning, aching, and stabbing dysesthesias and contact allodynia. Physical findings consistent with diabetic neuropathy may be absent. Symptoms resolve slowly, usually within months of achieving improved glucose control.

In formulating a list of differential diagnoses for acute and chronic sensorimotor neuropathy, similar symptoms may be caused by drug use, such as alcohol, nitrofurantoin, and isoniazid, or exposure to certain heavy metals. Other illnesses, such as pernicious anemia (vitamin B_{12} deficiency), chronic inflammatory demyelinating polyneuropathy, hypothyroidism, underlying neoplasms, Sjögren's syndrome, or uremia, need to be excluded through a thorough history, physical examination, and laboratory testing [16].

In the medical history, the clinician should question the patient about the use of drugs (prescription and recreational) and alcohol, looking for signs or symptoms of substance abuse, and exposure to toxins in the environment (insecticides) or in the place of work (solvents). Because some sensorimotor diseases are hereditary, a family medical history must be included.

Based on the history, the clinician may perform a complete physical examination. In every case, the careful examination of the lower extremities is mandatory. Because DSPN usually affects the small fibers and then the large nerve fibers, the physical examination must include vibratory sensation (using a 128-Hz tuning fork); light touch perception with a 5.07 (10-g) monofilament; pressure; temperature and pain sensation; dorsalis pedal pulses; ankle reflexes; and a thorough skin and nail examination. When using the 5.07 monofilament, the clinician places it on one of the 10 designated areas of the foot and then applies enough force to the monofilament to make it buckle (Fig. 1). Loss of monofilament perception and reduced vibratory perception indicate a foot at risk for developing ulcerations [17]. Because advanced stages of peripheral neuropathy can affect gait and balance, the clinician must pay particular attention as the patient walks and changes body position.

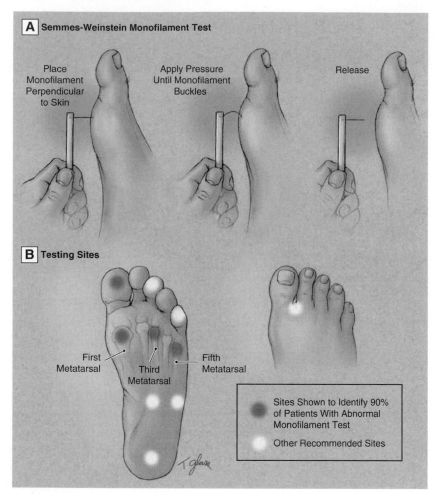

Fig. 1. Monofilament test for light touch sensation. (*A*) The 5.07 Semmes-Weinstein monofil-ament consists of a plastic handle supporting a nylon filament. The filament is placed perpen-dicular to the skin and pressure is applied until the filament buckles. The filament is held in place for approximately 1 second, then released. Inability to perceive the 10g of force it applies is clinically significant large-fiber neuropathy. (*B*) Testing 10 sites (as shown) evaluates all der-matomes of the foot and may improve the sensitivity and specificity compared with testing a sin-gle site. (*From* Singh N, Armstrong DG, Lipsky BA. Preventing foot ulcers in patients with diabetes. JAMA 2005;293:217–28, with permission. © 2005 American Medical Association. All rights reserved.)

Laboratory tests for the initial investigation of DSPN may include a com-plete blood count, erythrocyte sedimentation rate, vitamin B_{12} and folate levels, renal and liver function panels, and a thyroid-stimulating hormone level [16]. Other tests may be added specific to the findings of the history and physical examination.

Two types of electrodiagnostic tests are used to evaluate peripheral neuropathy: nerve conduction studies and needle electromyography. Nerve conduction studies can evaluate both sensory and motor nerves. In these studies amplitude, distal latency, and conduction velocity are recorded [18].

Use of the electromyography testing varies among clinical settings. It is invasive and usually uncomfortable for the patient. It is a sensitive indicator of axonal degeneration and the dying back of nerve fibers that occurs in many types of diabetic neuropathy. Routine use of electromyography as a diagnostic tool in peripheral neuropathy, however, is not universally recommended. Electromyography testing lacks the ability to evaluate unmyelinated C-fibers whose relatively slow conduction is not reflected in the standard electrophysiologic tests. Electromyography testing can be negative despite signs and symptoms indicative of peripheral neuropathy caused by C-fiber pathology. The alterations in the unmyelinated C-fiber are best seen in a 3-mm punch biopsy of the epidermis [19]. The use of electromyography testing is better suited to determine the presence of diabetic polyradiculopathy, amyotrophy, plexopathy, or other peripheral nerve disorders.

The American Diabetes Association recommends that the first step in the management of patients with DSPN is to optimize glucose control and avoid extreme fluctuations in glucose levels [20]. The management of neuropathic pain has been a clinical challenge for patients and providers for many years. Neuropathic pain can present in varying degrees with neurosensory signs manifesting as negative and positive phenomena [21]. Stimulus can evoke a pain perception that is either normal; reduced; or greatly exaggerated (hyperalgesia). Pain can also be evoked by a nonpainful stimulus, such as the touch of bed sheets (allodynia). Patients may describe spontaneous pain that burns, is knife-like, or feels like crawling insects on the legs. Numbness, or loss of sensation with "feet that feel like cement blocks," interferes with normal function and places the patient at risk for further foot trauma.

Achieving neuropathic pain control is difficult. The goal of neuropathic pain therapy is to reduce symptomalogy so that the patient is able to function. Unfortunately, most therapeutic strategies have only been able to reduce pain 20% to 30% as measured against placebo, not eradicate the pain. Some of this is caused by undertreatment by health care providers who are concerned with possible pain medication addictions, but the major reason is lack of effective therapeutic agents that reduce pain without impairing the patient's ability to function. Currently, there are five Food and Drug Administration–approved medications that are indicated for neuropathic pain treatment: carbamazepine for trigeminal neuralgia, gabapentin and transdermal lidocaine for postherpetic neuralgia, duloxetine for diabetic neuropathy, and pregabalin for diabetic neuropathy and postherpetic neuralgia [21]. An algorithm for the use of medications in the management of symptomatic DSPN is illustrated in Figure 2.

Symptomatic neuropathy

↓

Exclude nondiabetic etiologies

↓

Stabilize glycemic control

(insulin not always required in type 2 diabetes)

↓

Tricyclic drugs

(e.g., Amitriptyline 25–150 mg before bed)

↓

Anticonvulsants

(e.g., Gabapentin, typical dose 1.8 g/day)

↓

Opioid or opioid-like drug

(e.g., Tramadol, Oxycodone)

↓

Consider pain clinic referral

Fig. 2. Algorithm for management of symptomatic DSPN. Note that nonpharmacological, topical, or physical therapies might be useful at any stage. These include acupuncture, capsaicin, glyceryl trinitrate spray/patches, etc. (*From* Boulton AJM, Vinik AI, Arezzo JC. et al. Diabetic neuropathies: a statement by the American Diabetes Association. Diabetes Care 2005; 28:956–62. © 2005 American Diabetes Association. Reprinted with permission from the American Diabetes Association.)

The tricyclic antidepressants were among the first medications to show efficacy in relieving neuropathic pain. Amitriptyline, desipramine, and nortriptyline have all been used with good effect. Because this class of drugs can cause lethargy and drowsiness, the recommended time of administration is bedtime. The usual dosing pattern is to initiate at a low dose and gradually increase every 4 to 7 days as tolerated. Patients need to be educated on the possible adverse effects of the medication, which can mimic hypoglycemia or hyperglycemia symptoms: dry mouth, dizziness, blurred vision, constipation, urinary retention, sedation, cognitive impairment, and orthostatic hypotension. Care should be taken not to use this class of medications in those with cardiovascular disease, such as congestive heart failure, recent myocardial infarction, seizures, and urinary tract obstruction.

Although the serotonin reuptake inhibitors class of antidepressants is better tolerated than the tricyclic antidepressants, they are also less effective in neuropathic pain management [22]. Newer antidepressants medications,

such as the norepinephrine-specific reuptake inhibitors venlafaxine and duloxetine, have been used in the treatment of neuropathic pain with good results. Of these two drugs, duloxetine is approved for use with neuropathic pain. The starting dose for pain management is 30 mg every day, which is then titrated to 60 mg every day. In clinical trials 60 mg twice a day was prescribed with little to no additional benefit [23]. Common side effects include nausea, dizziness, somnolence, dry mouth, constipation, hyperhidrosis, decreased appetite, and asthenia.

The group of medications referred to as the "anticonvulsants" includes two alpha2-delta ligands: gabapentin and pregabalin. Both have been effective in treating neuropathic pain in clinical trials. Gabapentin is usually started with a low dosage once a day and then titrated to twice, and then three times a day as the dosage increases. During this titration the health care provider must be on the alert for adverse effects, such as somnolence, gait and balance disturbances, gastrointestinal complaints, and peripheral edema. It may take a number of weeks before an efficacious dose is reached (1800–3600 mg per day) [22]. Pregabalin has a similar adverse effect profile but titration time seems to be more rapid based on patient tolerance. Most patients start with 100 to 150 mg per day, given in divided doses, which is titrated as tolerated to a maximum of 300 mg [24].

Carbamazepine is an anticonvulsant used with less frequency because of its side effect profile. Thrombocytopenia, hypofibrinogenemia, aplastic anemia, cardiac toxicity, and Stevens-Johnson syndrome are possible adverse effects associated with carbamazepine [25].

In clinical studies, anticonvulsant topiramate demonstrated the ability to restore C-fiber nerve function by increasing dendrite length and intraepidermal nerve fiber density. Patients reported improved C-fiber function indicated by greater sensory perception to pin prick and touch or pressure [26]. Topiramate has side effects similar to the other anticonvulsants, however, and must be titrated very slowly. The initial dose is 15 to 25 mg/day not to exceed 100 mg/day.

The use of opioid analgesics in diabetic peripheral neuropathy is controversial. In this class of drugs, tramadol has been shown to be safe and effective when used at dosages of 50 to 100 mg every day. In general, adverse effects were moderate to mild and included dizziness, fatigue, dry mouth, and constipation [22].

Topical agents used for pain management in DSPN have an advantage over systemic agents in that the risks of any drug-to-drug interactions are minimized [27]. In those with cardiac conditions who are unable safely to use a number of the oral medications, peripheral analgesia offers a means for pain relief.

Of the topical agents, capsaicin cream and Lidoderm patches are effective in lessened neuropathic pain. Capsaicin cream works by desensitizing the C-fibers by depleting the neurotransmitter substance P. For a low-cost alternative, patients can make their own equally effective cream by adding cayenne pepper to cold cream. To be effective, it must be applied to the skin of

the painful area three to four times per day and it may take several weeks before pain relief is achieved. The patient must be reminded to wear gloves when applying the capsaicin cream and informed of the application schedule and time to efficacy. During the initial period of cream application, many patients experience a burning sensation deemed intolerable causing them to abandon this treatment before efficacy can be achieved. In those who are able to continue the therapy, the burning sensation diminishes with repeated use [27].

Clinical studies using Lidoderm patch 5% demonstrated improved symptoms of DSPN with reduced intensity of pain [28]. Up to three patches may be applied once daily to the painful site and worn during a 12-hour period. During the subsequent 12 hours the patches must be removed. The only side effects noted have been skin sensitivity and erythema, and in some cases a mild rash at the site of patch application.

Anecdotal clinical reports support the usefulness of acupuncture in relieving neuropathic pain. Whether this is an actual or a placebo effect has yet to be determined.

In searching for the cause of neuropathic pain, numerous pathophysiologic changes have been considered. The scientific consensus is that no one alteration, but rather a combination of factors contributes to the pain syndrome. It is reasonable to assume that the best pain management program uses a combination of topical and oral agents to achieve the best outcomes. Given the problematic nature of pain management in DSPN, combinations of complementary drug therapies may be the next step in treatment.

The importance of foot care education

Patient education in preventive foot care is a critical component in the management of DSPN. Patients with peripheral neuropathy, particularly those with insensate feet, are at highest risk for foot injuries that can lead to infection and ultimately the loss of a limb. Lower-extremity amputations occur 10 to 30 times more often in persons with diabetes as compared with the general population [29]. The risk of ulceration is proportional to the number of risk factors. Sumpio [30] states that risk is increased by 1.7 in persons with isolated peripheral neuropathy, by 12 in those with peripheral neuropathy and foot deformity, and by 36 in those with peripheral neuropathy, deformity, and previous amputation, as compared with persons without risk factors. Patients with 10 years or more duration of diabetes, poorly controlled glucose levels, or with cardiovascular, retinal, or renal complications are at highest risk for ulceration [31]. In 1999, the estimated cost of treating a diabetic foot ulcer was $28,000 [3].

Given these facts, foot care education is a cost-effective practice, one that must be incorporated into every diabetes clinical assessment [32]. Table 1 lists the essential components of foot care education.

Table 1
Foot care guidelines

Action	Rationale
Wear shoes and stockings that fit well	Poorly fitting footwear causes a shearing force and pressure points that lead to ulcerations
Never walk barefoot	The unprotected foot is at increased risk for injury
Examine feet daily	Decreased sensation to the feet may result in trauma or infection; visual inspection is necessary to identify foot problems
Wash and dry feet well using a mild soap	Clean, dry feet are less likely to develop infections (fungal); soaking feet promotes skin maceration and breakdown
Moisturize dry skin	Supple skin is at less risk for breakdown; use a nonperfumed emollient cream
Use foot powder as needed	Excessively moist feet encourage fungus growth; do not allow powder to cake between the toes
Trim toenails to the contour of the toe; do not clip into the corners; sharp edges may be smoothed with an emery board	Avoiding injury to the nail bed and preventing ingrown toenails reduces risk of infection; if the patient cannot adequately reach or see the toenails, a podiatry referral is indicated
Never self-treat corns or calluses	Over-the-counter remedies contain caustic chemicals that can burn or injure the skin
Do not use any form of external heat, such as heating pads, hot water bottles	Insensate feet cannot determine temperature resulting in burns, frostbite, and other thermal injuries
Wear adequate footwear in cold weather	
Seek the attention of a health care provider at the first sign of foot trauma, injury, or infection	Immediate care lessens the severity of outcome
Stop smoking	Improvement in vascular health aids in recovery from trauma and infection
Improve glucose control	Euglycemic control improves healing
Remind the health care provider to do a foot examination at each visit	Early discovery of decreased sensation, lesions, or infection reduces risk for ulceration or amputation

Focal and multifocal neuropathies

Most mononeuropathies have a sudden onset and effect median, ulnar, radial, and common peroneal nerves [20]. The pain and dysfunction affecting these nerves is usually associated with entrapment. Electrophysiology studies are used to identify blocks in conduction at the entrapment sites. Some focal neuropathies, such as carpal tunnel syndrome, may need surgery or decompression to relieve the entrapment. The risk of developing carpal tunnel syndrome is 2.2 to 2.5 higher in persons with diabetes compared with the general population [33].

Although rare, cranial neuropathies do occur and can present in a fashion similar to Bell's palsy. Cranial nerves II, IV, VI, and VII are typically involved and the underlying cause may be a microvascular nerve infarct. Diabetic sixth nerve palsies are unilateral and present with diplopia, papillary sparing, and weakness of eye abduction. Unlike trochlear or fourth nerve palsy where diplopia is constant and improved by tilting the head away from the affected eye, sixth nerve palsies improve in weeks to months with full recovery [33]. Patients should be advised to wear a patch over the affected eye to reduce corneal irritation and dry eye.

Diabetic amyotrophy presents with unilateral or bilateral weakness and atrophy in the proximal thigh muscles. Typically, it occurs in older, type 2 patients who present with severe pain, usually in the buttocks, and dysmobility. When observing the patient, it is clear that moving from a sitting to a standing position is very difficult and the patient uses their upper extremities to climb up their body or to push out of the chair. In some cases, nerve biopsy has shown an immune-mediated epineurial microvasculitis [20]. If the symptoms are very severe, the clinician needs to evaluate the patient for spinal stenosis. Pain management with gabapentin and tramadol is effective. Resolution of the symptoms occurs in 2 to 3 years.

Truncal neuropathy or radiculopathy presents with acute unilateral or bilateral pain and hyperesthesia following a thoracic or abdominal dermatome or in a girdle-like distribution. The pain, which can be severe, is of a burning, tearing, boring, or jabbing nature. Patients may describe a hypersensitivity of the skin overlying the area of the dermatome. It is not uncommon for the patient to have a loss of appetite and subsequent weight loss of 20 to 25 lb. Radiculopathy typically occurs in patients older than age 50 and duration of disease is not a principle factor. Although the patient can appear quite ill, the diagnostic evaluation for underlying conditions is negative. Pain management and improvement in glucose control are essential components of therapy. The pain resolves in 16 to 24 months after onset.

Diabetic autonomic neuropathies

Diabetic autonomic neuropathy (DAN) has an insidious onset yet can affect every part of the body. It results in significant morbidity and may lead

to mortality [20]. Although subclinical involvement may be widespread, the patient may present with symptoms involving only one organ. The cardiovascular system, gastrointestinal tract, genitourinary system, sweat glands, adrenal medullary system, and the ocular pupil are the organ systems usually affected by DAN. The changes in the autonomic nervous system may be related to function or to organic changes where nerve fibers are compromised or lost. Because the autonomic control for organ systems can be divided into sympathetic and parasympathetic response, diagnosis, treatment, and prognosis can be very difficult. This accounts for the wide variation in the estimates of the number of persons with DAN. If DAN is defined as diminished function of the autonomic nervous system, then the proportion of those with DAN rises to approximately 90% [34]. As in sensorimotor neuropathy, the history and clinical examination must focus on the differential diagnoses for each of the presenting signs and symptoms. The differential diagnoses for the various types of autonomic neuropathy are listed in Table 2.

Table 2
Differential diagnoses for autonomic neuropathies

Type of diabetic autonomic neuropathy	Differential diagnosis
Cardiovascular: tachycardia, exercise intolerance, orthostatic hypotension, silent myocardial infarction, arrhythmias	Orthostatic tachycardia Idiopathic orthostatic hypotension Pheochromocytoma Hypovolemia Congestive heart failure Shy-Drager syndrome Medications
Gastrointestinal: esophageal dysfunction, gastroparesis, diarrhea, constipation, fecal incontinence	Gastric or intestinal obstruction Gastritis Ketoacidosis Medications Bezoars Biliary disease Bacterial overgrowth Pancreatic exocrine insufficiency Gastric and duodenal ulcers
Genitourinary: neurogenic bladder, erectile dysfunction, retrograde ejaculation, female sexual disorder	Alcohol or drug abuse Genital or pelvic surgery Medications Psychogenic sexual issues Atherosclerotic vascular disease Hormonal abnormalities
Neurovascular: heat intolerance, anhidrosis, gustatory sweating, impaired blood flow to the skin	Thyroid disease Amyloidosis Medications
Metabolic: hypoglycemic unawareness	Medications (eg, β-blockers)
Pupillary: decreased diameter of dark-adapted pupil, Argyll Robertsons type pupil	Medications Neoplasms Syphilis

Cardiovascular autonomic neuropathy is the most important form of DAN because of the life-threatening consequences associated with this dysfunction. Reduced cardiovascular autonomic function was strongly associated with increased risk of silent myocardial ischemia and mortality [35]. The presence of cardiovascular autonomic neuropathy indicates the likelihood that DAN affects other organs and alerts the clinician to investigate further. Diagnostic testing for alterations in the cardiovascular system requires three simple procedures that can be performed in an office setting: (1) beat-to-beat heart rate variations, (2) heart rate response to standing, and (3) heart rate response to the Valsalva maneuver [36]. Other findings, such as resting heart rate above 100 beats per minute or fall in the systolic blood pressure of greater than 20 mm Hg from lying to standing, is an indication of cardiovascular autonomic neuropathy.

Patients may present with dizziness related to orthostatic hypotension or report exercise intolerance. In the clinical setting, erratic blood pressure response or prolonged time to down-regulation during cardiac stress testing may indicate cardiovascular autonomic neuropathy in an otherwise unsymptomatic patient. Patients at high risk for silent ischemia have an altered heart rate at maximum oxygen consumption [37]. Patients with cardiovascular autonomic neuropathy experiencing cardiac ischemia may present with mild to moderate symptoms, such as cough, nausea and vomiting, dyspepsia, dyspnea, and fatigue. The abnormal distribution of cardiac sympathetic innervation in cardiovascular autonomic neuropathy may lead to arrhythmias, with or without the presence of ischemia. Prolonged QT interval on an EKG is a marker for possible neuropathy and risk for arrhythmias [38]. Intraoperative cardiac lability associated with cardiovascular autonomic neuropathy places the diabetic patient at risk for surgical procedures requiring general anesthesia.

Early diagnosis of cardiovascular autonomic neuropathy allows the health care provider to be proactive in preventing end-organ damage. Overall risk can be reduced by 70% with the use of angiotensin-converting enzyme inhibitors and β-blockers, even in normotensive individuals; aspirin therapy; and physiologic management of blood pressure, lipid, and glucose control [35].

Orthostatic hypotension causes dizziness, interferes with the patient's function, and places him or her at risk for falls. Using gradient compression stockings and increasing water consumption achieves a reduction in these bothersome symptoms. In severe cases, a low dose of fludrocortisone, a mineralocorticoid, can be prescribed to increase blood pressure. Care must be taken when using this drug, however, because it can potentiate congestive heart failure and edema.

Gastrointestinal manifestations of DAN can affect the entire gastrointestinal tract from the esophagus to the large colon. In general, dysmotility caused by DAN can produce dysphagia, abdominal pain and bloating, nausea and vomiting, malabsorption, fecal incontinence, and constipation. The symptoms can range from mild to severe.

Esophageal dysfunction may affect as many as 30% of persons with diabetes, yet the actual clinical presentation is relatively uncommon [36]. Because esophageal peristalsis and diminished sphincter pressures are the most likely to be affected, the presentation of esophageal dysmotility resembles gastric reflux disease. Impaired gastric emptying further disposes the patient to reflux. Esophageal motility testing can determine if the symptoms are related to autonomic neuropathy.

Gastroparesis should be suspected in patients with erratic glucose control. The delayed emptying of the stomach results in postprandial hypoglycemia followed by hyperglycemia hours after the food has been ingested. Patients report early satiety, epigastric pain, cramping, bloating, and nausea. Undigested food may be present in emesis and feces.

Because hyperglycemia retards gastric emptying and reduces gastrointestinal motility, the first step in managing gastrointestinal autonomic neuropathies is to improve glucose control [39]. Reduced fiber and fat in the diet improves gastric emptying and avoids the formation of bezoars in the stomach. Frequent small meals of a soft consistency may help with absorption of nutrients. If necessary, liquid dietary supplements may be used to increase vitamin and mineral consumption. When treating hypoglycemia, the patient needs to use a rapidly absorbed liquid or glucose gel. Honey, fruit juices, and skim milk are also appropriate selections. The time to response to the hypoglycemic treatment may be prolonged in patients with gastroparesis. When the patient does not respond to oral treatment, family members must know how to administer subcutaneous glucagon.

The gastric emptying study is the most commonly used diagnostic test for gastroparesis. Endoscopy and barium studies may be used in selected cases at the discretion of the gastroenterologist.

Metoclopramide and domperidone are two drugs that are effective in the treatment of gastroparesis. Only metoclopramide is currently available in the United States. Both drugs work to reduce antiemetic activity. Because metoclopramide is a cholinergic drug, it has more central nervous side effects (tardive dyskinesias and parkinsonism) than domperidone. The medications are typically given four times per day, at meals and at bedtime [35]. Erythromycin, a commonly used macrolide antibiotic, improves gastric emptying and is taken three times a day, 30 minutes before the meal. Over time the effectiveness of this treatment may wane.

In dire cases, gastrostomy tubes may be placed to ensure the patient is receiving sufficient nutrition. A new therapy that uses a gastric electrical stimulation device is being studied and used through the Food and Drug Administration humanitarian device exemption. It is surgically implanted and the early reports are promising.

Diabetic diarrhea has a low prevalence (3.7%) and is more commonly seen in patients with type 1 than type 2 diabetes [35]. A number of factors may contribute to this disorder: diminished pancreatic enzyme secretion, bacterial overgrowth caused by dysmobility, malabsorption, and bile acid

complications. Diarrhea associated with autonomic neuropathy is typically sudden, explosive, and nocturnal. It can be cyclical or intermittent. Patients may suffer with up to 20 bowel movements per day and at times become incontinent. If the patient is incontinent, the clinician may need to investigate the competency of the internal and external anal sphincter.

For patients who become dehydrated, maintaining adequate hydration is critical. Once the cause of the diarrhea has been identified, treatment can begin. If the cause is bacterial overgrowth, a broad-spectrum antibiotic, such as doxycycline, is effective. The use of cholestyramine to aid in the reduction of bile salts can reduce the incidence of diarrhea. In some cases, antidiarrheals may be necessary to reduce the number of stoolings and to prevent dehydration. These drugs are used with extreme caution to prevent the occurrence of toxic megacolon. Some patients benefit from the use of clonidine, which lessens diarrhea but can pose problems with postural hypotension. Clinicians prescribing clonidine need to be alert for changes in blood pressure associated with use of this drug.

Constipation occurs as a result of bowel dysmotility. Complications of severe constipation include perforation, ulceration, and fecal impaction. Some of the medications used to treat the other neuropathies can cause constipation, particularly the opioids, calcium channel blockers, and some of the tricyclic antidepressants. Because colon cancers can present in a similar manner, patients should be encouraged to have colorectal examinations performed consistent with routine health maintenance.

Lactulose, hydrophilic colloid laxatives, and stool softeners may help to correct constipation. Stimulant laxatives, such as those containing senna, should be used with extreme caution. Healthy diet, exercise, and adequate hydration are essential to bowel regularity.

At times, constipation alternates with diarrhea. The reduced peristaltic action in the bowel predisposes the patient to bacterial overgrowth. Diarrhea then occurs in response to the bacterial overgrowth. Once the bowel recovers, constipation returns. This cycling continues to occur as long as the constipation remains untreated.

Genitourinary autonomic neuropathies encompass sexual dysfunction and cystopathy. Overflow incontinence occurs when the bladder no longer is able to empty completely and the sensation of bladder fullness is lost. Not only does this lead to embarrassment for the patient, it can cause recurrent bladder infections and vesicoureteric reflux with renal damage [36]. If a patient has more than two urinary tract infections in a year, the possibility of neurogenic bladder should be explored and the patient referred to urology services.

The goal of treatment for neurogenic bladder is to improve bladder emptying and prevent urinary tract infections. To this end, the patient can be educated in Credé's maneuver, a manual method to initiate urination and bladder emptying, on a 3- to 4-hour schedule. By pressing on the bladder in a downward motion with both hands and leaning forward the patient mechanically compresses the bladder assisting the flow of urine. In extreme

cases, the patient must self-catheterize to relieve bladder fullness. Medication, such as bethanechol, can be helpful for an underactive bladder.

Sexual dysfunction in men, such as retrograde ejaculation, erectile dysfunction (ED), and diminished libido, and dyspareunia and diminished vaginal lubrication in women, is associated with DAN. Of these dysfunctions, the most prevalent is ED. Approximately 35% to 75% of males with type 1 or type 2 diabetes have ED and studies indicate that ED develops 5 to 10 years earlier in men with diabetes [40]. Many men with ED do not disclose this problem to the health care provider because of embarrassment or fear of ridicule. Furthermore, many clinicians do not include sexual function in a routine assessment. The prevalence of ED among men with diabetes may be much higher than currently estimated.

ED is a condition defined as the consistent inability to attain and maintain an erection adequate for sexual intercourse, occurring over a period of months [41]. ED results from accelerated large vessel atherosclerosis, microvascular arterial disease, autonomic neuropathy, dyslipidemia, concomitant hypertension, and prominent endothelial dysfunction, making it a marker for generalized vascular disease [41]. The presence of ED should alert the health care provider that the patient is at increased risk for cardiovascular events and the appropriate screening must be done.

Clinical evidence correlates ED with increased hemoglobin A_{1C} and decreased glycemic control. Almost 100% of patients with diabetic neuropathy develop ED [41].

For patients with type 2, ED may be a presenting symptom of diabetes, whereas patients with type 1 may develop ED 8 to 10 years postdiagnosis. Frequently, the patient has spent 6 to 18 months before the medical visit self-treating with over-the counter or folklore remedies and herbal supplements without improvement.

In a comprehensive assessment for ED, the clinician must evaluate gonadal health, medication usage, recreational drug and alcohol intake, and psychologic status. Patients with diabetes take many medications to treat comorbid conditions, many of which affect sexual function. Medications for hypertension, depression, glaucoma, and neuropathic pain may be necessary for the patient's overall health and have deleterious effects if discontinued. When prescribing these medications, the clinician should alert the patient to the possibility of sexual side effects and when possible work toward substituting agents that are less likely to cause ED.

The first task is to determine if the sexual dysfunction is biologic or psychologic in origin. A detailed patient history must include past pelvic or abdominal surgeries; prostate gland or endocrine issues (particularly those related to testosterone); and cardiovascular health. During the sexual health history, the clinician must discuss the patient's ability to achieve and maintain an erection, any history of retrograde ejaculation, self-initiated treatments that the patient has tried in the past, and the impact ED has had on intimate relationships. Discussing such intimate topics may be

uncomfortable for the patient. The provider must try to minimize this by addressing this subject in a factual manner and identifying it as one of many medical complications of diabetes. Some patients broach the subject by requesting a prescription for one of the oral medications that treat ED, giving the clinician an opportunity to evaluate the problem further. The use of a written questionnaire can facilitate the acquisition of information critical for diagnosis and treatment in a manner that is less problematic for the patient [42]. One such questionnaire, the International Index of Erectile Function, is made up of 15 questions with Likert scale responses ranging from 0 to 5 and provides a broad measure of sexual function [43].

If the patient experiences an erection in response to increased hormonal levels in the early morning but has difficulty achieving an erection during intercourse, the organic function is intact. A nocturnal penile tumescence device can also assess penile response during sleep. This noninvasive test, which records penile erection much like an EKG reading, is done in the privacy of the patient's home. Conversely, if the patient reports penile flaccidity in the early morning hours, organic disease is present.

In addition to a physical examination to rule out any other underlying conditions that could cause ED, such as renal or liver disease, multiple sclerosis, spinal injuries, or prostate disease, diagnostic laboratory testing to assess the patient's hormonal status should be ordered. Chemistry profiles, thyroid studies, and prolactin and ferritin levels must also be included.

Controlling glucose levels, weight loss, and moderate exercise may all benefit the patient in men with moderate ED. In other cases, the oral phosphodiesterase type 5 inhibitors have greatly improved ED management. The three medications in this category (sildenafil, tadalafil, and vardenafil) prevent the breakdown of cyclic $3',5'$ guanosine monophosphate, a chemical that helps to prolong and improve smooth muscle relaxation. Without this muscle relaxation, the vasodilatation and engorgement of the cavernosal tissue essential to achieving and maintaining an erection does not occur. Although response rate to these medications in men with diabetes is not as robust as those in the general population, 50% to 70% have a good effect. Sildenafil and vardenafil are shorter-acting agents that once ingested are available in the system for 4 hours. Tadalafil has a longer half-life, with availability up to 36 hours, allowing for more spontaneity and flexibility in timing. It is important to note that all of these medications require arousal for the chemical response to result in an erection. The common adverse effects include headache, nasal congestion, and dyspepsia, all relating to the inhibition of phosphodiesterase type 5 [44]. In general, the medications are well tolerated. Patients using oral nitrates must never be prescribed phosphodiesterase type 5 inhibitors. α-Blockers are contraindicated with sildenafil and vardenafil. Patients with prolonged QTc interval changes, those taking antiarrhythmics, such as procainamide or amiodarone, may not use vardenafil.

Alprostadil, given by intracavernosal injection, is considered the gold standard treatment for ED. It has α-blocking properties and works to relax smooth muscle. Although it is 80% to 90% effective, approximately 50% of users stop after the first year because of injection pain, loss of effect, or lack of interest [43]. Intraurethral alprostadil, although avoiding the pain of injection, still causes urethral pain in approximately 30% of the users. The drug achieved a satisfactory response, however, in patients approximately 70% of the time [45].

Vacuum-constriction devices have a 75% success rate with diabetic men. It may also be used as an adjunct with oral therapies. Skin bruising, cumbersome use, and lack of spontaneity are the chief problems reported with this therapy.

Patients who are interested in implantable penile prostheses must be screened carefully to avoid the risk of poor outcomes. The underlying diseases (neurologic, vascular, and endothelial) that lead to ED also result in less successful outcomes in men with diabetes. Increased rates of infection and the removal of a failed device can further compromise the patient's health.

Female sexual dysfunction in women with diabetes usually consists of problems with arousal, lubrication, sexual pain, and orgasmic dysfunction. These problems are multifactorial in origin involving biologic, psychologic, and social determinants [46]. Although studies of female sexual dysfunction in women with diabetes are limited, it is estimated that 18% to 27% of women with type 1 diabetes and 42% of women with type 2 diabetes experience sexual health problems [47]. Women with more diabetic complications have more sexual dysfunction. Poor glucose control can contribute to vaginal candidiasis. Menopausal women experience tissue fragility and vaginal dryness. Partner relationships, depression, and stress of disease all affect female sexuality. The questions in need of study focus on the compounding effect of diabetes on female sexual dysfunction. At this time, treatment consists of vaginal lubricating gels and estrogen creams for symptomatic relief.

Gustatory sweating, anhidrosis, and hypoglycemic unawareness make up the metabolic autonomic neuropathies. Of these, hypoglycemic unawareness has the most detrimental affect on the patient's safety and quality of life. The relationship between autonomic neuropathy and hypoglycemic unawareness is complex. Although not all hypoglycemic unawareness is caused by autonomic changes, Vinik and colleagues [35] refer to a hypoglycemic-induced autonomic failure that occurs after recent antecedent hypoglycemia. A dangerous cycle of hypoglycemic unawareness that leads to a further decrease in counterregulatory hormone response to hypoglycemia occurs most often in individuals who are in strict glycemic control. Studies show that the epinephrine response to hypoglycemia is attenuated by the presence of autonomic neuropathy.

In patients with hypoglycemic unawareness parameters for glucose control must be designed for patient safety. Patients should self-monitor glucose

levels frequently: before meals, at bedtime, with activity, before operating a motor vehicle, and at any suspected symptom of hypoglycemia. Prevention of hypoglycemia is paramount. The patient must not skip meals but instead eat small meals more frequently and snack before activity. At times, patients learn to recognize new, more subtle symptoms of hypoglycemia and treat them accordingly.

Gustatory sweating, a profuse diaphoresis of the face, head, and neck, is often brought on by the ingestion of a strong tasting, spicy, or acidy food that causes salivation. Treatment consists of avoiding the offending foods. Anhidrosis, a diminished or absent response by the sweat glands, causes feet and hands to be more susceptible to the formation of fissures. These dry, cracked crevices of the skin acts as portals for infection, can be extremely tender, and are difficult to heal. Use of emollients, such as lotions containing urea, moisturize and protect skin and should be applied at least once a day.

Summary

During the lifetime of a person with diabetes the likelihood of experiencing diabetes-related neuropathy is almost assured. All of the neuropathic complications affect quality of life for the person with diabetes and can be among the most difficult conditions for the health care provider to diagnose, treat, and manage. Although medical and nursing science has made great strides in many aspects of diabetes management, the conditions that comprise the diabetic neuropathies present an ongoing challenge. Sensorimotor disorders can lead to loss of function and ultimately amputations. Autonomic neuropathies, such as those affecting the cardiovascular system, can be debilitating or cause sudden death. It behooves the conscientious health care provider to assist patients in the aggressive management of diabetes to prevent or minimize the occurrence of these life-threatening complications.

References

[1] Currie CJ, Morgan CL, Peters JR. The epidemiology and cost of inpatient care for peripheral vascular disease, infection, neuropathy, and ulceration in diabetes. Diabetes Care 1998;21:42.
[2] Vinik AI, Holland MT, Le Beau JM. Diabetic neuropathies. Diabetes Care 1992;15:1926–75.
[3] Pirart J. Diabetes mellitus and its degenerative complications: a prospective study of 4,400 patients observed between 1947 and 1973. Diabetes Care 1978;1:168.
[4] Kelkar P. Diabetic neuropathy. Semin Neurol 2005;25:168–73.
[5] Shaw JE, Zimmet PZ. The epidemiology of diabetic neuropathy. Diabetes Rev 1999;7: 245–52.
[6] Oates PJ. Polyol pathway and diabetic peripheral neuropathy. Int Rev Neurobiol 2002;50: 325–92.
[7] Masson EA, Boulton AJM. Aldose reductase inhibitors in the treatment of diabetic neuropathy: a review of rationale and clinical evidence. Drugs 1990;39:190–202.
[8] Kelkar P, Parry GJ. Mononeuritis multiplex in diabetes: evidence for underlying immune pathogenesis. J Neurol Neurosurg Psychiatry 2003;74:803–6.

[9] Consensus Statement. Report and recommendation of the San Antonio conference on diabetic neuropathy. American Diabetes Association /American Academy of Neurology. Diabetes Care 1988;11:592–7.

[10] Vinik AI, Mehrabyan A. Diabetic neuropathies. Med Clin North Am 2004;88:947–99.

[11] Vinik AI. Neuropathy: new concepts in treatment and evaluation. South Med J 2002;95: 21–3.

[12] National Center for Chronic Disease Prevention and Health Promotion. The prevention and treatment of complications of diabetes mellitus: a guide for primary care practitioners. Available at:www.cdc.gov/diabetes/pubs/complications/neuro.htmAccessed November 10, 2002.

[13] Hanson PH, Schumaker P, Debugne TH, et al. Evaluation of somatic and autonomic small fibers neuropathy in diabetes. Am J Phys Med Rehabil 1992;71:44–7.

[14] Mc Arthur JC, Stocks EA, Hauer P, et al. Epidermal nerve fiber density: normative reference range and diagnostic efficiency. Arch Neurol 1998;55:1513–20.

[15] Bloomgarden Z. Report on the American Diabetes Association 61st Scientific Sessions in Philadelphia, PA. Diabetes Care 2002;25:1085–94.

[16] Hughes RA. Peripheral neuropathy. BMJ 2002;324:466–9.

[17] Abbott CA, Carrington AL, Ashe H, et al. The North-West Diabetes Foot Care Study: incidence of, and risk factors for, new diabetic foot ulceration in a community based cohort. Diabet Med 2002;19:377–84.

[18] Daube JR. Electrophysiological testing in diabetic neuropathy. In: Dyck PJ, Thomas PK, editors. Diabetic neuropathy. 2nd edition. Philadelphia: WB Saunders; 1999. p. 222–38.

[19] McCarthy BG, Hsieh ST, Stocks A. Cutaneous innervation in sensory neuropathies: evaluation by skin biopsy. Neurology 1995;45:1848–55.

[20] Boulton AJM, Vinik AI, Arezzo JC, et al. Diabetic neuropathies. Diabetes Care 2005;28: 956–63.

[21] Backonja MM. Defining neuropathic pain. Anesth Analg 2003;97:785–90.

[22] Duby JJ, Campbell RK, Setter SM, et al. Diabetic neuropathy: an intensive review. Am J Health Syst Pharm 2004;61:160–76.

[23] Wernicke JF, Lu Y, Waninger A, et al. Duloxetine at doses of 60 mg QD nad 60 mg BID is effective treatment of diabetic neuropathic pain [abstract]. New York: APA; 2004.

[24] Rosenstock J, Tuchman M, LaMoreaux L, et al. Pregabalin for the treatment of painful diabetic peripheral neuropathy: a double-blind, placebo-controlled trial. Pain 2004;110: 628–38.

[25] Mangan MM. Diabetic neuropathy: clinical evaluation and pain management. Clinician Reviews 1999;9:61–78.

[26] Vinik A, Pittenger G, Anderson A, et al. Topiramate improves C-fiber neuropathy and features of dysmetabolic syndrome in type 2 diabetes [abstract A130]. In: Program and abstracts of the 63rd Scientific Sessions of the American Diabetes Association, New Orleans, June 13–17, 2003. Alexandria (VA): American Diabetes Association.

[27] Argoff CE. Targeted topical peripheral analgesics in the management of pain. Curr Pain Headache Rep 2003;7:34–8.

[28] Galer BS, Jensen MP, Ma T. The lidocaine patch 5% effectively treats all neuropathic pain qualities: results of a randomized, double-blind, vehicle-controlled, 3-week efficacy study with the use of the Neuropathic Pain Scale. Clin J Pain 2002;18:297–301.

[29] Trautner C, Haastert B, Giani G, et al. Incidence of lower limb amputations and diabetes. Diabetes Care 1996;19:1006–9.

[30] Sumpio BE. Foot ulcers. N Engl J Med 2000;343:787–92.

[31] American Diabetes Association. Preventive foot care in people with diabetes. Diabetes Care 1999;22(Suppl 1):S54–5.

[32] Ramsey SD, Newton K, Blough D, et al. Incidence, outcomes, and cost of foot ulcers in patients with diabetes. Diabetes Care 1999;22:382–7.

[33] Donofrio PD. Diabetic neuropathy. In: Leahy JL, Clark NG, Cefalu WT, editors. Medical management of diabetes mellitus. New York: Marcel Decker; 2000. p. 479–97.

[34] Prendergast JJ. Diabetic autonomic neuropathy. Practical Diabetology 2001;20:7–14.

[35] Vinik AI, Maser RE, Mitchell BD, et al. Diabetic autonomic neuropathy. Diabetes Care 2003;26:1553–79.

[36] Vinik AI, Erbas T, Pfeifer MA, et al. Diabetic autonomic neuropathy. In: Porte D, Sherwin RS, Baron A, editors. Ellenberg and Rifkin's diabetes mellitus. 6th edition. New York: McGraw-Hill; 2003. p. 789–822.

[37] Vinik AI, Johnson BF, Pfeifer M. Heart rate response to exercise is a poor indicator of VO2 max in patients with cardiac autonomic dysfunction [abstract 1207]. Diabetes 1997;46:316A.

[38] Bloomgarden ZT. Diabetic retinopathy and neuropathy. Diabetes Care 2005;28:963–70.

[39] Unger J. Diabetic neuropathy; early clues, effective management. Consultant 2004;14: 1549–56.

[40] Romeo JH, Seftel AD, Madhun ZT, et al. Sexual function in men with type 2 diabetes: association with glycemic control. J Urol 2000;163:788–91.

[41] Thethi TK, Osafu-Adjaye NO, Fonseca VA. Erectile dysfunction. Clinical Diabetes 2005;23: 105–13.

[42] Rice D, Jack L. Use of an assessment tool to enhance diabetes educators' ability to identify erectile dysfunction. Diabetes Educ 2006;32:373–80.

[43] Fonseca V, Seftel A, Denne J, et al. Impact of diabetes mellitus on the severity of erectile dysfunction and response to treatment: analysis of data from the tadalafil clinical trials. Diabetologia 2004;47:1914–23.

[44] Basu A, Ryder RE. New treatment options for erectile dysfunction in patients with diabetes mellitus. Drugs 2004;64:2667–88.

[45] Padma-Nathan H, Hellstrom WJ, et al. Treatment of men with erectile dysfunction with transurethral alprostadil. Medicated Urethral System for Erection (MUSE) Study Group. N Engl J Med 1997;336:1–7.

[46] Brown JS, Wessells H, Chancellor MB, et al. Urologic complications of diabetes. Diabetes Care 2005;28:177–85.

[47] Enzlin P, Mathieu C, Van den Bruel A, et al. Sexual dysfunction in women with type 1 diabetes: a controlled study. Diabetes Care 2002;25:672–7.

ELSEVIER
SAUNDERS

NURSING
CLINICS
OF NORTH AMERICA

Nurs Clin N Am 41 (2006) 719–736

Microvascular Complications of Diabetes

Marjorie Cypress, MSN, C-ANP, CDE[a],*,
Donna Tomky, MSN, C-ANP, CDE[b]

[a]University of New Mexico College of Nursing, 3501 Camino Aplauso NW,
Albuquerque, NM 87107, USA
[b]Division of Endocrinology and Metabolism, Lovelace Sandia Health Systems,
5400 Gibson Blvd, SE, Albuquerque, NM 87108, USA

Of all the complications associated with diabetes mellitus, perhaps the most devastating to people are those involving the microvasculature, which primarily involve the retina, kidneys, and the nervous system. Microvascular damage may also affect gingival and cutaneous tissues. The complications arising from damage to these vessels affect the quality of life of those affected. Microvascular complications are the result of chronic hyperglycemia on cells, tissues, and blood vessels, exacerbated by uncontrolled hypertension, and have a natural history that can result in debilitating consequences. Several studies over the past 10 years, however, including the Diabetes Control and Complications Trial [1] (DCCT) and United Kingdom Prospective Diabetes Study [2] have demonstrated that glycemic control, along with blood pressure control, can prevent, delay the onset, or slow the progression of microvascular disease. Glycemic control (defined as hemoglobin $A_{1c} < 7\%$) is not easily attained, as demonstrated by a decline in hemoglobin $A_{1C} < 7\%$ from 44.5% in the years 1988 to 1994, to only 35.8% in the years 1999 to 2000 [3]. Diabetic retinopathy (DR) remains the leading cause of blindness in people 20 to 64 years of age [4], and leads to 12,000 to 24,000 new cases of blindness in the United States each year. Diabetic nephropathy accounted for 40% of new cases of end-stage renal disease (ESRD) in the United States in the year 2000 [4]. Nearly 64% of patients with diabetes may have gingival infections compared with 50% of those without diabetes [5], and people with diabetes may experience a number of dermatologic disorders along with increased risk for foot ulcers. This article discusses

---

* Corresponding author.
E-mail address: mcypress@salud.unm.edu (M. Cypress).

0029-6465/06/$ - see front matter © 2006 Elsevier Inc. All rights reserved.
doi:10.1016/j.cnur.2006.07.009   *nursing.theclinics.com*

the proposed etiology and natural history of microvascular complications of diabetes, specifically DR and diabetic nephropathy; oral and skin manifestations; assessment; detection; and treatment interventions. With this knowledge, nurses can be instrumental in helping to identify people at high risk for these complications, prevent, screen, and intervene early.

Risk factors for microvascular complications

Although hyperglycemia and hypertension are major risk factors for vascular complications, dyslipidemia, obesity, smoking, and physical inactivity have been implicated as comorbid factors that may accelerate vascular damage (for microvascular and macrovascular) disease. Hyperglycemia, particularly with blood glucose concentrations highest after meals [6], is an independent risk factor for vascular complications of type 2 diabetes. Control of fasting and mealtime hyperglycemia with optimal pharmacologic therapies and eating behaviors are important for overall glycemic control and reducing vascular complications. Hypertension is twice as common in people with type 2 diabetes, compared with those without diabetes, and was shown to be present in 85% of people with nephropathy [7]. The coexistence of diabetes and hypertension is associated with an increase in the risk of retinopathy, renal failure, and cardiovascular disease. An increase of 5 mm Hg in systolic or diastolic blood pressure increases the risk of cardiovascular disease by 20% to 30%; a diastolic blood pressure above 70 mm Hg increases the risk of retinopathy; and ESRD is five to six times more common in the person with diabetes and hypertension [7]. Despite the fact that research has demonstrated a decrease in the risk of developing microvascular complications or slowing the progression with glucose and blood pressure control, poor control of both persists. In the National Health and Nutrition Examination Survey only 35.8% of people with diabetes attained hemoglobin A_{1C} levels <7% [3]. In 2003, self-reported rates of hypertension were 52.4 and rates of high blood cholesterol were reported to be 50.8 per 100 diabetic population [8]. In addition, 23.4% of people with diabetes noted they currently smoked, 80.6% were reported to be overweight or obese, and 35.7% of the surveyed diabetic population was physically inactive [8]. There are also ethnic and racial disparities in the risk of microvascular complications [9–11]. Mexican Americans are twice as likely and non-Hispanic blacks are almost 50% more likely to develop DR than non-Hispanic whites. Non-Hispanic blacks are 2.6 to 5.6 times as likely, Mexican Americans 4.5 to 6.6 times as likely, and Native Americans 6 times more likely to develop diabetic nephropathy than non-Hispanic whites [12]. Although there may be a myriad of factors contributing, poor preventive care practices among individuals and health care professionals are identified [11,13].

Preventive strategies

Although there are specific treatment interventions for diabetic eye and kidney disease, the strategy common to all treatment interventions is control of blood glucose (hemoglobin A_{1c}), blood pressure, and lipids. These have been labeled the ABCs (hemoglobin A_{1C}, blood pressure, and cholesterol) of diabetes management by the American Diabetes Association. In the Epidemiology of Diabetic Interventions and Complications study, individuals with type 1 diabetes who had experienced periods of good glycemic control but whose control had deteriorated somewhat years later still showed a sustained preventive effect of developing retinopathy and nephropathy [14]. Hypertension control has also been shown to decrease the risk for developing microvascular disease [15], and there is evidence that links diabetic dyslipidemia with retinopathy and nephropathy [16]. Smoking and poor metabolic control increase the risk of periodontal disease. Besides pharmacologic therapies, healthy lifestyle habits, such as healthy eating and being physically active, are mainstays of treatment. Diabetes self-management education is crucial to the prevention of diabetic complications.

Pathophysiology

Altered glucose metabolism, as the result of chronic hyperglycemia, is thought to cause a number of changes in the blood vessels. The association between hyperglycemia and diabetic complications is believed to be caused by the effect that high levels of glucose have on several metabolic pathways. Four specific pathways that have been identified are (1) glycation of proteins, (2) the polyol or sorbitol pathway, (3) the protein kinase C pathway, and (4) the hexosamine pathway [17]. These altered pathways form glucotoxins that cause alterations in gene expression and abnormal protein function. The effect is cellular dysfunction and damage, specifically in abnormal angiogenesis, abnormal cell growth and survival, hyperpermeability of cells, capillary basement membrane thickening, abnormal blood flow through the vasculature, increased leukocyte adhesions, and thrombosis [18]. Recently, the role of oxidative stress has been implicated as the unifying mechanism responsible for the microvascular complications of diabetes. All of the pathway defects are believed to lead to oxidative stress, which produces reactive oxygen species or free radicals that cause cellular damage [19].

The polyol or sorbitol pathway metabolizes glucose into sorbitol via the enzyme aldose reductase. Aldose reductase uses nicotinamide adenine dicnucleotide in this pathway. Nicotinamide adenine dicnucleotide is also involved in the synthesis of nitric oxide, a key vasodilator in the microcirculation. When the amount of intracellular glucose increases, nicotinamide adenine dicnucleotide is diverted from its role in synthesizing nitric oxide. With less available nicotinamide adenine dicnucleotide in the cell, formation of nitric oxide decreases, causing vasoconstriction and decreased blood

supply [17]. Glycation of proteins produces advanced glycated end products (AGE). Circulating AGEs accumulate in the arterial walls, kidney mesangium, glomerulus, and basement membranes, leading to capillary basement membrane thickening. Low-density lipoproteins and immunoglobulins become trapped in artery walls, leading to oxidation and inflammation of the vessel wall. AGEs affect endothelial cells and stimulate macrophages to secrete factors that lead to enhanced cell permeability, increased fibroblast formation, and have procoagulant effects. The AGEs also cause the cells to become more rigid, impairing cell adhesion and axonal transport through the neuron [20]. AGEs in the kidney lead to leaking of protein through capillary basement membrane thickening, and alter function and structure of the microvessels. Protein kinase C is another glucose pathway that regulates vascular functions by specific enzymes. In the environment of hyperglycemia, the protein kinase C enzyme is activated and does not perform normally. This results in decreased amounts of nitric oxide leading to vasoconstriction. Growth factor-β1 and plasminogen activator inhibitor-1 are also increased [17]. This can result in changes to the renal and retinal blood flow, contractility of vessels, vascular permeability, vascular inflammation, decreased fibrinolysis, and resultant vascular occlusion. Increased glucose flux through the hexosamine pathway causes a diversion in the pathway such that pathologic changes occur resulting in increased growth factor-β1 and plasminogen activator inhibitor-1, both damaging to blood vessels. All of these pathway defects are believed to lead to oxidative stress. The free radicals produced by this affect the microvessels leading to the retina, kidney, and nervous system

Retinopathy

DR is an extremely common complication of diabetes affecting virtually all people with diabetes. Not all cases of DR result in blindness, although 33% to 87% of legal blindness occurring in people with diabetes is directly attributable to DR [21]. The natural history of DR is a progression from mild nonproliferative DR, in which there is increased vascular permeability, to moderate to severe nonproliferative DR, to proliferative DR, which is characterized by growth of new blood vessels on the retina. Macular edema may also occur by leaking blood vessels, with retinal thickening. People with more severe disease can develop vitreous hemorrhage and retinal detachment. Because diabetes-related blindness is preventable, early detection and intervention is crucial to saving vision; there is ample evidence that demonstrates improvement with surgical treatments.

Epidemiology

After 20 years of diabetes, almost all people with type 1 diabetes and over 60% of those with type 2 diabetes have some kind of DR [21]. Duration of diabetes is a major predictor for the development and progression of DR.

There is also evidence that DR may begin before the diagnosis of diabetes is made, because DR has been found in people with impaired glucose tolerance and impaired fasting glucose [22].

Pathophysiology

The proposed mechanisms for DR include alterations in the polyol and protein kinase C pathways, resulting in oxidative stress. An increase in vascular endothelial growth factor, believed to induce proliferation of retinal capillary cells, may also contribute and lead to the development of macula edema from fibrous bands that accompany new vessel growth in the retina [23]. Initial nonproliferative DR is characterized by microaneurysms. These are outpouchings along the vessel wall that may become small dot, blot, or flame hemorrhages seen on a retinal eye examination. Over time, with less perfusion, ischemia results and appears as venous beading, dilated capillary vessels, and hemorrhages. Table 1 is a summary of the International Clinical Diabetic Retinopathy Disease Severity Scale with management options [24].

Macular edema may exist along with nonproliferative DR or proliferative DR. This results from increased permeability of blood vessels that leak fluid and exudates into the macula. Because the macula is the area of central vision, this can lead to visual impairment. Vitreous hemorrhage occurs when the newly formed, friable blood vessels break and bleed into the vitreous body. Patients may complain of an oily, pink haze or total blockage of vision. Retinal detachment can also result from the breakage and leaking of new blood vessels in the retina. Adhesions and fibrous bands pull the layers of the retina apart, and cause detachment from the eye wall [25].

Assessment, detection, and screening

Because early intervention may prevent vision loss, it is essential that the diagnosis of DR be made early. A frightening symptom experienced by many people with diabetes is blurring of the vision. This is not DR but tends to occur with extremely high blood glucose levels, and may initially get worse with improved glucose control. Because this is usually the result of osmotic changes within the eye, patients should be reassured that with more prolonged glycemic control, these symptoms improve. Any change in vision, however, should be evaluated.

Eye examinations by eye professionals in some studies have been shown to have a higher sensitivity to detecting abnormalities than noneye professionals. Newer technologies, however, such as digital retinal imaging have been used in the primary care setting and have demonstrated increases in surveillance and treatment [26]. Although nonmydriatic retinal cameras are sometimes used for screening, they are affected by cataracts and glaucoma, which may limit their use as a universal screening tool. They may be useful, however, in situations where dilation is not possible. A systematic review to evaluate the effectiveness of screening and monitoring tests for DR

Table 1
International Clinical Diabetic Retinopathy Disease Severity Scale with management options

Proposed disease severity level	Findings on dilated retinal examination	Management options
No apparent retinopathy	No abnormalities	Optimize therapy to control glucose, blood pressure, and lipids
Mild non proliferative DR	Microaneurysms only	Optimize therapy to control glucose, blood pressure, and lipids
Moderate nonproliferative DR	More than microaneurysms but less than severe nonproliferative DR	Refer to ophthalmologist; optimize therapy to control glucose, blood pressure, and lipids
Severe non proliferative DR	Any of the following: extensive intraretinal hemorrhages in each of 4 quadrants, venous beading in 2+ quadrants, prominent intraretinal microvascular abnormalities in 1+ quadrant, and no signs of proliferative DR	Consider scatter (panretinal) laser treatment for patients with T2DM; optimize therapy to control glucose, blood pressure, and lipids
Proliferative DR	One or both of the following: neovascularization, neovascularization, vitreous-preretinal hemorrhage	Strongly consider panretinal laser treatment without delay for patients with vitreous hemorrhage or neovascularization; optimize therapy for glucose, blood pressure, and lipids

Abbreviations: DR, diabetic retinopathy; TZDM, type 2 diabetes mellitus.
Adapted from American Academy of Ophthalmology. Diabetic retinopathy preferred practice pattern. Available at: www.aao.org/education/library/ppp/upload/Diabetic-Retinopathy.pdf.

concluded that the use of mydriatic retinal photographs with additional use of ophthalmoscopy if photographs are ungradeable, is the most effective test [27].

The American Academy of Ophthalmology's examination recommendations for people with diabetes include [24] visual acuity, intraocular pressure, dilated fundoscopic examination, and evaluation of the peripheral retina and vitreous. Other ancillary tests may include color fundus photography, fluorescein angiography, ultrasonography, and optical coherence tomography. Color fundus photography is more reproducible than a clinical examination and can be used to monitor progression of disease and response to treatment. Fluorescein angiography is commonly used as a guide for treating macular edema, and can identify areas of macular capillary nonperfusion. Ultrasonography may be useful in cases where there are opacities, such as cataracts or vitreous hemorrhage. Newer techniques are being

used to improve diagnostic sensitivity. Optical coherence tomography provides images by projecting a pair of near-infrared light beams into the eye, and is being used to measure and monitor retinal thickness and retinal structures [21]. There is also a laser Doppler flow meter that measures retinal blood flow, and a noninvasive method for measuring retinal oxygenation through functional MRI [23].

The American Diabetes Association [12] clinical practice guidelines state that an ophthalmologist or optometrist who is knowledgeable and experienced in diagnosing DR and is aware of its management should perform the eye examination. Patients who have been identified with a specific risk of visual loss should be promptly referred to an ophthalmologist or optometrist who is knowledgeable and experienced in the management and treatment of DR. The American Diabetes Association advises annual dilated retinal examinations for individuals with type 1 diabetes within 3 to 5 years after the diagnosis of diabetes once the patient is 10 years of age or older, and for individuals with type 2 diabetes at the time of diagnosis. It is not uncommon for DR to be present on the diagnosis of type 2 diabetes mellitus because DR is asymptomatic in its early stages and may not manifest in visual changes until there is actual loss of vision. Because type 2 diabetes may be undiagnosed for many years, retinal damage can be progressing and remain untreated for years.

It is recommended that women with diabetes who wish to become pregnant receive a dilated eye examination before conception and during the first trimester. For those individuals who already have diagnosed DR, the American Academy of Ophthalmology [24] recommends annual eye examinations for those with normal or mild nonproliferative DR, 6- to 12-month examinations for those with moderate nonproliferative DR and no macular edema, and more frequent follow-up and treatment for those with mild to moderate nonproliferative DR with macular edema.

Intervention and prevention

Treatment for DR includes medical, laser, and surgical interventions. Medical treatment begins with intensification of medical therapies to control blood glucose, blood pressure, and lipids. Glycemic control is known to benefit the outcome of DR. In the DCCT, for every 1% lowering of hemoglobin A_{1C}, there was approximately a 35% risk reduction in the development or progression of DR. In addition, these risk-reduction benefits seen in the intensive management group have shown a sustained benefit 7 years after the DCCT, even when hemoglobin A_{1C} levels have increased [14]. Progression of DR is associated with hypertension, and in the United Kingdom Prospective Diabetes Study, patients who maintained blood pressures < 150/85 mm Hg with an angiotensin-converting enzyme inhibitor or β-blocker had a 34% reduction in progression to retinopathy and a 47% reduced risk of deterioration in visual acuity compared to those with blood pressure between

150/85 and 180/105 mm Hg [15]. Although whether the effect of intensively lowering lipid levels reduces the severity of DR is not known, the existence of hard exudates has been associated with elevated low density lipoprotein levels [28]. The Action to Control Cardiovascular Risk in Diabetes trial will be evaluating the effect of lipid lowering on both microvascular and macrovascular diabetes complications (www.accordtrial.org).

Laser photocoagulation is the standard treatment for proliferative DR and clinically significant macular edema. The treatment involves placing laser burns either throughout the peripheral fundus to specific leaking microaneurysms or in a grid pattern to areas of edema from diffuse capillary leakage. This treatment has been found to be efficacious, particularly for severe nonproliferative DR and proliferative DR.

Nephropathy

Diabetic nephropathy is a major microvascular complication with considerable medical and economic impact among persons with diabetes. Estimates of diabetic nephropathy defined by increased urinary albumin excretion in the absence of other renal diseases are approximately 40% of type 1 and type 2 patients with diabetes [29]. Diabetic kidney disease is the most common cause of ESRD (or kidney failure requiring dialysis or transplantation) in the United States, Japan, and Europe [30] and is associated with increased cardiovascular mortality [29].

Epidemiology

The rising incidence of ESRD is caused by the increasing prevalence of type 2 diabetes; the extended life span due to improved treatment of diabetes comorbid conditions; and because patients with diabetic ESRD are now being accepted for treatment in ESRD programs who formerly had been excluded [31]. Over 40% of new cases of ESRD were attributable to diabetes and costs for treatment were in excess of $18 billion annually [30]. Native Americans, Hispanics (especially Mexican Americans), and African Americans have the highest rates of ESRD. Nephropathy percentage rate is somewhat lower in type 2 diabetes probably because of the greater prevalence of being older and dying from cardiovascular complications. Nevertheless, more that half of diabetes patients reaching ESRD have type 2 diabetes. Recent studies have now demonstrated, however, that the onset and course of diabetic nephropathy can be ameliorated with early screening and interventions.

Pathophysiology

Diabetic nephropathy, or more recently termed "diabetic kidney disease," consists of a host of changes in the kidney [32]. At the severe end

of this spectrum is overt (or clinically apparent) diabetic nephropathy, which is characterized by persistent proteinuria, hypertension, and a progressive decline in kidney function that often leads to chronic kidney disease ultimately requiring renal replacement therapies (ie, hemodialysis, peritoneal dialysis, or transplantation), or premature mortality from cardiovascular disease [31]. Chronic kidney disease is defined as kidney damage or glomerular filtration rate (GFR) <60 mL/min/1.73 m^2 for 3 months or more, irrespective of cause [33]. Toward the milder end of the spectrum is microalbuminuria whereby appropriate and timely clinical intervention may delay or prevent the progression to kidney failure [34].

Altered renal hemodynamics, metabolic factors, and inflammatory responses occur within the kidney during exposure to hyperglycemia. It is thought that sustained high concentrations of glucose may be directly toxic to cells, altering cell growth, gene, and protein expression, increasing extracellular matrix and growth factor production [30]. In addition, glucose may induce its effects indirectly through the formation of metabolic derivatives, such as oxidants and AGEs [17]. The formation of AGEs may cause damage to cells by modifying extracellular matrix proteins and cellular proteins [35]. AGE-mediated pathways and the renin angiotensin system, oxidative stress, protein kinase C, and growth factors all are thought to play significant roles in the development and progression of diabetic kidney disease [36].

Severe proteinuria is thought to be both a marker of significant glomerular damage and serve to speed the progression of diabetic and other proteinuric kidney diseases. Animal studies and correlative human studies indicate that exposure of the tubular cells to high concentrations of filtered proteins and growth factors produces a tubulointerstitial inflammatory response that leads to progressive interstitial fibrosis. As a result, clinicians are using angiotensin-converting enzyme inhibitors and angiotensin receptor blockers for therapy in reducing proteinuria [30]. Less than 40% of patients develop diabetic nephropathy; other factors other than hyperglycemia are thought to be involved. Those factors are thought to be related to genetics, because of the tendency for diabetic nephropathy to cluster in families and in ethnic groups, such as the Pima Indians [30].

Assessment, detection, and screening

Screening, detection, and treatment are critical to ameliorate early diabetic nephropathy. The American Diabetes Association clinical practice guidelines recommend annual screening of microalbuminuria in type1 patients with diabetes duration ≥ 5 years and in all type 2 diabetes patients starting at diagnosis and during pregnancy [12]. The prevalence of microalbuminuria before 5 years in type 1 patients with patients with sustained poor glycemic and lipid control, however, and high normal blood pressure levels and puberty are additive risk factors [29]. Screening for microalbuminuria can be performed by three methods: (1) measurement of the albumin-to-creatinine ratio in

a random spot collection; (2) 24-hour collection with creatinine, allowing the simultaneous measurement of creatinine clearance; and (3) timed (eg, 1 hour or overnight) collection. Classification of microalbuminuria and macroalbuminuria is found in Table 2.

The Kidney Disease Outcomes Quality Initiative guidelines assist in identifying individuals at earlier stages than currently possible with measuring serum creatinine alone [37]. The serum creatinine should be measured at least annually for the estimation of GFR in all adults with diabetes regardless of the degree of urine albumin excretion [12]. The serum creatinine alone is an insensitive marker for kidney disease, whereas GFR measures the kidneys' ability to filter waste products from the blood and provides a more accurate method for staging chronic kidney disease. Although urinary albumin excretion measurement is the standard for diagnosing diabetic nephropathy, there are some type 1 or type 2 diabetes patients who have decreased GFR in the presence of normal urinary albumin excretion [29]. Both GFR estimates and urinary albumin excretion measurements should be done routinely for proper screening of diabetic nephropathy. The recommended equation by the National Kidney Foundation is the Modified Diet in Renal Disease Study, or access online the public domain calculator to estimate GFR at (www.kidney.org/klsprofessionals/gfr_calculator.cfm). Further staging and treatment of chronic kidney disease is done based on estimated GFR (Table 3).

Intervention and prevention

Medical interventions are more effective with the greatest impact if instituted in the very early course of renal disease. The goal of treatment is to prevent the progression from microalbuminuria to macroalbuminuria, slow the decline in renal function in patients with macroalbuminuria, and prevent the occurrence of cardiovascular events [29]. Preventing diabetic kidney disease needs to start early on with glycemic control. Many

Table 2
Definitions of abnormalities in albumin excretion

Category	Spot collection (μg/mg creatinine)	24–h collection (mg/24 h)	Timed collection (μg/min)
Normal	<30	<30	<20
Microalbuminuria	30–299	30–299	20–199
Clinical albuminuria	>300	>300	>200

Because of variability in urinary albumin excretion, two of three specimens collected within a 3- to 6-mo period should be abnormal before considering a patient to have crossed one of these diagnostic thresholds. Exercise within 24 h, infection, fever, congestive heart failure, marked hyperglycemia, marked hypertension, pyuria, and hematuria may elevate urinary albumin excretion over baseline values.

Adapted from ADA Position Statement. Nephropathy in diabetes. Diabetes Care 2004; 27(S1):S79–83.

Table 3
Stages of chronic kidney disease

Stage	Description	GFR mL/min/1.73 m^2	Action
0	Individuals at risk (diabetes)		Screen annually and treat diabetes and comorbid conditions
1	Kidney damage with normal or ↑ GFR	≥90	Interventions to slow progression, reduction of cardiovascular disease risk[a]
2	Kidney damage with mild ↓ GFR	60–89	Estimation of progression[a]
3	Moderate ↓ GFR	30–59	Evaluation and treatment of complications[a]
4	Severe ↓ GFR	15–29	Preparation for kidney-replacement therapy[a]
5	Kidney failure	<15 or dialysis	Replacement therapy[a]

Abbreviation: GFR, glomerular filtration rate.
[a] Includes actions from preceding stages.
Data from K/DOQI clinical practice guidelines for chronic kidney disease: evaluation, classification, and stratification. Kidney Disease Outcome Quality Initiative. Am J Kidney Dis 2002;39(Suppl 2):S1–246.

therapeutic options are available to treat diabetes effectively for controlling preprandial and postprandial hyperglycemia. The Epidemiology of Diabetes Interventions and Complications study, another 8 years of follow-up of the DCCT cohort, demonstrated the persistent beneficial effects on albumin excretion and the reduced incidence of hypertension. These findings suggest that previous intensive treatment of diabetes with near-normal glycemia has an extended benefit in delaying progression of diabetic nephropathy [38]. Referring to a diabetes team of endocrinologists and diabetes educators can assist with intensive skill training, education, and management to improve glycemic control.

Hypertension control is paramount in retarding the progression of diabetic kidney disease. In general, hypertension in patients with both types of diabetes is associated with an expanded plasma volume, increased peripheral vascular resistance, and low renin activity, but other causes, such as renal vascular disease, must be ruled out and if present surgically treated. Appropriate antihypertensive intervention can significantly increase the life expectancy in type 1 diabetes by 50% reduction in mortality and need for renal replacement therapy 16 years after the development of overt nephropathy [29]. The goal of antihypertensive therapy for nonpregnant adult diabetes patients is to decrease and maintain blood pressure <130/80 mm Hg [29]. Multifactorial interventions for improvement in outcomes should consist of lifestyle modifications including weight loss, reduction in sodium and alcohol, smoking cessation, low-dose aspirin, lipid-lowering agents, and increased physical activity. Many studies have shown that angiotensin-converting enzyme inhibitors and angiotensin receptor blockers can reduce the level of albuminuria and the rate of progression

of renal disease to a greater degree than other antihypertensive agents for both hypertensive and normotensive patients [12].

Dietary protein restriction showed reduction in hyperfiltration in animals. Since then, human studies failed to show a clear benefit of protein restriction [39]. The general consensus, however, is to prescribe a protein intake of approximately the adult Recommended Dietary Allowance of 0.8 g. kg^{-1} day^{-1} (approximately 10% of daily calories) in the patient with overt nephropathy [12].

Cutaneous and oral manifestations of microvascular complications

Overview

Cutaneous and oral manifestations seen in diabetes mellitus are not always recognized as part of microvascular complications. The skin and gums, however, may be subject to some of the same endothelial vascular damage that is believed responsible for DR and diabetic kidney disease. There is conflicting evidence whether the skin and oral diseases seen in people with diabetes are specifically related to microvascular damage from hyperglycemia; however, there is an association between these diseases and the presence of DR and diabetic kidney disease [40]. The same abnormalities (accumulation of sorbitol, AGEs, oxidative stress, and protein kinase C activation) all may contribute to some skin lesions [40]. The chief oral lesion seen in diabetes is periodontal disease. It is hypothesized that hyperglycemia, along with elevated lipoproteins and triglycerides, leads to the formation of AGEs, which affect macrophage production and lead to inflammation, tissue destruction, and alveolar bone loss [41]. There are a wide range of oral problems and skin lesions that are often seen in people with diabetes. This discussion, however, is limited to those disorders that are believed related to microangiopathy.

Characteristics, detection, and interventions: periodontal disease

People with type 1 and type 2 diabetes have a higher prevalence, extent, and severity of periodontal disease [42]. Almost one third of people with diabetes have severe periodontal disease with loss of attachment of the gums to the teeth measuring 5 mm or more [4]. In addition, periodontal disease was found to be linked to mortality and nephropathy in people with diabetes [43]. Hyperglycemia by itself increases the risk for infections in the mouth. In diabetes and periodontitis, there is greater periodontal tissue destruction in people with poor metabolic control, but also poorer metabolic control of diabetes leads to greater destruction [42]. Periodontal disease is an infectious and inflammatory disease affecting the hard and soft tissues surrounding the teeth. It begins with inflammation of the gingival tissue, which may lead to bacterial infections and may, without treatment, progress to irreversible periodontal disease consisting of bone loss and tooth mobility.

An examination of the mouth may reveal reddened swollen, bleeding gingiva; pain; foul odor; receding gums; and loose teeth [44]. Prevention in the form of glycemic control, smoking cessation, and dental hygiene is foremost. Treatment begins, however, with improving metabolic control to decrease the risk of infection, good nutrition, antibiotics, antimicrobial rinses, and frequent dental visits. Diabetes self-management education should stress the importance of daily brushing and flossing, along with metabolic control.

Characteristics, detection and interventions: cutaneous manifestations

Foot ulcers are commonly associated with diabetes and have a multifactorial etiology. A combination of altered foot biomechanics, diabetic neuropathy, and vessel ischemia is often responsible. Decreased capillary perfusion leads to ischemia, tissue death, inability of the capillaries to vasodilate in response to injury, and poor wound healing. Capillary basement membrane thickening limits the ability of the white blood cells to migrate to the site of injury, and damage to the microvasculature impairs tissue oxygenation. Prevention consists of management of all the traditional risk factors for vascular disease. In addition, meticulous foot hygiene is essential. Treatment for diabetic ulcers often consists of proper fitting or customized shoes, non–weight bearing, antibiotics, and sometimes hyperbaric oxygen therapy to correct the poor oxygenation of the tissues and induce healing [40].

Diabetic dermopathy, with a prevalence rate of > 50%, is the most common skin lesion seen in diabetes [40]. It is more common in men, and increases in frequency with increased age and duration of diabetes. The presence of diabetic dermopathy has been found to increase with each of the three microvascular complications (DR, nephropathy, and neuropathy), but also in relation to the number of complications in each patient [45]. Typically, diabetic dermopathy is seen as small, round or oval brown or red macules on both shins and is believed to be related to poorly vascularized skin. Patients may complain of darkened areas of skin on the lower legs, without any pain, itching, history of trauma, or rash. Although there is a relationship to metabolic control, there is no real effective treatment for diabetic dermopathy. Microscopic examination of the nail bed capillaries in people with diabetes and periungual erythema has shown dilation and tortuosity of the venous vessels. Although people with connective tissue disorders also commonly have periungual erythema, the capillary changes are different than those seen in diabetes. Other nail bed disorders believed to be related to microangiopathy are onycholysis, splinter hemorrhages, and yellow nail discoloration [40].

Diabetes thick skin may manifest as scleroderma-like changes in the hand, or more thickened skin that begins in the face and neck and spreads to the upper body, back, and shoulders. Both lead to stiffness and limited mobility, and are strongly associated with retinopathy and nephropathy.

Glycation of skin collagen and skin hypoxia may be caused by microvascular changes [40]. The lesions are tiny pebble-like papules that become confluent, and may cause decreased skin flexibility and back discomfort [46]. Diabetic thick skin in the fingers and hands is seen in 39% of people with type 1 diabetes. During examination, asking patients to hold their hands in a prayer position may reveal an inability to press the hands tightly together. Treatment effectiveness is limited but may consist of improving glucose control, use of topical steroids, penicillamine, intralesional insulin, low-dose methotrexate, bath psoralen plus UVA, and pentoxifylline.

Necrobiosis lipoidica diabeticorum is a granulomatous lesion characterized by erythematous papules and plaques with a depressed waxy yellow brown center, and is generally asymptomatic. The plaque may result, however, in thinning of the skin and increase the risk of ulcer. The etiology is controversial because there are some pathologic changes involving endothelial cells of the capillaries, but there is significant evidence that it is an antibody-mediated vasculitis [40]. Treatment is varied and may consist of topical or injected steroids, UVA light, cyclosporine, laser therapy to reduce bleeding and improve appearance, and specialized wound care [46].

Summary

The microvascular complications of diabetes are serious, and can be life threatening. Many are preventable through glycemic, blood pressure, and lipid control, along with good diabetes self-management practices. Education is essential, and nurses can be great advocates for patients by promoting healthy practices and working as part of the health care team to prevent and decrease the progression of these diseases if they are present. Diabetes can affect the entire body, and timely screening, along with following guidelines for monitoring frequency, and target ranges for management can improve the health of people with diabetes. Table 4 provides a list of recommendations for screening and target values.

Future therapies and implications

Glycemic control, although demonstrated to be effective in preventing microvascular complications and slowing progression, has been difficult to achieve. Scientists have focused on finding agents that can interfere with those metabolic pathways believed to produce glucotoxins and oxidative stress. Aldose reductase inhibitors, which block the polyol pathway, were shown to lack efficacy and be toxic. Aminoguanadine, an AGE inhibitor, is being explored in small trials [20]. Current interest has focused on protein kinase C inhibitors, specifically the protein kinase C-β inhibitor, roboxistaurin. Roboxistaurin has been shown in rodent models to prevent and reverse vascular dysfunction [47]. A recent, although small study, demonstrated that roboxistaurin reduced albuminuria and maintained estimated

Table 4
Guidelines for screening and targets for control

Risk factor	Measurement	Monitoring frequency	Targets for control and management
Glycemic control	Hemoglobin A_{1c}	Every 3–6 mo	<7.0% ADA <6.5% AACE
Hypertension	Blood pressure	Every visit	<130/80 mm Hg
Dyslipidemia	Cholesterol and lipids	At least annually	LDL < 100 mg/dL; very high risk LDL < 70 mg/dL HDL > 40 mg/dL Trig < 150 mg/dL
Retinopathy	Dilated eye Examination	At least annually	Detection, staging, and treatment
Nephropathy	Urine microalbumin serum creatinine	At least annually	<30 μg/mg <1.5 mg/dL[a]
Peripheral neuropathy	Monofilament and inspection	At least annually	No foot ulceration or amputation
Cardiovascular disease	Aspirin therapy	Every visit	75–162 mg/d preventive measure for adults
Smoking	Tobacco use	Every visit	Smoking cessation
Obesity	Weight	Every visit	Weight management or loss

Abbreviations: AACE, American Association of Clinical Endocrinologists; ADA, American Diabetes Association; HDL, high-density liproprotein; LDL, low-density lipoprotein.

[a] Depends on laboratory normal range.

GFR in people with type 2 diabetes [48]. Other agents directed against vascular endothelial growth factor, such as corticosteroids, are being investigated, and there are reports that vitrectomy may be helpful in eyes with refractive macular edema [21]. With current and new therapies on the horizon, nurses can play a vital role in primary and secondary prevention of these debilitating complications.

Nurses can be instrumental with motivating, training, and educating individuals in healthy behaviors that are critical to living well with diabetes. Focusing on healthy eating, being physically active, monitoring blood glucose or blood pressure, taking and administering medications, problem solving for sick days, hyperglycemia, or hypoglycemia, reducing risks for complications, and healthy coping are self-management behaviors that contribute to improved health outcomes [49]. Community nurses, diabetes nurse educators, nurse specialists, and nurse practitioners have all been found to be effective in screening, detection, and treatment of diabetic complications [50–53]. Nurse case management was demonstrated to be effective in improving adherence with diabetes services and had a favorable effect on short-term glucose control trends [54,55]. More research is needed for effects of long-term management of diabetes complications that require focus on

the ABCs of risk reduction, and strategies that can motivate and maintain healthy lifestyles.

References

[1] DCCT Research Group. The effect of intensive treatment of diabetes on the development and progression of long-term complications in insulin-dependent-diabetes mellitus. N Engl J Med 1993;329:977–86.
[2] UK Prospective Diabetes Study Group. Intensive blood-glucose control with sulphonylureas or insulin compared with conventional treatment and risk of complications in patients with type 2 diabetes (UKPDS 33). UK prospective diabetes study (UKPDS) group. Lancet 1998;352:837–53.
[3] Koro CE, Bowlin SJ, Bourgeois N, et al. Glycemic control from 1988 to 2000 among US adults diagnosed with type 2 diabetes: a preliminary report. Diabetes Care 2004;27: 17–20.
[4] Centers for Disease Control. National diabetes fact sheet, United States 2005. Available at: www.cdc.gov/diabetes/pubs/factsheet05. Accessed February 16, 2006.
[5] Ryan ME, Carnu O, Kramer A. The influence of diabetes on periodontal tissue. J Am Dent Assoc 2003;134:34S–40S.
[6] Home P. Contributions of basal and post-prandial hyperglycemia to micro- and macrovascular complications in people with type 2 diabetes. Curr Med Res Opin 2005;21:989–98.
[7] Dandona P, Chaudhuri A, Aljada A. Endothelial dysfunction and hypertension in diabetes mellitus. Med Clin North Am 2004;88:911 31.
[8] CDC. Risk factors for complications: national diabetes surveillance system. Available at: www.cdc.gov/diabetes/statistics/comp/us.htm. Accessed January 23, 2006.
[9] Harris MI, Klein R, Cowie CC, et al. Is the risk of diabetic retinopathy greater in non Hispanic blacks and Mexican Americans than in non-Hispanic whites with type 2 diabetes? A US population study. Diabetes Care 1998;21:1230–5.
[10] Harris MI, Eastman RC, Cowie CC, et al. Racial and ethnic differences in glycemic control of adults with type 2 diabetes. Diabetes Care 1999;22:403–8.
[11] Harris MI. Racial and ethnic differences in health care access and health outcomes for adults with type 2 diabetes. Diabetes Care 2001;24:454–9.
[12] American Diabetes Association. Standards of medical care in diabetes: 2006 position statement. Diabetes Care 2006;29:S4–42.
[13] Institute of Medicine. Unequal treatment: confronting racial and ethnic disparities in health care 2002. Washington: National Academy of Sciences; 2002.
[14] Writing team for the Diabetes Control and Complications Trial/Epidemiology of Diabetes Interventions and Complications Research Group. Effect of intensive therapy on the microvascular complications of type 1 diabetes mellitus. JAMA 2002;287:2563–9.
[15] The UKPDS Study Group. Tight blood pressure control and risk of macrovascular and microvascular complications in type 2 diabetes: the UKPDS report no. 38. BMJ 1998;317: 703–13.
[16] Jenkins AJ, Rowley KG, Lyons TJ, et al. Lipoproteins and diabetic microvascular complications. Curr Pharm Des 2004;10:3395–418.
[17] Brownlee M. Biochemistry and molecular cell biology of diabetic complications. Nature 2001;414:813–20.
[18] Sheetz MJ, King GL. Molecular understanding of hyperglycemia's adverse effects for diabetic complications. JAMA 2002;288:2579–88.
[19] Brownlee M. The pathobiology of diabetic complications: a unifying mechanism. Diabetes 2005;54:1615–25.
[20] Feldman EL. Etiology of diabetic microvascular disease and scientific rationale for new therapeutic targets. Advanced Studies in Medicine 2005;5:S138–43.

[21] Fong DS, Aiello LP, Ferris FL, et al. Diabetic retinopathy (technical review). Diabetes Care 2004;27:2540–53.
[22] van Leiden HA, Dekker JM, Moll AC, et al. Risk factors for incident retinopathy in a diabetic and nondiabetic population: the Hoorn study. Arch Ophthalmol 2003;121:245–51.
[23] Frank RN. Medical progress: diabetic retinopathy. N Engl J Med 2004;350:48–58.
[24] American Academy of Ophthalmology. Preferred practice patterns: diabetic retinopathy. Available at: www.aao.org/education/library/ppp/upload/Diabetic-Retinopathy.pdf. Accessed February 12, 2006.
[25] Phelps R. Ocular changes with diabetes. In: Childs B, Cypress M, Spollett G, editors. Complete nurse's guide to diabetes care. Alexandria (VA): American Diabetes Association; 2005. p. 113–21.
[26] Wilson C, Horton M, Cavallerano J, et al. Addition of primary care-based retinal imaging technology to an existing eye care professional referral program increased the rate of surveillance and treatment of diabetic retinopathy. Diabetes Care 2005;28:318–22.
[27] Hutchinson A, McIntosh A, Peters J, et al. Effectiveness of screening and monitoring tests for diabetic retinopathy: a systematic review. Diabet Med 2000;17:495–506.
[28] Klein BE, Klein R, McBride PE, et al. Cardiovascular disease, mortality and retinal microvascular characteristics in type 1 diabetes: Wisconsin epidemiology study of diabetic retinopathy. Arch Intern Med 2004;164:1917–24.
[29] Gross JL, de Azevcdo MJ, Silverberg SP, et al. Diabetic nephropathy: diagnosis, prevention, and treatment. Diabetes Care 2005;28:164–76.
[30] Rabkin R. Diabetic nephropathy. Clin Cornerstone 2003;5:1–11.
[31] Molitch M, DeFronzo R, Franz M, et al. Nephropathy in diabetes. Diabetes Care 2004;27: S79–83.
[32] National Kidney Foundation. K/DOQI Clinical practice guidelines. Available at: www. kidney.org/professional/kdoqi/guidelines_ckd/toc.htm. Accessed December 1, 2005.
[33] Levey AS, Eckardt K, Tsukamoto Y, et al. Definition and classification of chronic kidney disease: a position statement from kidney disease. Improving global outcomes. Kidney Int 2005;67:2089–100.
[34] Coonrod B, Ernst KL. Nephropathy. In: Franz M, editor. A core curriculum for diabetes educators: diabetes and its complications. 5th edition. Chicago: AADE; 2003. p. 153–88.
[35] Viassara H, Palace MR. Diabetes and advanced glycation endproducts. J Intern Med 2002; 251:87–101.
[36] Coughlan MT, Cooper ME, Forbes JM. Can advanced glycation end product inhibitors modulate more than one pathway to enhance renoprotection in diabetes. Ann N Y Acad Sci 2005;1043:750–8.
[37] Levin A, Stevens LA. Executing change in the management of chronic kidney disease: perspectives on guidelines and practice. Med Clin North Am 2005;89:701–9.
[38] Nathan D. Sustained effect of intensive treatment of type 1 diabetes mellitus on development and progression of diabetic nephropathy: the Epidemiology of Diabetes Interventions and Complications (EDIC) study. JAMA 2003;290:2159–67.
[39] Waugh NR, Robertson AM. Protein restriction for diabetic renal disease. Cochrane Database Syst Rev 2002;2:CD02181.
[40] Ngo BT, Hayes KD, DiMiao DJ, et al. Manifestations of cutaneous diabetic microangiopathy. Am J Clin Dermatol 2005;6:225–37.
[41] Iacopino AM. Diabetic periodontitis: possible lipid-induced defect in tissue repair through alterations of macrophage phenotype and function. Oral Dis 1995;1:214–29.
[42] Borrell LN, Papapanou PN. Analytical epidemiology of periodontitis. J Clin Periodontol 2005;32:132–58.
[43] Saremi A, Nelson RG, Tullock-Reid M, et al. Periodontal disease and mortality in type 2 diabetes. Diabetes Care 2005;28:27–32.
[44] Stegeman CA. Oral manifestations of diabetes. Home Healthc Nurse 2005;23:233–42.

[45] Shemer A, Bergman R, Linn S, et al. Diabetic dermopathy and internal complications in diabetes mellitus. Int J Dermatol 1998;37:113–5.
[46] Spollett G. Dermatological changes associated with diabetes. In: Childs BP, Cypress M, Spollett G, editors. Complete nurse's guide to diabetes care. Alexandria (VA): ADA; 2005. p. 146–54.
[47] He Z, King GL. Can protein kinase C B-selective inhibitor, ruboxistaurin, stop vascular complications in diabetic patients? Diabetes Care 2005;28:2803–5.
[48] Tuttle KR, Bakris GL, Toto RD, et al. The effect of ruboxistaurin on nephropathy in type 2 diabetes. Diabetes Care 2005;28:2686–90.
[49] Mulcahy K, Maryniuk M, Peeples M, et al. Technical review: diabetes self management education outcome measures. Diab Educ 2003;29:768.
[50] Walker R. Diabetic retinopathy: protecting the vision of people with diabetes. Br J Community Nurs 2004;9:545–7.
[51] Seaman S. The role of the nurse specialist in the care of patients with diabetic foot ulcers. Foot Ankle Int 2005;26:19–26.
[52] Stern E, Benbassat CA, Goldfracht M. Impact of a two-arm educational program for improving diabetes care in primary care centres. Int J Clin Pract 2005;59:1126–30.
[53] Hensley RD, Jones AK, Williams AG, et al. One-year clinical outcomes for Louisiana residents diagnosed with type 2 diabetes and hypertension. J Am Acad Nurse Pract 2005;17: 363–9.
[54] Wilson C, Curtis J, Lipke S, et al. Nurse case manager effectiveness and case load in a large clinical practice: implications for workforce development. Diabet Med 2005;22:1116–20.
[55] Adiseshiah M. Effective care of patients with type 2 diabetes and dyslipidemia: a nurse's perspective. Diabetes Res Clin Pract 2005;68·S23–7.

ELSEVIER
SAUNDERS

Nurs Clin N Am 41 (2006) 737–744

NURSING
CLINICS
OF NORTH AMERICA

Index

Note: Page numbers of article titles are in **boldface** type.

0029-6465/06/$ - see front matter © 2006 Elsevier Inc. All rights reserved.
doi:10.1016/S0029-6465(06)00088-0

nursing.theclinics.com

Moving?

Make sure your subscription moves with you!

To notify us of your new address, find your **Clinics Account Number** (located on your mailing label above your name), and contact customer service at:

E-mail: elspcs@elsevier.com

800-654-2452 (subscribers in the U.S. & Canada)
407-345-4000 (subscribers outside of the U.S. & Canada)

Fax number: 407-363-9661

Elsevier Periodicals Customer Service
6277 Sea Harbor Drive
Orlando, FL 32887-4800

*To ensure uninterrupted delivery of your subscription, please notify us at least 4 weeks in advance of move.

United States Postal Service
Statement of Ownership, Management, and Circulation

1. Publication Title	2. Publication Number	3. Filing Date
Nursing Clinics of North America	5 9 8 - 9 6 0 0	9/15/06

4. Issue Frequency	5. Number of Issues Published Annually	6. Annual Subscription Price
Mar, Jun, Sep, Dec	4	$105.00

7. Complete Mailing Address of Known Office of Publication (Not printer) (Street, city, county, state, and ZIP+4)

Elsevier Inc.
360 Park Avenue South
New York, NY 10010-1710

Contact Person
Sarah Carmichael
Telephone
(215) 239-3681

8. Complete Mailing Address of Headquarters or General Business Office of Publisher (Not printer)

Elsevier Inc., 360 Park Avenue South, New York, NY 10010-1710

9. Full Names and Complete Mailing Addresses of Publisher, Editor, and Managing Editor (Do not leave blank)
Publisher (Name and complete mailing address)

John Schrefer, Elsevier Inc., 1600 John F. Kennedy Blvd., Suite 1800, Philadelphia, PA 19103-2899

Editor (Name and complete mailing address)

Alexandra Gavenda, Elsevier Inc., 1600 John F. Kennedy Blvd., Suite 1800, Philadelphia, PA 19103-2899

Managing Editor (Name and complete mailing address)

Catherine Bewick, Elsevier Inc., 1600 John F. Kennedy Blvd., Suite 1800, Philadelphia, PA 19103-2899

10. Owner (Do not leave blank. If the publication is owned by a corporation, give the name and address of the corporation immediately followed by the names and addresses of all stockholders owning or holding 1 percent or more of the total amount of stock. If not owned by a corporation, give the names and addresses of the individual owners. If owned by a partnership or other unincorporated firm, give its name and address as well as those of each individual owner. If the publication is published by a nonprofit organization, give its name and address.)

Full Name	Complete Mailing Address
Wholly owned subsidiary of	4520 East-West Highway
Reed/Elsevier Inc., US holdings	Bethesda, MD 20814

11. Known Bondholders, Mortgagees, and Other Security Holders Owning or Holding 1 Percent or More of Total Amount of Bonds, Mortgages, or Other Securities. If none, check box ▶ None

Full Name	Complete Mailing Address
N/A	

12. Tax Status (For completion by nonprofit organizations authorized to mail at nonprofit rates) (Check one)
The purpose, function, and nonprofit status of this organization and the exempt status for federal income tax purposes:
☐ Has Not Changed During Preceding 12 Months
☐ Has Changed During Preceding 12 Months (Publisher must submit explanation of change with this statement)

(See Instructions on Reverse)

PS Form 3526, October 1999

---

13. Publication Title		14. Issue Date for Circulation Data Below
Nursing Clinics of North America		September, 2006

15.	Extent and Nature of Circulation		Average No. Copies Each Issue During Preceding 12 Months	No. Copies of Single Issue Published Nearest to Filing Date
a.	Total Number of Copies (Net press run)		4,000	3,900
b. Paid and/or Requested Circulation	(1)	Paid/Requested Outside-County Mail Subscriptions Stated on Form 3541. (Include advertiser's proof and exchange copies)	2,445	2,331
	(2)	Paid In-County Subscriptions Stated on Form 3541 (Include advertiser's proof and exchange copies)		
	(3)	Sales Through Dealers and Carriers, Street Vendors, Counter Sales, and Other Non-USPS Paid Distribution	579	563
	(4)	Other Classes Mailed Through the USPS		
c.	Total Paid and/or Requested Circulation [Sum of 15b. (1), (2), (3), and (4)] ▶		3,024	2,894
d. Free Distribution by Mail (Samples, complimentary, and other free)	(1)	Outside-County as Stated on Form 3541	111	116
	(2)	In-County as Stated on Form 3541		
	(3)	Other Classes Mailed Through the USPS		
e.	Free Distribution Outside the Mail (Carriers or other means)			
f.	Total Free Distribution (Sum of 15d. and 15e.) ▶		111	116
g.	Total Distribution (Sum of 15c. and 15f) ▶		3,135	3,010
h.	Copies not Distributed		865	890
i.	Total (Sum of 15g. and h.) ▶		4,000	3,900
j.	Percent Paid and/or Requested Circulation (15c. divided by 15g. times 100)		96.46%	96.15%

16. Publication of Statement of Ownership
☐ Publication required. Will be printed in the December 2006 issue of this publication.
☐ Publication not required.

17. Signature and Title of Editor, Publisher, Business Manager, or Owner

Jesy Sancira — Executive Director of Subscription Services

Date 15/06

I certify that all information furnished on this form is true and complete. I understand that anyone who furnishes false or misleading information on this form or who omits material or information requested on the form may be subject to criminal sanctions (including fines and imprisonment) and/or civil sanctions (including civil penalties).

Instructions to Publishers

1. Complete and file one copy of this form with your postmaster annually on or before October 1. Keep a copy of the completed form for your records.
2. In cases where the stockholder or security holder is a trustee, include in items 10 and 11 the name of the person or corporation for whom the trustee is acting. Also include the names and addresses of individuals who are stockholders who own or hold 1 percent or more of the total amount of bonds, mortgages, or other securities of the publishing corporation. In item 11, if none, check the box. Use blank sheets if more space is required.
3. Be sure to furnish all circulation information called for in item 15. Free circulation must be shown in items 15d, e, and f.
4. Item 15h., Copies not Distributed, must include (1) newsstand copies originally stated on Form 3541, and returned to the publisher, (2) estimated returns from news agents, and (3), copies for office use, leftovers, spoiled, and all other copies not distributed.
5. If the publication had Periodicals authorization as a general or requester publication, this Statement of Ownership, Management, and Circulation must be published; it must be printed in any issue in October or, if the publication is not published during October, the first issue printed after October.
6. In item 16, indicate the date of the issue in which this Statement of Ownership will be published.
7. Item 17 must be signed.
   Failure to file or publish a statement of ownership may lead to suspension of Periodicals authorization.

PS Form 3526, October 1999 (Reverse)